FAMILY THERAPY AND FAMILY MEDICINE

THE GUILFORD FAMILY THERAPY SERIES
ALAN S. GURMAN, EDITOR

Aesthetics of Change
BRADFORD P. KEENEY

Family Therapy in Schizophrenia
WILLIAM R. MCFARLANE, EDITOR

Mastering Resistance: A Practical Guide to Family Therapy
CAROL M. ANDERSON AND SUSAN STEWART

Family Therapy and Family Medicine: Toward the Primary Care of Families
WILLIAM J. DOHERTY AND MACARAN A. BAIRD

Ethnicity and Family Therapy
MONICA MCGOLDRICK, JOHN K. PEARCE, AND JOSEPH GIORDANO, EDITORS

Patterns of Brief Family Therapy: An Ecosystemic Approach
STEVE DE SHAZER

The Family Therapy of Drug Abuse and Addiction
M. DUNCAN STANTON, THOMAS C. TODD, AND ASSOCIATES

From Psyche to System: The Evolving Therapy of Carl Whitaker
JOHN R. NEILL AND DAVID P. KNISKERN, EDITORS

Normal Family Processes
FROMA WALSH, EDITOR

Helping Couples Change: A Social Learning Approach to Marital Therapy
RICHARD B. STUART

FAMILY THERAPY AND FAMILY MEDICINE
Toward the Primary Care of Families

WILLIAM J. DOHERTY

Department of Family Practice
The University of Iowa

MACARAN A. BAIRD

Community Clinic
Wabasha, Minnesota

THE GUILFORD PRESS
New York   London

©1983 William J. Doherty and Macaran A. Baird

Published by The Guilford Press
A Division of Guilford Publications, Inc.
200 Park Avenue South, New York, N.Y. 10003

Printed in the United States of America

LIBRARY OF CONGRESS CATALOGING IN PUBLICATION DATA
Doherty, William J. (William Joseph), 1945–
    Family therapy and family medicine.

    (The Guilford family therapy series)
    Includes index.
    1. Family psychotherapy.   2. Family medicine.
I. Baird, Macaran A.   II. Title.   III. Series.
[DNLM: 1. Family practice.   2. Family therapy.
3. Primary health care. WM 430.5.F2 D655f]
RC488.5.D63   616.89′156   82-3135
ISBN 0-89862-041-4   AACR2

ACKNOWLEDGMENTS

We wish to thank a number of colleagues who have read and commented on parts of the manuscript: Paul Williamson, MD, Elizabeth Burns, MD, Robert Rakel, MD, Reuben Widmer, MD, Joseph McGrath, MD, John Verby, MD, William Clements, PhD, Jeri Hepworth, PhD, Israela Meyerstein, ACSW, Denise LeBlanc, MA, Terrence McCormally, MD, and Stephen Taplin, MD. We profited enormously from their suggestions. Our special thanks to Claudia Hallas, who typed and retyped a number of drafts of the book just prior to the advent of word processing in the Department of Family Practice.

v

PREFACE

This is a book about treating patients in their family and social contexts. Like people, a book has a social context and a social history, which in this case began when we met in 1979 at a family therapy meeting. Mac Baird was a family practice residency graduate trained in family therapy and working for a year and a half to implement a family-oriented medical practice in rural Minnesota. Bill Doherty was a family therapist new to the family practice faculty at The University of Iowa's College of Medicine. We realized immediately that we needed each other: Mac needed Bill's links to the wider family therapy profession and to academic family medicine, and Bill needed Mac's grounding in the world of private practice family medicine. For personal reasons as well as professional, we began a long-distance friendship and partnership.

In the winter of 1980 we decided to submit a conference abstract to the American Association for Marriage and Family Therapy. After the abstract was accepted, we met and telephoned regularly until the meeting in Toronto in November 1980, where we presented a workshop on family therapy and family medicine. About the same time, Alan Gurman wrote to Bill inviting him and a family physician colleague of his choice to write a book on family therapy and family medicine for The Guilford Family Therapy Series. The writing team was already in place.

The social context of this book also includes several family physician/ therapists with whom we have become acquainted and who share our enthusiasm for family-oriented family medicine. Janet Seely from Montreal; Randy Rissman from Woodstock, New York; and Jim McCoy from Chicago all participated with us in the ground-breaking Skidmore College Conference on Family Therapy and Family Medicine, held in August 1981. To this list should be added Yves Talbot, a pediatrician turned family physician, who has been Bill Doherty's friend and link to the medical world for 7 years. Yves and Janet Seely have been steering a similar path to ours at McGill University in Montreal. While inevitably there are some differences in style and substance between us and these colleagues, we nevertheless feel part of an important new movement in family medicine. In a nutshell, this movement applies the family systems perspective developed by family therapists to the emerging field of family medicine.

In addition to having a social context, a book has a purpose and an intended audience. Our purpose is to create a model for primary care family-oriented treatment that will be theoretically coherent, helpful for families, practical for practicing family physicians—and different from specialized family therapy. We try to show how a family systems approach can be applied to a wide range of problems that patients bring to their family doctors. Since the effectiveness of this approach in the primary care arena remains to be demonstrated, we hope that this book stimulates the needed research. Patient compliance may be the area most ripe for such a research breakthrough, and Chapter 9 delineates a testable procedure for enhancing patient compliance through family compliance counseling.

This book has three audiences: a primary audience of family physicians, a secondary audience of other physicians and health care professionals who are interested in treating patients in a family context, and an eavesdropping audience of family therapists who wish to learn more about the world of family physicians in order to work more closely with them. Although we believe that the latter two groups (other health care professionals and family therapists) can benefit from the book, the prospective reader should nevertheless realize that our basic primary model is designed for the family physician who interacts with, treats, and coordinates the care of all members of the family.

Original in our approach, we think, is a new way to understand the delivery of family-oriented treatment for psychosocial problems. Just as the delivery of biomedical treatment is divided into primary, secondary, and tertiary levels, we believe that family treatment can be divided in most parts of the country into at least two levels—primary and specialized. Family therapists, who come from a variety of disciplines and receive supervised training in family treatment, serve as the specialists for family-related problems, while family physicians (and certain other health care professionals, school counselors, and clergy) serve as the principal primary care providers.

We use the terms "primary care family counseling" and "specialized family therapy" to distinguish between these two levels of treatment. (In areas of the country where family therapy training centers are functioning, a level for tertiary care family treatment can be added to the list.) These distinctions serve two purposes: first, to denote family physicians' important and distinctive role in family treatment, as opposed to viewing them as watered-down and inadequate family therapists or as biomedical specialists who should leave all psychosocial problems to therapists or psychiatrists; and second, to underline the natural link between family physicians and family therapists for both referral and consultation. Family therapists and family physicians should be partners in the delivery of comprehensive, multilevel care to families.

The body of the book begins with a discussion of the issues facing family medicine as it tries to incorporate a family approach to medical education, and offers some background information on the contemporary American family. Chapter 2 is the heart of the book; it presents an overview of the basic concepts and the basic model, in particular introducing the notion of the therapeutic triangle in medical care. Chapter 3 gives a nontechnical introduction to the family systems approach to family treatment and describes in more detail Salvador Minuchin's structural family therapy approach. Chapters 4–6 deal with several stages in our primary care counseling model: observing and assessing families; forming therapeutic contracts and assembling families in the office or hospital; and guidelines for deciding when to refer to a therapist and when to treat in a primary care mode. Chapter 7 is another core chapter; it presents four main functions of primary care family counseling (education, prevention, support, and challenge) and describes a number of basic primary care family counseling techniques.

The remaining chapters apply the primary care model to a number of common problems in family practice: stress-related medical disorders, patient compliance, marital and sexual problems, parent–child problems, chemical dependency or substance abuse, depression, and anxiety. We have used case examples and counseling vignettes liberally in this part of the book. Since each of these chapters represents an application of our basic assessment and treatment approach, the reader will find some repetition of major concepts throughout these discussions. The final chapter deals with practical issues in implementing a family-oriented approach to health care: support systems for the physician; creation of a family-oriented service network; scheduling and time issues; fees; and self-protection of the physician from overload and overinvolvement in primary care family counseling.

Our procedure for planning and writing the book was as follows: We planned each chapter collaboratively, and then Doherty was responsible for drafting Chapters 1–11 and Baird for Chapters 12–16. We then commented on each other's drafts until we agreed on a final version. Many of the new concepts in the book emerged from our discussions. Some things we each brought into the partnership: Doherty had developed the notion of the therapeutic triangle and had done patient compliance research; Baird already had much practical experience in family-oriented medical care, particularly in treating chemical dependency and in using community resources. The result is a different book than either of us could have written alone. Our collaboration has been consistently rewarding and at times exhilarating. We

wish the same for family physicians and family therapists who work together
to give comprehensive care to patients and families.

WILLIAM J. DOHERTY, PHD
MACARAN A. BAIRD, MD

CONTENTS

FAMILY THERAPY AND FAMILY MEDICINE

1 IN SEARCH OF THE FAMILY IN FAMILY MEDICINE

Unlike most other medical specialties, which rose out of scientific and technological developments, the new specialty of family medicine was founded on an *idea*—or a set of *ideals*. John Geyman, a leader in the field of family medicine, has summed up this ideological mission as follows:

> It is axiomatic that the specialty of family practice is involved in the comprehensive, ongoing care of individual patients and their families, and that the knowledge and skills required by the family physician include a broad range of clinical competencies. It is likewise axiomatic that the family is the basic unit of care in family practice, but involved herein is a profound conceptual shift extending well beyond the care of the "whole patient" to the care of the *family*, not just the individual, as the patient. Although this point is part of the everyday language of the developing discipline of family medicine, a gap usually exists between this conceptual goal and actual practice, including teaching practices with intended commitment to this goal. (Geyman, 1977, p. 571)

Thus, a profound philosophical difference between general practice prior to 1970 and the emerging field of family practice lies in the emphasis on *family*.

In the field of psychotherapy during the 1950s and 1960s, the emerging discipline of family therapy also struggled with the "profound conceptual shift" toward viewing the family as the treatment unit. Family therapy arose partly out of the frustration of psychotherapists with fragmented, individually oriented treatment of children's psychiatric disturbances (Olson, 1970)—just as family medicine was created in the late 1960s as a response to impersonal and fragmented medical care practices. Since family therapy has had more time to develop its conceptual framework for family treatment, it has much to offer family medicine in its own search for the family. Similarly, family medicine, as a comprehensive primary care field not limited to either physical or psychosocial problems alone, can serve as a powerful partner to the discipline of family therapy. The two fields are natural allies.

1

THE CASE FOR A FAMILY ORIENTATION IN HEALTH CARE

Every discipline needs to delineate its area of knowledge and its basic methodology, and then must struggle with the limits of this paradigm. As George Engel (1977) articulated in his classic article in *Science*, modern medicine has opted for molecular biology as its knowledge base: Disease is accounted for by deviation from the norm of measurable biological variables and is supposedly independent of social behavior. The methodology of this biomedical model may be characterized as that of the applied scientist: The physician gathers data through history and objective assessment, formulates and tests diagnostic hypotheses, and treats disease primarily by chemical and surgical interventions. Data are then gathered on the results of the treatment, and further objective decisions are made. Despite its enormous contributions, Engel maintains that the biomedical model ignores crucial aspects of health and health care. Instead, he calls for a biopsychosocial model that emphasizes the unity of body, mind, and social context.

THE BREADTH OF MEDICAL CARE

The issue of the scope or breadth of medical care orientations is stated graphically in Fig. 1-1. The figure presents a continuum ranging from a narrow disease orientation through a personalistic orientation to a social orientation. In the disease orientation, the physician is concerned almost exclusively with a liver patient's *liver* ("How's the cirrhosis in Room 210?"). The more humanistically oriented physician asks the nurse and the patient not only about the diseased liver but about whether the patient has expressed fears of dying or any second thoughts about alcohol use. The physician with a social orientation may ask all the above questions, but also inquires about the reactions of the patient's family and the meaning of the illness in the

FIG. 1-1. THE BREADTH OF MEDICAL CARE ORIENTATIONS.

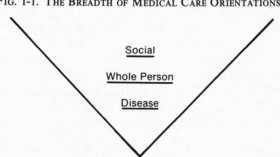

Social

Whole Person

Disease

patient's culture. It should be noted that as one moves along the continuum towards more breadth, nothing is lost and something new is added. That is, the socially oriented physician is no less concerned with the diseased organ than with the patient's feelings. In fact, sound clinical skills are the rock-bottom foundation for a family–social orientation to medical care. No patient should be exposed to physicians whose social skills mask clinical incompetence. Optimally, the family physicians should have the knowledge and skills to be helpful at all points on the continuum. Given the heavy emphasis applied to the disease orientation in medical education, however, it is difficult enough for physicians to embrace a personalistic approach to medical care. To integrate a social orientation with the other two is a profound achievement for a practicing physician. The rest of this section of the chapter reviews some of the reasons why this higher integration is needed for optimal patient care. The argument is posed as a family curriculum for medical education, the family being the primary social group of most patients.

Tenets in a Family Curriculum in Medical Education

1. *The family is the primary social context for health care.* In addition to being the agent of the genetic transmission of disease, the family is a major source of the following aspects of health and illness:

a. *The transmission of infectious diseases.* Studies like Dingle, Badger, and Jordon's (1964) 3-year investigation of 60 families have documented the clustering of contagious diseases in family groups and the relationship between disease incidence and the age and school status of children.

b. *Health behaviors such as nutrition, hygiene, and medicine taking.* In a study of over 2700 individuals living in almost 800 families, Osterweis, Bush, and Zuckerman (1979) found that other family members' medicine use was a strong predictor of each individual's medicine use, a better predictor even than the individual's level of morbidity.

c. *Psychosocial stress affecting health.* In a classic study that followed 16 families over a 1-year period, Meyer and Haggerty (1962) found that 36% of beta-strep illnesses were associated with some acute stress affecting the family; furthermore, families high in chronic stress had members with the highest number of streptococcal acquisitions, illnesses, and antistreptolysin-*O* titer rises.

d. *Social support for preventing illness and recovering from illness.* In a large prospective study in Israel, Medalie, Snyder, Groen, Neufeld, Goldbourt, and Riss (1973) found that reported family problems were a strong predictor of the development of angina pectoris over a 5-year period, with men who reported the fewest family problems developing angina at about one-third the rate of those who reported the most family problems. Wives' love and support apparently served as a risk-lowering factor even in the presence of other known high-risk factors for developing angina (Medalie & Goldbourt, 1976).

e. *Definitions of health and illness events.* Medical sociologists such as Kasl and Cobb (1966) have documented the pivotal role of family and other social influences in defining the nature and seriousness of symptoms.

f. *Decisions on health care utilization.* Most illness episodes are treated within the family context (Albert, Kosa, & Haggerty, 1967), and decisions about home versus medical/professional treatment are usually negotiated among family members (Litman, 1974).

g. *The social group most immediately affected by illness and medical treatment.* An extensive literature has examined the unsettling effects of illness—particularly chronic illness—on the family (Bruhn, 1977; Pattison & Anderson, 1978).

The next three curriculum items are extensions of the first item's emphasis on the family as the primary social context of health care.

2. *Patients' individual problems are also family problems.* In some cases family dysfunction may be seen as an *etiological* factor in the patient's distress; in other cases it may be useful to view the family as the social group most damaged by the patient's problem, or as the group that must be mobilized to help the patient recover from the problem. In treating psychosocial problems and stress-related illness, these three perspectives can be combined into a "systems" orientation that views the patient and the family as both "actors" and "reactors" in creating and responding to the problem. The fundamental point of this curriculum item is that when individual patients have biopsychosocial problems, the family also needs attention, because it too is involved and hurting.

3. *The patient's family is potentially the physician's greatest ally in treatment.* As compliance researchers have forcefully articulated, patient noncompliance with medical regimens is a leading cause of disease, disability, and death (Haynes, Taylor, & Sackett, 1979). Family support has been shown in a number of studies (reviewed in Chapter 9) to be an important predictor of the patient's level of cooperation with physician advice. Spouses remind—or do not remind—patients to take their pills. Parents make sure their children take their medicine—or neglect to do so after the first few days of a 10-day regimen. Furthermore, in this era of short hospitalization, patients recuperate from serious illness more at home than at the hospital. And the treatment of a serious chronic illness such as kidney disease requires massive family cooperation. We argue that a wise physician in any specialty will view the patient's family as a treatment ally and partner, to be cultivated in the same way that a consultant or a referral source should be. The physician needs them and they need the physician—and the patient needs both the physician and a family.

4. *The physician's family is present during every patient interview.* No physician is completely objective when dealing with patients' personal problems. It is impossible for a physician to listen to a woman complain of her husband's inattentiveness without being influenced by his or her own experiences with parents and/or spouse. Likewise, a child out of control in the office brings to the fore the physician's own cherished notions of proper child-rearing practices. The key to not imposing idiosyncratic values on patients is to be willing to acknowledge and confront one's own experience-laden values and biases. Dealing with one's own family issues in this way holds great potential for personal development—as well as, at times, for personal discomfort.

5. *Primary care family-oriented treatment can be an effective way to help patients and families.* Unfortunately, the research evidence for this effectiveness in the primary care setting is virtually nonexistent. Until recently, most family therapy outcome research—like biomedical research—has been conducted in specialized treatment settings. Primary care family-oriented treatment is just beginning to emerge as an identifiable treatment modality separate from family therapy and individually oriented medicine. Once the theory and processes of family-oriented care are delineated, family medicine researchers must demonstrate the efficacy of the approach. The demonstration of the efficacy of *specialized family therapy,* on the other hand, has been under way heavily since 1970, and the initial results—despite difficult problems with outcome measurement and control-group designs—are encouraging for those in the primary care area. Gurman and Kniskern (1978) reviewed over 200 studies of the effectiveness of marital and family therapy. Gross improvement rates across studies were 65% for marital therapy and 73% for family therapy. The most impressive medically related outcomes have been reported for Minuchin, Rosman, and Baker's (1978) family treatment of anorexia nervosa, brittle juvenile diabetes, and uncontrolled juvenile asthma. Using objective measures such as weight gain, blood sugar levels, respiratory functioning, and rehospitalizations, this team reported improvement sustained over several years for 80 to 90% of patients. Thus, although primary care family treatment has not yet demonstrated its effectiveness, specialized family therapy is making important strides in that direction.

6. *Family-oriented medical care requires sophistication beyond the normal training of physicians.* As the continuum depicted in Fig. 1-1 suggests, the most comprehensive care involves the combination of the biological, the humanistic, and the social aspects of medicine. This comprehensive bio-psychosocial approach requires *sophistication,* a label that our culture typically—and unfortunately—assigns to individuals who specialize quite narrowly. The physician who can handle the whole continuum of care is a sophisticated practitioner, though with less depth at any one level than the subspecialist. The generalist's unique terrain is the whole terrain. The family-

oriented physician, who is neither a cardiologist nor a family therapist nor a community social worker, must blend all of these roles when a middle-aged man goes on disability because of coronary artery disease. Part of this sophistication comes from the recognition of one's limits as a generalist. These limits are drawn not by the relatively clear demarcation of an organ system (the cardiologist knows the ears are not the business of cardiology), but by a self-assessment of the family physician's own training and the experience with the problem. Only an overspecialized culture fails to recognize the sophistication of such comprehensive health care.

THE PLURALISTIC AND CHANGING AMERICAN FAMILY

What is this thing called "family" that serves as the mission of family medicine? The meaning of "family" is quite clear only if it is not examined too closely. Doherty has enjoyed asking medical students and residents to write down a definition of the family. The answers range from "Mom and Dad and two kids and a dog" to "two roommates who support each other emotionally." Is a married couple a "family" or just a couple who may become a family when they have children—that is, when they "start a family"? Are cohabitating couples "families" to each other? The Census Bureau steers clear of these subtleties by defining the family as two or more people who are related by blood, marriage, or adoption and who live in the same dwelling. Clear enough, perhaps. But this definition leaves out Grandma, who may live next door but may really run the family. It also leaves children out of the family when they move out to their own apartments, even though the parents may still pay the medical bills. If the Census Bureau definition is too restrictive, very loose definitions of the family are also unsatisfying; for example, the Pittsburgh Pirates declared themselves a "family" during their 1979 world championship season, although presumably they were merely teammates the next season.

One way to bring sense to this confusion is to think of the term "family" as having multiple definitions, all appropriate in some contexts and for some purposes. "Structural" definitions of the family refer to legal categories of membership, emphasizing first the primary marital and parental ties and then the relationships of extended kin. Structural definitions are helpful for gathering demographic and genetic information and for providing clear guidance on issues such as gaining permission for medical treatment from "next of kin." "Functional" definitions of the family refer to the everyday interdependences among people. Thus, one's family consists of the handful of intimates who provide continuing social support and to whom one turns for physical and emotional assistance in time of trouble. An individual patient's functional family may be quite different from the structural family, although usually there is quite a bit of overlap between the two. "Metaphorical" definitions of the family refer to relationships that are characterized by emotional closeness and mutual support but that are more circumscribed than those in the functional family. Some groups *feel* like a family. Members of some academic departments and group medical practices, for example, refer to themselves collectively as a "family" in order to suggest close interpersonal bonds. But metaphorical families are usually not ongoing primary support groups for their members.

In the practice of family-oriented medicine, the physician needs to be concerned mostly with both the structural family and the functional family. Since the legal kin are more visible to the physician, special attention should be given to learning about the patient's functional family as well. When a patient is recuperating from an illness, who are the people who will provide the most help? Who is the patient's primary lay health consultant? Although the answers to these questions often point to members of the family who live in the same dwelling, at other times the crucial family members in the functional sense are grandparents or other relatives who do not reside in the patient's household, as well as lovers, close friends, or folk healers. The socially oriented physician is equipped to assess both of the patient's important families, the structural and the functional.

Although this discussion has emphasized that the functional family may be different from the structural family, relationships with spouses and blood relatives (the structural family) are in reality the cornerstones of physical and emotional security for most individuals. Most people in the United States live with relatives. According to the U.S. Bureau of the Census (1980), almost 90% of the population make their home with other family members, and 83% of all families in 1979 were maintained by a married couple. Thus, despite the increases in the number of single persons, daily face-to-face interaction with other family members is the most pervasive life context in American society.

A DEMOGRAPHIC UPDATE ON THE AMERICAN FAMILY

The American family has been undergoing dramatic changes in the second half of the 20th century while maintaining impressive areas of continuity. This section documents both the changes and the continuity, and ends with a graphic portrait of the American family that may be quite different from that held by many physicians.

1. *Despite the increase in nonmarital cohabitation and postponement of marriage, marriage continues to be a nearly universal experience for adults.* The United States is a marrying society. Paul Glick, Senior Demographer with the Population Division of the U.S. Bureau of the Census, calculates that the proportion of people who never marry has averaged only about 7% over the last 80 years (Glick, 1977). Thus, over 90% of American

adults marry at some point in their lives, although the median age at first marriage has been rising since the 1950s. Despite the enormous increase in nonmarital cohabitation during the 1970s, this life style does not seem to represent a permanent alternative to marriage for most young adults; they usually get married or break up within a couple of years (Macklin, 1978).

2. *Although there are signs of a small increase in voluntary childlessness, over 90% of married couples bear children.* The proportion of couples who bear a child has actually increased from the early 1900s, when the figure was about 78%, to the 1970s, when it was about 90% (Glick, 1977). If one considers the numbers of couples with fertility problems, the 90% figure implies a substantial endorsement of parenthood, despite a small increase during the 1970s of young wives who say they want no children (U.S. Bureau of the Census, 1978).

3. *Married couples are living longer and bearing fewer children, thus extending the couple-alone period of the family life cycle.* The most striking change in American parenthood has been that parents are having fewer children. American couples marrying in the 1970s expected to have an average of only two children, down from an actual average of three to four children that held from the early 1900s through the 1950s (Glick, 1977). In addition, couples are waiting longer after they are married to have their first child, from 14 months in the early 1960s to 24 months in the late 1970s (U.S. Bureau of the Census, 1979b). Coupled with the increased life expectancy of Americans, this lower fertility rate has lengthened by 14 years the period in which the average couple lives together without children (Glick, 1977, 1979).

4. *Divorce rates have reached historically high levels in the 1970s and 1980s.* The divorce rate in the United States has shown a striking increase since the late 1960s. Earlier, there had been a peaking of the divorce rate after World War II, followed by a period of relative stability. In 1970 there were 708,000 divorces, a rate of 15 divorces for every 1000 married women. This means that 1.5% of existing marriages ended in divorce during 1970. In 1978, divorces numbered 1,122,000, a rate of 22 divorces per 1000 married women, indicating that 2.2% of marriages ended in divorce that year (U.S. Bureau of the Census, 1979c). Thus, the divorce rate increased 48% from 1970 to 1978. Divorce figures since 1978 indicate the rate of divorces is continuing to climb in the early 1980s, although the rate of increase per year has slowed down. If current divorce rates persist, some demographers estimate that future generations of married couples will have a likelihood of divorce greater than 50%. Along with the increase in divorce has been the increase in single parenthood. Single-parent families headed by a woman increased 55% during the 1960s and another 78% from 1970 to 1978 (U.S. Bureau of the Census, 1979c).

5. *The dual-earner couple has become the norm in American society.* In 1978, there were more dual-earner couples (both partners working) than couples in which only the husband was employed. This included 51% of all

wives aged 18–24, 43% of all mothers, and 41% of mothers with a child 2 years of age or younger (U.S. Bureau of the Census, 1979a).

THE REAL AMERICAN FAMILY

Several years ago the U.S. Bureau of Labor Statistics presented a graphic breakdown of American households (Fig. 1-2), which demonstrates the minority status of the so-called "typical" American family—consisting of a father who works, a mother who stays home, and one or more children. Although this pattern seems still true for most physicians' families, it represents a minority experience in today's world. In fact, there are more single-parent families than "typical" American families in the American world that the family physicians are being trained to serve.

FIG. 1-2. THE REAL AMERICAN FAMILY. FROM NEWS RELEASE, BUREAU OF LABOR STATISTICS, MARCH 8, 1977.

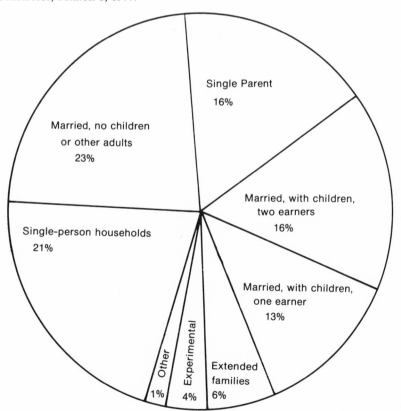

CONCLUSION

In choosing the word "family" to describe a medical specialty, family medicine has taken on a conceptual and clinical challenge of large proportions. It is attempting to replace the prevailing paradigm of medicine with a revolutionary alternative. Unfortunately, the outlines of that revolution are still vague. We argue in this book that a *family systems framework* offers the best available clinical blueprint for the family medicine revolution. The next chapter summarizes our model for primary care family-centered treatment.

2 A MODEL FOR THE PRIMARY CARE OF FAMILIES

This chapter presents a model for understanding the physician–patient–family relationship and for providing family-oriented treatment. The need for new models or blueprints in this area is clear. Despite the best intentions and the firmest ideological convictions, family medicine's delivery of family-oriented care is still quite limited in practice. The reasons for this gap are varied and complex, but one of the needs is for an ádequate conceptual framework for understanding the physician's relationship to the family.

A review of the literature on family medicine suggests that the field has borrowed a systems view of the family from the social and behavioral sciences (Bauman & Grace, 1977; Ransom & Massad, 1978; Smilkstein, 1980; Worby & Gerard, 1978). Bewildering new terms confront the physician who delves into this family medicine/family systems literature—terms such as "family homeostasis," "family adaptability," and "subsystem boundaries." All of these concepts are important for a theory of family interaction, but they are not always useful in helping a physician make practical decisions about helping a family. Awareness of family dynamics is of questionable usefulness without concrete plans of action. Unfortunately, many of the plans of action developed for family treatment come from specialists in family therapy who function outside the primary care sector. Most family physicians are understandably reluctant to employ powerful family therapy techniques without special training. The result is that the family systems perspective tends to be more popular in academic family medicine than in applied family practice.

If family systems theory has not lived up to its potential in family medicine, part of the reason is that the family has been viewed as separate from the physician's involvement in the system. The physician tends to be seen as an *observer* of family processes (like a sociologist), rather than as a *participant* in family processes. As family therapists such as Minuchin (1974)

11

and Haley (1976) have emphasized, the central unit in family treatment is not the family alone, but the therapeutic system, which includes both the family and the helping professional. The starting point for a model of the family physician's role in helping families, then, is that *the physician is part of the system.*

THE THERAPEUTIC TRIANGLE IN FAMILY PRACTICE

The fundamental point to be made in this discussion is that the physician–patient relationship is multilateral rather than bilateral. Although most physician–patient encounters occur on a one-to-one basis, the therapeutic system operates in units of at least three members—the patient, a member of the patient's family or social support system, and the physician. This therapeutic triangle is outlined in Fig. 2-1. Of course, there are other members of the therapeutic system such as nurses, referring physicians, and other family members and friends, but a three-part system is the most basic building block for viewing multilateral relationships (Haley, 1976).

THE ILLUSION OF THE DYAD IN MEDICAL PRACTICE

Modern medicine has frequently been accused of treating the disease but ignoring the patient as a person. The field of family medicine was created in part to provide an antidote to this problem. Medical schools are now offering limited training in communication skills to increase physicians' sensitivity to patients' emotional needs as well as to their physical needs. The holistic medicine movement is attempting a reintegration of the body and the mind in health care delivery—promoting, in other words, the care of the whole person. These developments represent progress from the impoverished model of the disease-oriented physician. However, much of the writing in this "humanistic" approach to medical care ignores the social context of the physician–patient relationship. This view of the medical relationship as strictly one-to-one can be termed "the illusion of the dyad in medical practice." Except in the most extreme form of episodic care, family members are involved in what transpires between the physician and the patient. Therefore, medical practice occurs in triads rather than in dyads. As documented in the previous chapter, family members influence the patient's selection of a health care practitioner, expectations for appropriate care, and evaluation of the diagnosis and the prescribed treatment. Metaphorically, the family is the "ghost in the room" when the physician is interacting with a solitary patient. These influences occur even if the physician has not treated other family members; hence, every physician who deals with patients—family physician or not—is involved in therapeutic triangles.

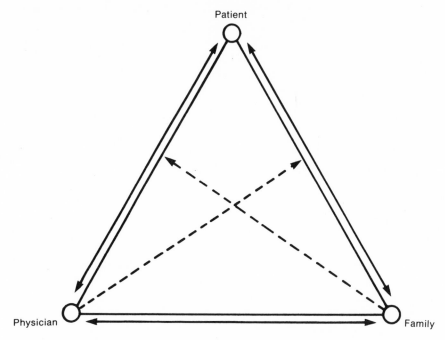

FIG. 2-1. THE THERAPEUTIC TRIANGLE IN MEDICINE.

IMPLICATIONS OF A TRIANGULAR PERSPECTIVE

The clinical potential to be gained from viewing the therapeutic system as a triangle is most available to the family physician who has regular access to both the patient and the patient's key social support person(s). (For convenience, this person or persons are referred to as the "family.") Of the three relationships in the therapeutic triangle in Fig. 2-1, the physician–patient relationship has received the most attention from physicians and researchers alike. Other implications of the triangular perspective that have not received much attention are highlighted in this discussion.

THE FAMILY'S SUPPORT OF THE PATIENT

Family physicians who overlook the therapeutic role of the family are *failing to use* full-time physician's assistants. While physicians typically diagnose and prescribe in the office, medical treatment is usually carried out at home in the family setting. Even when hospital treatment is involved, the current trend is toward brief acute care in the hospital and early release to the home setting for continued care and recuperation. Hygiene, nutrition, medication taking, exercise, rest—all of these physician-prescribed activities are performed with the support of the family. An extensive literature attests to the importance of the family in the patient's recovery from chronic illness (see the review by Pattison & Anderson, 1978). The family's involvement is equally important, moreover, in the treatment of patients' psychosocial problems. Particularly when the patient is not highly motivated to change a behavior pattern, as in alcoholism and obesity, the physician may be powerless to effect an improvement without the involvement of other family members. In general, outside the acute care setting of the office and hospital, the physician has relatively limited influence over the patient's cooperation with the treatment plan. The family has potentially the greatest influence. Mobilizing cooperative efforts among all three parts of the therapeutic triangle— patient, family, and physician—should yield the greatest likelihood of success with both medical treatment and life style change.

THE PHYSICIAN–FAMILY RELATIONSHIP

The quality of the physician's relationship with the patient's family may be a crucial influence on the amount of cooperation that occurs between the physician and the patient. The clearest illustration of this point is the therapeutic triangle consisting of the physician, the child, and the parent. Korsch and Negrette (1972) found that the likelihood of a child receiving proper at-home care after a clinic visit was affected by the mother's feelings about how much interest the physician showed in her as a person. Physicians who related well to the child but not to the mother ended up with poorer cooperation from the family. For adult treatment, it also seems likely that a positive physician–family relationship will enable the physician to gain important information about the patient's condition and to enlist the family's support in the treatment program. Generally, one would expect that the more serious or chronic the disease and the more difficult the therapeutic regimen, the more important the physician–family relationship would become.

THE PHYSICIAN'S SUPPORT OF THE PATIENT–FAMILY RELATIONSHIP

The dotted line connecting the physician to the midpoint between the patient and the family represents the ways in which the physician supports (or undermines) that patient–family relationship. In the field of human development, Urie Bronfenbrenner (1979) has stressed that the quality of primary dyadic relationships (like parent–child or husband–wife) is influenced by the support given to these relationships by significant outsiders. For example, the mother–child relationship depends on the support of the father; marital relationships are strengthened or weakened by the influence of in-laws. Robert Ryder and his colleagues (Ryder, Kafka, & Olson, 1971) likewise found evidence for the pivotal influence of family and friends on the development of a couple's relationship during courtship and early marriage. As a significant outsider in family relationships, the family physician inevitably has an effect for good or ill. For example, by supporting the family in dealing with the chronic illness of a member, the physician may help maintain the quality of the family bonds during a period of stress. On the other hand, if a physician actively or passively takes the side of a dissatisfied and anxious wife, but does not help her and her husband address their problems, then that physician is unintentionally undermining the marital relationship. *There is an irony here: The most positive and intense physician–patient relationships may serve to weaken family relationships if the physician is unaware of being involved in a triangle.*

THE FAMILY'S SUPPORT OF THE PHYSICIAN–PATIENT RELATIONSHIP

Just as the physician is implicated in family relationships, the family is continually either supporting or undermining the physician's relationship with the patient, as suggested by the dotted line in Fig. 2-1. In order to protect the interests of its members, the family evaluates the competence and concern of the physician. A diagnosis of serious illness, an uncertain or mistaken diagnosis, the suggestion by the physician that the symptoms have a nonorganic origin, a treatment plan that is not working—these are circumstances in which the patient's trust in the physician may be tested. The triangular model suggests that an important element in the continuation of a trusting and constructive physician–patient relationship will be the family's support of the physician's role. These are examples of family responses that support the physician–patient relationship: "Dr. Smith usually knows what he is doing. Remember the time he caught Johnny's meningitis?" "Why don't you ask the doctor about whether these pills ought to make you sleepy? I'm sure she'll try to find something else you can take." These are examples of undermining responses: "He's not a specialist, you know, so he's probably not up on diabetes." "She probably wouldn't listen to your complaints; she's too busy." Similarly, when the physician feels like withdrawing from a difficult patient, the family's active support of the physician may help keep the physician–patient relationship therapeutic and keep the patient in the physician's practice.

STAGES IN THE PRIMARY CARE OF FAMILIES

This part of the model discusses how family physicians can deal with patients' problems within a family context. Figure 2-2 outlines the stages and decision points along a continuum that begins with an individual patient

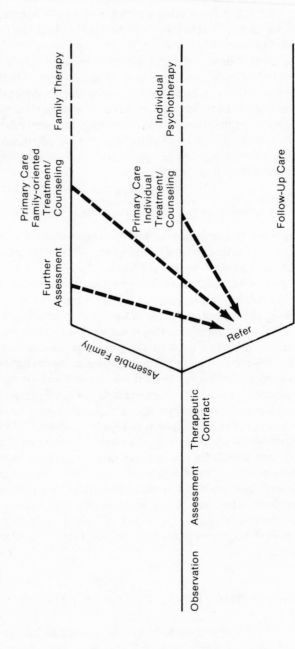

FIG. 2-2. STAGES AND OPTIONS IN FAMILY-ORIENTED TREATMENT.

presenting with a problem to the physician. The assessment and treatment processes are different in some important ways from those used by family therapists. For example, the family physician typically starts with one family member who presents with physical complaints or vague emotional complaints. The family therapist usually works from the outset with a couple or family who acknowledges a psychosocial problem of some sort. Physicians must assess the biomedical as well as the psychosocial context of the presenting problem; therapists specialize in the psychosocial context. The physician sometimes must persuade an individual that an organic complaint is associated with a psychological and social problem, whereas family therapists can assume the recognition of such problems. On the other hand, family physicians have opportunities not easily available to specialized therapists—namely to provide supportive, educational, and preventive services to patients and families without making artificial distinctions between physical problems and psychosocial problems. A myocardial infarction is a biopsychosocial event best treated by a family physician who is trained to provide comprehensive primary care.

Subsequent chapters in this book discuss each stage in the model in more detail. Here the discussion is general and introductory.

OBSERVATION

Observing patients and families in family practice is a process that occurs informally over an extended period of time. Individuals in the family come to the physician for episodic or continued care; the physician gradually accumulates not only objective information about each patient, but also an informal "feel" for the patient and family. In smaller communities, the family physician also encounters family members at the grocery store or the church. In addition, at times of birth and death, the physician is likely to observe directly how family members relate to each other. These observations, however, tend to lack the discipline that can be provided by a framework for understanding family dynamics. Using a model of family dynamics such as Minuchin's (1974), for example, the physician can more systematically observe the patterns of decision making in the family. Such information might be very useful when a medical or family problem arises at a later date. If the physician has observed that a grandmother has a powerful influence over child-rearing decisions, then the grandmother can be invited to the family conference called to discuss the child's serious medical condition. Finally, since the family physician is part of the family system in some important ways, observation of individual and family functioning should include an awareness of how the physician relates to family members and how they relate to their physician.

ASSESSMENT

Whereas the observation process occurs throughout the family physician's ongoing relationship with the patient and family, more formal assessment is likely to begin after an individual family member presents to the physician with a symptom or complaint. At this point the family physician calls upon past observations of the patient and family and tries to assess the present problem. The family physician equipped with a framework for assessing problems in their biopsychosocial context has the unique opportunity to help patients and families whose problems are still in their early stages. Biomedical and psychological assessment of the index patient are crucial steps in this overall assessment process. The focus of this book's chapter on assessment, however, is on assessment of family dysfunction and how the individual symptoms are associated with family interaction patterns. Family assessment categories must be designed for effective action. "Bad marriage," for example, is not a diagnosis that lends itself to a therapeutic intervention, whereas the diagnosis of a specific destructive marital pattern—for example, the wife becomes ill to get her husband's attention—may suggest the possibility of a therapeutic intervention aimed at having the couple deal more directly with the issues of attention and affection. Unfortunately, the field of family therapy has a confusing array of assessment models. The family physician should choose an assessment framework that lends itself to use in a conventional medical practice. Chapter 3 briefly describes the major current assessment models in family therapy and suggests an approach for the family physician based on the work of Minuchin (1974). (See also Minuchin & Fishman, 1981.)

FORMING A THERAPEUTIC CONTRACT

Forming a therapeutic contract is the process by which the physician and patient achieve joint recognition of a problem and agree to assess it further or to handle it in a particular way. The agreement may call for further tests, referral to a specialist in the problem area, specific treatment by the family physician, and/or assembling the family for further assessment or counseling about the problem. Sometimes the therapeutic contract is straightforward: The patient has the flu and agrees to stay home from work and drink lots of fluids. At other times, the therapeutic contract may be more complex: The patient probably has coronary artery disease; the physician seeks a consultation from a cardiologist and calls a family conference to discuss the diagnosis and treatment plan. If a patient presents with marital distress, the physician may suggest undertaking primary care marriage counseling with the patient and spouse, with the possibility of making a referral if the counseling is not proceeding well after several sessions. *The hallmark of a family-oriented physician will be that he or she will make the option of assembling the family a routine part of the therapeutic contract for a number of serious or chronic problems—traditional biomedical problems as well as explicitly psychosocial problems.* In subsequent chapters, we discuss criteria for deciding when to involve the family directly in assessment and treatment.

At times the therapeutic contract stage will require the high art of helping the patient view a physical symptom in its psychosocial context. The art calls for taking the physical symptom seriously while forging a treatment agreement that will introduce psychosocial factors that the patient is initially unready or unwilling to examine. To repeat, family physicians are uniquely situated to integrate at the primary care level the entire biopsychosocial terrain—body, mind, and social system. The therapeutic contract at its best helps patients perceive this same unity in their lives.

Referring versus Treating

The decision to treat or refer confronts family physicians daily over the whole range of biopsychosocial problems that patients bring to their physicians. Our focus is on the decision to offer primary care counseling or to refer to a therapist for psychosocial problems. Since we stress *family-oriented* treatment, the criteria for this decision include the physician's level of training and confidence in primary care family counseling, as well as the amount of available time and energy for treating the family. Most family physicians will choose to refer families with obviously serious problems. A more difficult decision is involved when the extent of the problem is not clear and the physician is uncertain as to whether primary care counseling or more intense family therapy is appropriate. At times, the physician will want to proceed with counseling only when a family therapist consultant is available. Generally, the physician should leave open the option to refer the patient and family if primary care counseling is not proceeding to the physician's or family's satisfaction.

After the decision is made to refer to a therapist, the physician's task is to select an appropriate therapist, to persuade patients and families to see the therapist, and to support the therapy once the referral has been achieved. After the therapy is completed, the family physician is also responsible for continued follow-up care of the patient and family.

Assembling the Family

The key difference between a family physician who *thinks* in family terms and one who *practices* a family approach is that the latter regularly sits down with families in the office and hospital. Assembling the family means calling a family conference with the patient and at least the spouse or one significant other, and sometimes with the entire nuclear or extended family. Assembling the relevant "family" also might mean inviting the patient's employer or pastor to the conference. Which family members to invite will depend on the nature and severity of the presenting problem. The physician's office and hospital settings must have accommodations suited for family meetings, and the office and hospital support staff must be oriented to this "unusual" practice. A few family physicians require family conferences before a family is admitted into the practice (Saalwaechter & Heinrichs, 1976). While this requirement may be optimal as a way to create a family-oriented practice, we think it is impractical on a large scale—and would be discouraging to many family physicians who would like to ease into a more family-centered approach.

In our model, the family physician decides whether to assemble the family after assessing the individual patient's problems in their biopsychosocial context. Generally, we believe that the physician should attempt to assemble the family when the patient is newly diagnosed with a serious acute or chronic illness, is not responding to or complying with treatment, is suffering a psychosocial problem, or is faced with making a life style change such as weight loss. A subsequent chapter lays out these criteria more systematically and presents practical ways of getting the family together as a group. A final note: We have found that holding family meetings of 20 to 30 minutes' duration two or three times a day does not unduly disrupt routine patient flow in the office. Hospital routines likewise can accommodate family conferences. Patients and families come to accept and expect such invitations to discuss their health and well-being.

MAKING A FURTHER ASSESSMENT

The best way to assess the family context of a problem is to meet with the family. Although a systems-oriented physician can learn much from interviewing an individual patient, a fully adequate assessment requires engaging the whole therapeutic triangle at the same time. During a family conference the physician can learn more about (1) the impact of the family on the patient's presenting problem; (2) the impact of the patient's presenting problem on the family; (3) the functioning of the family as a unit; and (4) the way in which the family relates to the physician in the therapeutic triangle. Often this information is needed for an intelligent referral of the whole family for treatment. In this case, the physician can share with the family an assessment of the presenting problems and make a convincing case for family treatment by a specialist in family therapy. If the assessment suggests a primary care approach, the physician can make a therapeutic contract with the whole family for primary care family counseling. Either way, constructive treatment has probably already begun through the process of engaging the family in the assessment process.

PRIMARY CARE TREATMENT: FAMILY ORIENTED VERSUS INDIVIDUAL

Following the therapeutic contract and any subsequent evaluation of the patient's problems, the family physician may choose to handle treatment in a primary care mode. The traditional approach has been to focus on medical treatment of the individual patient without direct involvement of the family, except in the case of serious illness or the patient's inability to fend for himself or herself. Similarly, psychosocial counseling generally is done with the index patient only. In Fig. 2-2, this is referred to as "primary care individual treatment/counseling," with "treatment" referring to the biomedical aspect and "counseling" to the psychosocial aspect of patient care. Frequently the biomedical treatment and the psychosocial counseling go hand in hand: The woman with headaches, for instance, is treated with pain medication and counseled about learning to relax and handle stress at home better.

We are proposing that this treatment of the individual patient should commonly be conducted with direct family involvement—hence the term "primary care family-oriented treatment/counseling." The family can be involved (if the patient and family wish) in both the biomedical and psychosocial aspects of treatment. Sometimes, the family can become involved in helping the patient adhere to the therapeutic regimen. When the family is directly involved in the etiology of the patient's problem (e.g., when an overwhelmed and undersupported mother presents with anxiety), then the family's interaction patterns may constitute the primary focus of treatment. The following sections of the chapter discuss further treatment options for the *psychosocial* aspects of patient care. But we want to reiterate that psychosocial counseling is woven inextricably into the *bio*psychosocial garment of family medicine.

OPTIONS FOR TREATING PSYCHOSOCIAL PROBLEMS IN FAMILY PRACTICE

Figure 2-3 diagrams the range of options available to the family physicians to help patients with psychosocial problems. Psychosocial problems represent the whole range of psychological and social difficulties experienced by patients and families (e.g., depression, anxiety, chemical dependency or substance abuse, marital distress, child behavior problems, sexual dysfunc-

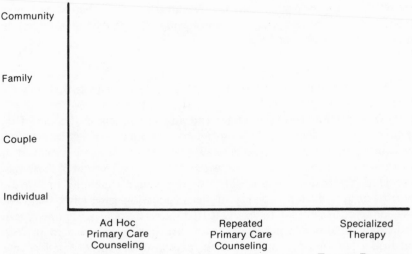

Community

Family

Couple

Individual

Ad Hoc	Repeated	Specialized
Primary Care	Primary Care	Therapy
Counseling	Counseling	

FIG. 2-3. OPTIONS FOR TREATING PSYCHOSOCIAL PROBLEMS IN FAMILY PRACTICE.

tion). Psychosocial problems can serve as both *causes* of physical illness and as *effects* of physical illness—and may also be unrelated to any physical illness. They can be idiosyncratic to a particular patient and family, or connected to patterns of stress facing the wider community. The typology in Fig. 2-3 is intended to represent the spectrum of treatment options available to family physicians after a therapeutic contract has been formed. The vertical axis represents the breadth of the treatment—that is, the number of persons (or institutions) with whom physicians directly work in helping patients with psychosocial problems: an individual patient alone, a couple, a family, or a community. "Couple" and "family" refer to persons in primary supporting relationships with one another; these persons are not necessarily legally married or in blood relationships. "Community" refers to the larger social environment, including the human services network, that may be used by the family physician to help patients with psychosocial problems.

Each level on the vertical axis in Fig. 2-3 encompasses the levels lower than itself. That is, counseling with couples can be used to help individuals as well as marriages; counseling with families can help couples and individuals as well as parent–child relationships. Similarly, interventions at the community level are aimed at mobilizing community resources—for example, Alcoholics Anonymous (AA) and spouse abuse centers—to help both individual patients and their families. A main assumption in this model is that the more a therapeutic intervention touches the significant social influences in a patient's life, the greater the potential benefit from the therapy. This is not to say that couples and families cannot benefit from psychotherapy conducted with one member, but the generalization of gains from individual psychotherapy to the marriage and family is precarious. It is much harder to move up the ladder when therapy is begun with the individual than it is to move down the ladder when therapy is begun with a larger social group such as the family.

The horizontal axis in the typology represents the depth of the treatment attempted by the physician. "Depth" refers to the amount of *change* the therapist attempts to bring about in the individual, couple, or family, as well as the *power* of the therapeutic techniques utilized or created. With reference to the community level of intervention, "depth" indicates the extent to which community resources are systematically utilized. This depth dimension is represented in Fig. 2-3 as a continuum ranging from one-shot or ad hoc counseling through repeated primary care counseling to specialized therapy. The first two categories are termed "primary care counseling" to denote an emphasis on support, education, and prevention of more serious problems, as opposed to specialized therapy's greater emphasis on more powerful intervention aimed at fundamental changes of rigid patterns. The dividing line between primary care counseling and specialized therapy is not clear in practice; therapy, for example, may be long-term, and counseling may be short-term. But the goals of therapy will generally be more ambitious, and the techniques will require more specialized training. These distinctions are developed in subsequent chapters. The important point to be made here is that each level of depth, from ad hoc counseling to therapy, has its contribution—and each has its drawbacks.

AD HOC COUNSELING

"Ad hoc counseling" refers to the one-time-only or episodic discussion between patient(s) and physician concerning a psychosocial problem. This discussion is often initiated by an individual patient as part of an office visit for an organic complaint. Based on his or her sensitivity, training, and available time, the physician tries to help the patient deal with the problem. This help may take the form of listening empathically, attempting to clarify the problem, making suggestions, or giving the patient outright advice. An ad hoc family counseling session might occur in a hospital emergency room. The counseling is ad hoc, however, because there is no follow-up unless the patient or family happens to bring up the problem again.

ADVANTAGES

Ad hoc counseling has several important uses. First, it is useful for the physician in gathering information about the patient and the family and in forming impressions about the nature of the presenting psychosocial problems. In other words, ad hoc counseling sessions are helpful in the observation and preliminary assessment stages of the family physician's involvement. This is especially true if the physician does not attempt to "solve" the patient's problem in 10 minutes, but rather shows a sympathetic openness to pursue the problems further if the patient wishes. Why is an ad hoc approach appropriate in some situations? It may be that the patient is not yet ready for more in-depth work on the problem but does want to "test the waters" with a family physician. If the physician makes the "water" comfortable enough, while respecting the patient's initial tentativeness, then the patient may decide at a later time to take the "plunge" and seek more systematic help with the problem. In addition to serving as a nonthreatening entree for serious psychosocial problems, ad hoc counseling alone may help to resolve certain less serious problems, especially those in early stages of development when brief, educational interventions may be effective. Sometimes, for instance, the physician can normalize an experience that the patient thinks may be abnormal, thereby preventing a full-blown negative reaction. Examples include counseling a new mother who is guilty about resenting the infant's demands, or a newly divorced man who is experiencing mood swings for the first time. In these situations, ad hoc counseling alone can sometimes be helpful, especially in the context of an ongoing physician–patient relationship.

LIMITATIONS

Ad hoc counseling alone is not helpful for serious problems, just as an episodic medical treatment is not normally effective for treating serious disease. What may be less obvious are the *risks* involved in the premature advice giving that often occurs in ad hoc counseling by physicians. A physician who would never prescribe a potent medication without a careful assessment of the patient's illness may give potent advice to a patient with psychosocial problems after a 10-minute conversation. There are two dangers here: First, the patient may feel as if the physician does not want to take the time needed to really help with the problem, and therefore may not seek further help for the problem; and second, the patient may follow the physician's advice and experience negative consequences that the physician will not find out about. Since the physician has not scheduled a follow-up session, the responsibility to "bother" the doctor again about the problem is the patient's. Unfortunately, too much counseling in physicians' offices is of the ad hoc, advice-giving type, with the focus on the individual patient rather than the patient in the context of social relationships.

REPEATED PRIMARY CARE COUNSELING

Most family physicians engage in multiple sessions of supportive counseling with patients who have psychosocial problems. Often this counseling accompanies treatment with psychotropic medication, in which case the primary weight of the treatment unfortunately tends to rest with the medication, while the physician monitors the patient's progress and offers emotional support or advice. The most common counseling is with individual patients presenting symptoms of depression or anxiety: The physician supports the patient while the medication takes effect. Less common are situations in which the patient and family are seen more than once for counseling about a psychosocial problem. This treatment approach—termed "primary care family counseling"—is the major focus of this book. Its main functions are support, education, prevention, and challenge. This primary care counseling turf lies somewhere between the common-sense approach of the old-time country doctor and the specialized interventions of the family therapist.

ADVANTAGES

Most people at some time in their lives can benefit from primary care counseling from a family physician. This treatment modality is most useful in helping individuals, couples, and families through temporary crises and disruptions—when they need short-term nurturance and education. Examples include the death of a family member, adjustment to life after a heart attack, adjustment to a marital disruption. At other times, more long-term but (less frequently scheduled) counseling is helpful to patients and family dealing with the chronic illness of a family member. In such cases, community resources may also be needed to help the family, and the physician can serve as the coordinator of such services. Primary care counseling can be quite helpful to patients and families who have the resources to deal with their problems, provided they are given adequate support. In addition, primary care counseling can be used to educate patients and families about the stresses and opportunities of family life, and thereby to prevent the occurrence of more severe problems. Finally, primary care counseling has the function of challenging patients and families—for example, by confronting them about serious problems and persuading them to enter specialized treatment.

LIMITATIONS

Like ad hoc counseling, primary care counseling is not effective for chronic, serious psychosocial problems, such as alcoholism, severe marital distress, child abuse, or chronic difficulties in dealing with social relationships. Family physicians who try to treat such serious problems with primary care counseling alone will quickly become frustrated. These patients and families need more intensive help.

Another contraindication for primary care counseling is a patient or family who appears quite resistant to trying new ways to solve problems. When the parents never successfully carry out the plans that the physician has helped them work out to deal with their child, the physician should consider shifting gears by proposing that the family undertake family therapy. In other words, unsuccessful supportive or educational counseling should signal the family physician to consider challenging the family members about a problem that may be more serious than they realized, and then making a referral to a family therapist.

One problem with primary care counseling as practiced by many physicians occurs when the counseling is conducted with only an individual patient. Here the physician/counselor may be unaware of the family dynamics involved in the patient's problem, as well as the implications of the counseling for the patient's family relationships. The unaware physician who develops a close relationship with a patient may unwittingly be creating conflict between the patient and a spouse. Or the physician may become "triangulated" into a family conflict by being used by one family member against another (e.g., "The doctor told me to take it easy around here and for you to help more"). Even the most benign-appearing supportive counseling has its hazards as well as its benefits.

Finally, the family physician who does much primary care family counseling will need a network of other family-oriented professionals for consultation and referral. Such networks are not always available and must be created.

THERAPY BY FAMILY PHYSICIANS

Therapy for psychosocial problems implies a conceptual framework and treatment plan that is outside the normal training of family physicians (thus, the dotted lines in Fig. 2-2), although more physicians are beginning to obtain such specialized training. The therapist—as distinguished from the primary care counselor—must know how to manage the intracacies of the therapist–patient or therapist–family relationship, especially how to deal with resistance to change. The family therapist in particular often takes the risk of temporarily destabilizing the family in order to make change possible —for example, by stirring up conflict in a conflict-avoidant couple. Therapy is like aggressively treating a serious illness in the same way that primary care counseling is like conservatively treating the symptoms of a patient whose body might eventually cure its own disease. Community-oriented therapy adds the additional impact of providing social supports and specialized services that no individual physician could offer alone.

ADVANTAGES

Therapy for psychosocial problems has the obvious advantage of being the most powerful nonchemical treatment at the disposal of the family physician. A family physician who is trained in family therapy has a sorely needed service to offer patients. The physician/therapist is already likely to have the confidence of the patient or family and to have an accessible data base about the family. Just as early treatment of serious disease is usually preferable to later treatment, family therapy initiated early by a family physician who sees problems in their infancy has a clear advantage over referral therapy. In addition, the family physician can manage in a "holistic" fashion both the psychosocial problems and any accompanying medical problems. It is hard to imagine more comprehensive care than that provided by a well-trained family physician/therapist who is also able to mobilize community resources to help families in stress.

LIMITATIONS

The chief limitation on family physicians' provision of psychotherapy or family therapy—more important than the practical problems—is the amount of training and ongoing consultation required to specialize in the therapy of psychosocial problems. Probably no residency training program in the country provides enough family therapy training in its curriculum in order to turn out family physician/therapists, although some residents do obtain this training through aggressive individual initiative. Like medical skills, the development of family therapy skills requires years of supervision. Thus, even a reasonably well-trained resident will need several additional years of guidance in family therapy after he or she begins to practice in a community. In addition, the family physician who does family therapy must have a supportive environment of colleagues with whom to share successes and failures; this work is emotionally quite demanding and at times unsettling to one's own personal relationships. Finally, there are important practical problems associated with family therapy in a physician's office, including issues of finding time in a busy practice, facilities, and fees. These constraints call for a less ambitious goal for family medicine in the psychosocial area, an approach we term "primary care family counseling."

SUMMARY

This chapter presents a conceptual framework for understanding the family physician's role in helping patients in a biopsychosocial context. The fundamental orientation of the model is that the physician–patient relationship is enacted in triangles rather than dyads, with third parties such as family members being implicated in all but the most episodic medical transactions. This orientation suggests that it is generally safe to assume family involvement in the problems that an individual patient brings to the physician. Thus, family physicians who wish to provide comprehensive care to patients are advised to obtain a working knowledge of family dynamics and insight into the physician's relationship with families.

The second part of the model delineates the stages of a family physician's involvement with individual and/or family problems. The model attempts to capture the unique nature of the family physician's relationship to families—a relationship quite different from that experienced by the specialist in family therapy. Family physicians have the opportunity to observe individuals and families over their natural histories and to assess their strengths and weaknesses in response to a variety of stresses. This longitudinal relationship gives the family physician a special role in the early diagnosis and treatment of psychosocial problems. The trust a family often has in its physician gives that physician a special opportunity to form a therapeutic contract aimed at getting such a family the help it may need. Skills in observing, assessing, and forming therapeutic contracts, as well as in facilitating appropriate referrals, are crucial for every family physician.

For family physicians who choose to address the psychosocial aspects of patient care actively, there is a range of possible interventions, from the traditional ad hoc counseling of individuals to full-fledged family therapy that also uses community resources. The most helpful and realistic treatment option for family physicians without special training in therapy is family-oriented primary care counseling, with the option to refer if more intensive therapy is needed. Tied by disciplinary speciality to neither a narrow biomedical nor a strictly psychosocial approach, family medicine is the ideal field to forge an integrated biopsychosocial model in both theory and clinical practice.

3 FAMILY SYSTEMS THEORY AND FAMILY THERAPY

This chapter presents a nontechnical introduction to family systems theory and family therapy. Most of these concepts are elaborated upon and exemplified frequently in later chapters. In addition, the chapter outlines the requirements for a family practice approach to family counseling, and summarizes the school of structural family therapy, from which our family assessment framework is largely derived.

FAMILY SYSTEMS THEORY

In struggling to understand the individual's symptoms in the context of the family, the pioneers of family therapy in the 1950s (many of whom were psychiatrists) borrowed ideas from the emerging discipline of general systems theory. The systems orientation is quite familiar to physicians from their training in biology. The heart, lungs, and blood vessels, for example, are viewed as interdependent parts of the cardiovascular system rather than simply as discrete organs. Disease in one part of the system affects the rest of the system; treatment of an individual organ must be conducted carefully in order to avoid undesirable effects on other parts of the body. The human body, then, is a biological system with component subsystems. The interdependence of these subsystems can make medical treatment frustratingly complex, as in the case of drugs that kill tumors but also shut down the body's immune responses. Physicians, then, are no strangers to the systems approach to biological organisms, but generally they are not accustomed to viewing social groups such as families in systems terms. *Assessing and treating families requires such a framework.* Following are several core family systems axioms that family therapists have adapted from general systems theory:

1. *The family is more than a collection of individuals.* This proposition is synonymous with the notion that the whole is greater than the sum of its parts. On a practical basis, this means that a physician cannot understand a marriage simply by knowing the two partners individually, and that change or stress affecting one family member affects the whole family. Since physicians usually deal with individuals one at a time, they must guard against understanding the *family members* while missing the family.

2. *Families have repeating interaction patterns that regulate members' behavior.* All families develop implicit rules for daily living. These may be viewed as family "rituals"—often not articulated—that give regularity to the family's life. On the mundane level, families have repeated mealtime patterns (who sits where, who cooks, who cleans up) and customary ways to handle bathroom privacy (open door versus closed door). The rule-like quality of these repeated interaction patterns may be visible only when someone violates the custom (e.g., by sitting in someone else's chair at dinner or by entering the bathroom without knocking). Families tend to have stable patterns of handling decisions, of celebrating holidays, and of relating to outside professionals such as physicians. On a less benign level, families also may develop troublesome rule-like interaction patterns, such as the following: (a) family members may interrupt one another's conversations at any time; (b) the father is to be kept in the dark about the children's misbehavior; (c) one child is to be singled out for blame when something goes wrong (the family scapegoat), while another child is consistently praised; (d) the wife of an alcoholic is expected to make excuses for his lapses from responsibility; and (e) the only way to get attention from other family members is to become ill. Analysis of these interaction patterns is the chief assessment tool of most family therapists.

3. *Individuals' symptoms may have a function within the family.* A physical or psychosocial symptom may become incorporated into the family interaction patterns in such a way that it seems essential for the family's harmony and regularity. A brittle diabetic's precarious health may help hold the parents' precarious marriage together. Or a marital union may be based on the caretaker–patient roles of the spouses, with one partner's illness serving as the counterpart to the other partner's overprotectiveness and feelings of self-competence. On a practical level, a history of repeated psychosomatic or psychosocial prroblems and a failure to cooperate with medical treatment should alert the physician to the possibility that the patient's symptoms are serving hidden purposes in the family—purposes that the family is almost always unaware of. Stated differently, there is a "fit" between the symptoms and the family's needs. Family therapy may be required to help the family change this dysfunctional interaction pattern. On the other hand, when the symptoms are of recent origin, it is possible that the family has not yet stabilized around these problems. In such cases, primary

care family counseling—as opposed to family therapy—may be sufficient to help the patient and the family through the temporary difficulty. *Such an early family counseling intervention by the physician may prevent the symptoms from becoming entrenched in the family and thereby becoming much more difficult to treat.*

4. *The ability to adapt to change is the hallmark of healthy family functioning.* Change is the ever-present challenge to families: change as individual members get older; as the family adds and loses members; as the social, political, and geographic environment changes; as the health of members waxes and wanes. Family therapists stress the importance of the family's flexibility or adaptability in the face of such changes. When the husband and wife become parents for the first time, they must learn to juggle parental and marital roles without sacrificing either. When adolescents struggle for autonomy, the parents must learn different ways of being parents. When older children begin to marry, the parents must learn the new role of "in-laws." These are some of the normal transitions of the family's career—transitions that some families handle quite well but that leave other families paralyzed and in conflict.

In addition to life cycle transitions, illness may challenge a family's ability to adapt to new circumstances. When the father or mother in the family becomes incapacitated for an extended period, the coping resources of the family must allow for a reshuffling of roles (e.g., who earns the primary income, who does the primary housekeeping and child care). Illness events also test the flexibility of the extended family, as when a grandmother can no longer live on her own without help: Are her children now able to "parent" their mother, and will she permit this role reversal? When a family is not able to handle a major change, one member may develop symptoms and go to the doctor to get help for the family. The family physician with a family systems orientation may be able to discover that this patient is the "squeaky wheel" for the rest of the family. This discussion of family adaptability may be summed up in a saying attributed to Ludwig von Bertalanffy, the biologist who founded general systems theory: "System sickness is system rigidity."

5. *There are no victims and victimizers in families: Family members share joint responsibility for their problems.* One of the blind spots of many professionals is the tendency to view family problems in "good guy/bad guy" terms. The alcoholic husband is viewed as the cause of marital problems, with the wife relegated to the role of passive victim. The emotionally disturbed child is seen as the necessary product of poor parenting, or the parents are regarded as afflicted with an "impossible" child. The quiet but anxious husband is pitied for having to suffer with an aggressive, domineering wife. The nurturant, trusting wife is consoled because her unfeeling husband is too busy to pay enough attention to her. A closer look at the family system in

each case will most likely reveal that the so-called "victim" is playing as active a role as the so-called "victimizer" is. *Family members are both actors and reactors, especially in maintaining chronic problems.* There are no family villains.

A common example of complementary roles is the following alcoholic marital pattern: The alcoholic husband misses work because of his drinking; his wife calls in an excuse to his employer; the husband takes this as implicit acceptance of his drinking; she comes to treat him more and more like an irresponsible child; being treated this way makes him feel worse about himself. There are no good guys and bad guys in this drama—just fellow actors and fellow sufferers. Similarly, the "overprotected" child will struggle to maintain this status even after the parents try to change their ways. This aspect of the systems perspective is what family therapists call "circular causality," a repeating sequence of actions that creates or sustains a problem. The following vignette exemplifies the application of a circular causality model to a psychosomatic disorder:

> A 5-year-old girl who has suffered various respiratory ailments since infancy is finally diagnosed as having asthma. [*Note*: the family dynamics have not *caused* her asthma.] Her parents are quite concerned about her breathing and are faithful in administering the medication. Soon after the asthma treatment begins, the girl gets angry at her parents for not letting her watch television and works herself into an asthmatic attack. The terrified parents call the physician to say that their daughter cannot breathe and must be seen and then they take the child to the emergency room. The daughter recovers after treatment and returns home for an ice cream treat and some television to settle her down. She gradually becomes more skilled at inducing attacks, while her parents become more emotionally reactive to her illness episodes. They start to disagree about how to handle the problem, with the father accusing the mother of spoiling the girl and the mother telling the father that he is callous. If the cycle does not soon stabilize, the family—and the girl—become quite dysfunctional. The physician who comes upon this family in the emergency room is likely to emphasize *either* the overreactiveness of the parents *or* the manipulations of the girl. The family systems perspective would take *both* factors into account and would try to break the vicious circle without blaming anyone for the mess they unintentionally created. Helping this family would also involve an assessment of the physician's role in this family system.

If one phrase could be used to capture the family systems approach, it would be "the interactional context" of human behavior and human problems (Watzlawick & Weakland, 1977). A central metaphor would be that of "the dance": Family members move with one another in complementary ways that lead to healthful or hurtful consequences for individuals and the family group. Family systems theory emphasizes the interconnectedness of human beings in their intimate environment.

MODELS OF FAMILY THERAPY

Although most family therapists would agree on the preceding tenets of family systems theory, there is nevertheless wide divergence in the field on the best way to treat dysfunctional families. The *Handbook of Family Therapy* (Gurman & Kniskern, 1981) contains chapters on 15 different approaches to marital and family therapy. Fortunately or unfortunately for the family physician, there is no evidence that one school of family therapy is generally more effective than another, although some approaches have established firm grounding in treating selected disorders (Gurman & Kniskern, 1981, Chapter 20). Since family medicine has yet to establish its own approach to family counseling and family therapy, we must borrow from the established theories. But just as tertiary medical care practices are often not appropriate in family practice offices, so too family therapy approaches must be adapted and distilled for use by the family physician. This is the task of the subsequent chapters in this book. For now, we briefly discuss some commonalities and differences among models of family therapy.

COMMONALITIES

Most family therapists try to gain access to the entire family system (at least to those members residing in the same household) or to both married partners in the case of marital therapy. Family therapists assess the family system as a whole rather than piecemeal through separate interviews with individual members, although sometimes members may be interviewed individually as well. In addition to assessing the family at the systems level, family therapists of all persuasions attempt to help the family modify its *dysfunctional interaction patterns*. Thus, family therapists tend to be more concerned with the *process* of the family's interaction (e.g., the ways in which the family makes decisions or responds to stress) than with the *content* of the family's specific conflicts (e.g., arguments over money or child-rearing practices). Novice counselors/therapists tend to get caught up in the content of the specific family issues and lose sight of the underlying structural or process issues that are keeping the family dysfunctional. In line with this focus on interaction patterns, family therapists try to keep themselves out of coalitions with one family member against another; they do not allow themselves to be used by one member to gain points on another. All family therapists try to get family members to communicate clearly with one another, beginning with the principle of speaking only for self and not for anyone else. Finally, most family therapists are actively involved in structuring the therapy sessions by shaping goals, confronting dysfunctional patterns, and intervening to clear up confused communication. Few family therapists succeed by remaining passive in the face of powerful family interaction patterns.

DIFFERENCES

One of the principal differences among family therapy approaches lies in the attention paid to individual family members' psychological development. Some schools—for example, Murray Bowen's (1978) approach—emphasize that the level of the family's functioning depends on the psychological development of the parents. Thus, in addition to helping family members change their interaction patterns, some family therapists engage in long-term therapy aimed at helping the spouses handle their own feelings in a more deliberate way. Other schools of family therapy—for example, Minuchin (1974) and the Palo Alto group (Bodin, 1981)—deemphasize the role of individual psychological development and focus almost exclusively on helping families change the way they *behave* or interact. In the same way, some schools stress the historical roots of family dysfunction and treat three-generational family systems (grandparents–parents–children), while other schools emphasize the role of the here-and-now interaction patterns and pay little attention to historical causes. In the area of assessment, some approaches gather rather extensive background information about the family, whereas other approaches obtain a brief outline of family history and then a careful description of the presenting problem. Some therapies emphasize a wide range of family problems, while others treat a more narrow band of problems such as marital dysfunction or parent–child problems.

REQUIREMENTS FOR A PRIMARY CARE APPROACH TO FAMILY COUNSELING

A primary purpose of this book is to derive from family therapy's Tower of Babel a coherent framework for family physicians. Following are some important requirements for a primary care approach:

1. In Jay Haley's (1980) terms, the theory of family dynamics and family counseling should be *simple enough* for an average family physician, but *comprehensive enough* to cover many of the problems that physicians will encounter.
2. The treatment should be problem-focused rather than aimed at a thorough overhaul of individual and family functioning.
3. The treatment should be short-term. A year of weekly sessions is not feasible for most family physicians. Reasonable progress should be achievable within six sessions for problems that lend themselves to a primary care intervention.
4. The treatment should not require two counselors. Since the availability of a cotherapist is unlikely, family physicians should avoid strict allegiance to treatment approaches like Masters and Johnson's

(1970) sex therapy and Whitaker's symbolic–experiential family therapy (Whitaker & Keith, 1981), both of which strongly urge the use of cotherapy teams.

5. The treatment should have reasonably low risk for the physician and the family. For example, the treatment should avoid strong confrontation of family members' intrapsychic defenses and should avoid saddling the family physician with expectations for a high degree of self-disclosure of feelings and experiences to the family.

6. The treatment should be usable by physicians of average psychological development. Some family therapy schools, such as Bowen's (1978), maintain that the success of their treatment depends to a major extent on the level of psychological maturity of the therapist. For Bowen, this maturity depends on how well the therapist has handled relationships with his or her family of origin. Other schools, such as Minuchin's (1974), do not explicitly require exceptional levels of psychological development. Although the role of the therapist's own family experiences and level of personal maturity is clearly an important issue, we nevertheless believe that many family physicians possess the personal resources to help many families in primary care treatment.

7. The treatment should have special relevance to psychosomatic or stress-related medical problems. The reason for this criterion should be obvious: Family physicians often encounter family problems presenting themselves as individuals' psychosomatic complaints.

If any of the established schools of family therapy fulfilled these seven criteria for primary care treatment, our task in this book would be simply to select this approach and explain it to family physicians. In fact, family therapy models have been designed for specialists who treat severe family dysfunctions, not for family physicians who have the time and training to develop only a modicum of skill in family treatment. An obvious example of the difference is that family physicians will not normally be able to devote the full hour or more assigned by therapists to treatment sessions. Furthermore, family physicians, unlike therapists, must attend to a broad range of the family's biopsychosocial needs over a long period of time, and will inevitably develop closer bonds with some family members than with others.

Because we believe that family medicine requires its own family treatment model, this book swears allegiance to no one school of family therapy. The family counseling techniques described in Chapter 7 are an eclectic combination derived from our background in family therapy and our clinical experience in primary care settings. Although our family *treatment* model is deliberately eclectic, we have adopted established family *assessment* categories based on the work of Salvador Minuchin and his colleagues (Minuchin, 1974; Minuchin & Fishman, 1981). Minuchin's structural family therapy approach to family assessment fits the criterion of being simple enough but comprehensive enough for use in family medicine. More than any other family assessment approach, it has been applied to the assessment of psychosomatic problems in families (Minuchin *et al.*, 1978). The approach does not require an elaborate data base or extensive history taking. It is problem-focused while remaining sensitive to underlying family dynamics. Although some family physicians may want to gather more information about the family than Minuchin's model calls for, his framework does provide enough basic information to begin planning treatment. Finally, there is an element of personal taste here: We ourselves use Minuchin's assessment categories (modified somewhat, as shown in Chapter 4) and find it compatible with our preferences for treating families.

The next section briefly introduces some of the principal concepts of structural family therapy, with detailed discussion left for future chapters.

MINUCHIN'S THEORY OF FAMILY DYNAMICS

Structural family therapy (Minuchin, 1974) has four basic notions in its theory of family dynamics: transactional patterns, adaptation, family subsystems, and boundaries.

TRANSACTIONAL PATTERNS

"Transactional patterns" are the repeating sequences of family interaction: who relates to whom, how, and when. This notion is identical to the previously discussed family systems concept of repeating interaction patterns, and in subsequent chapters we use the more common term "interaction patterns." Transactional patterns take the form of family rules developed over time in explicit and implicit contracts. Minuchin observes that transactional patterns serve the function of maintaining the family's stability.

ADAPTATION

"Adaptation" refers to the availability of alternative transactional patterns and to the family's ability to mobilize these alternatives when necessary. Just as transactional patterns help the family maintain its homeostasis or stability, the family's adaptability helps it change in the face of external and internal pressures. Like other family systems theorists, Minuchin believes that family dysfunction is often a product of poor adaptability, as in the typical case of a family's inability to adjust to the father's illness: The mother takes on a greater wage-earning burden, but the father does not adjust to a home-bound role, a situation leading to marital strain and sometimes child abuse when the father gets frustrated in his new "mothering" role.

SUBSYSTEMS

"Subsystems" in a family are the smaller units, such as the married couple and siblings; in addition, each individual family member can be seen as a subsystem of the larger unit. According to Minuchin, subsystems are the ways in which the family system differentiates and carries out its functions of mutual support, nurturance, regulation, and socialization of its members. For example, nurturance and socialization of children are the function of the parental subsystem; adult mutual support is the function of the spouse subsystem. Minuchin believes that participation in both family and non-family subsystems is a principal vehicle for children to develop a sense of identity and to learn interpersonal skills. A girl, for instance, learns that she is a daughter, a sister, a student, a member of the basketball team, a church member, a granddaughter, and a niece. In each case, the child is learning to participate in a subsystem with its own set of transactional boundaries.

BOUNDARIES

"Boundaries" of a subsystem are the rules defining who participates in a subsystem and how they participate. Boundaries are essential to protect the unique identity of the subsystem. The marital subsystem, then, must be clearly differentiated from the parent–child subsystem. The boundaries must be *clear* enough to prevent interferences, but *flexible* enough to allow contact across subsystems. Assessment of boundary clarity is central to structural family therapy. "Boundary clarity" represents a continuum from "disengaged" to "enmeshed," with clear boundaries in the middle. "Disengagement" is characterized by boundaries that are too rigid, as when the mother–child subsystem excludes the father's involvement in parenting. "Enmeshment" occurs when boundaries are diffuse or porous, as when the marital pair have no privacy from their children. According to Minuchin, most families have both enmeshed and disengaged subsystems at different parts of the family life cycle (e.g., for a time a breast-feeding mother and her infant may be enmeshed, with the father temporarily excluded; or an adolescent may be disengaged from the parental subsystem for a period of time). However, when a number of subsystems are functioning at the extremes of enmeshment, then the whole family will be overresponsive and overreactive to stress on individuals. Members are metaphorically in each other's skins, overinvolved in each other's feelings and experiences. A disengaged family, on the other hand, offers its members little protection and the children little guidance. In subsequent chapters, we use the more general term "cohesion" instead of "boundaries" to characterize the degree of closeness and distance between family members, with extremes being labeled "enmeshment" and "disengagement."

PSYCHOSOMATIC FAMILIES

Minuchin *et al.* (1978) postulate a typical family profile when a child has a psychosomatic disorder such as anorexia nervosa, brittle juvenile diabetes, or stress-induced asthma. Their research suggests that children with such disorders come from families whose transactional patterns are measurably different from those of families with seriously but nonpsychosomatically ill children. According to Minuchin and his colleagues, the four core characteristics of psychosomatic families are as follows:

1. Enmeshment—members are overly reactive to stress on one member and demonstrate a lack of individual autonomy.
2. Overprotectiveness—members are not permitted to handle their own problems.
3. Conflict avoidance—open airing of disagreement is not permitted, although covert conflict is rampant.
4. Rigidity—transactional patterns are repeated inflexibly, and change is resisted.

Although this family pattern has been documented only in a pediatric setting, we believe that it probably has relevance to adult psychosomatic disorders and to chemical dependency in adults. Such families are apt to overutilize family physicians' services and to try to incorporate the physicians into their dysfunctional style (i.e., to get the physicians to overreact and overprotect in treatment situations). Such families are typically warm and pleasant, grateful to their overinvolved physician—and will engulf you if you let them.

STRUCTURAL FAMILY THERAPY INTERVENTIONS

Although we urge family physicians not to view themselves as structural family therapists without special training, the following discussion gives background information on this approach to therapeutic intervention. A central assumption of structural family therapy is that family transactional patterns affect the inner process of individual members. Thus an effective way to help individuals change is to change their family context. The individual problems most often treated by structural family therapists are psychosomatic and acting-out problems of children and adolescents.

There are two general stages in structural family therapy. First is that of *joining the family*. The therapist must engage the family in order to change it. Joining consists partly of being sociable and gracious. This is what many physicians do with a new patient during a preliminary period of informal conversation. The second aspect of joining the family is to temporarily accept the family structures or transactional patterns. For example, in a family where the father is the titular head, the therapist will address him with special deference. Third, joining a family requires the therapist to temporarily adopt the family's overall mood and style: Some families are playful, others serious; some intellectual, others folksy. A skillful structural family therapist will learn to take on the tone of the family in order to be accepted by its members.

The second stage of structural family therapy is *restructuring the family*. The content of the restructuring is idiosyncratic to each family, but generally the therapist is quite active in trying to modify the family's dysfunctional interaction patterns and clarify boundaries. Special emphasis is usually placed on the parental subsystem. Parental conflict facilitates the development of coalitions of one parent with a child against the other parent. This often leads to dysfunctional behavior in the "triangled" child. Structural family therapists move to unite the parents in disciplining their children, even sometimes insisting that parents sit beside each other during the sessions. The disengaged parent may be given an assignment to check the child's homework every night. Other restructuring interventions include blocking family members from keeping secrets that others have the right to know; stopping interruption (one of the ways that families keep boundaries too diffuse is by interrupting conversations that two members are having with each other); and getting members to deal directly with their conflict rather than detouring it through another member (e.g., helping the couple to confront their disappointments in each other rather than focusing exclusively on the children's problems). Generally, structural family therapists actively orchestrate the family therapy sessions and move quickly to restructure the family.

Assessment in Minuchin's therapy goes hand in hand with intervention. The rigidity of the family, for example, might be assessed by observing how the family performs a therapeutic assignment given during the first session. The therapist gains diagnostic information by interacting with the family and probing the family's ability to change rather than by taking an elaborate history. Finally, structural family therapists typically begin therapy with the whole family—those who live under the same roof or who are important participants but who live elsewhere. Subsequent sessions may be conducted with the whole family or with particular subsystems of the family, especially with the mother and father. Part of a session may be spent with the whole family, while the other part is spent with the parents alone. The latter arrangement helps to strengthen the parental alliance by emphasizing their unique role and relationship.

CONCLUSION

Of the ideas presented in this chapter, three are crucial to the rest of the book:

1. Interaction patterns.
2. Adaptability.
3. Family enmeshment versus disengagement (family cohesion).

This new family systems vocabulary is necessary to conceptualize the shift from treating isolated individual patients to treating families. The analogy made earlier is to the difference between treating bodily organs in isolation and treating the body as an interconnected biological system. Families are interconnected social systems of staggering complexity. Even more complex is the larger social system that constitutes the family physician's vehicle for helping families—the physician–family relationship in the therapeutic triangle.

4 OBSERVING AND ASSESSING FAMILIES IN FAMILY PRACTICE

Observing and diagnosing physical signs and symptoms is a treacherous enough enterprise for most primary care physicians, despite their extensive training in organic medicine. Attending to emotional and psychological symptoms is trickier still, since physicians receive much less training in this area. The third component of a biopsychosocial assessment—a family and social assessment—requires a breathtaking leap beyond the traditional practice of medical diagnosis. The first problem in family assessment is how to organize and evaluate the enormous quantity of information about families that the family physician acquires in a daily office practice. Unlike family therapists who gather information about families through whole-family interviews, family physicians generally must gather data in piecemeal fashion through contacts with individual family members. In addressing the issues of observing and assessing family functioning, this chapter discusses three topics: first, observing family dynamics during routine medical care; second, detecting clinical "red flags" that suggest the presence of family dysfunction; and third, assessing family dysfunction after a presenting problem has been identified. Special attention is paid to the physician's role in the family system.

OBSERVING FAMILY DYNAMICS IN THE THERAPEUTIC TRIANGLE

The title of this section reflects a fundamental assumption of this book: that the physician is part of the "system." Hence, much of the data on a family's interaction comes not from the physician's observation of the family, nor from objective tests or assessment tools; rather, the crucial data emerge from the physician's week-to-week interchanges with family members. The family physician can learn much about a family before a family problem arises or before the family makes the problem known to the physician. Much of this information concerns how the family handles the health and illness of its members, and how the family relates to the physician. This information in turn will make more sense to a family physician who has a framework for understanding family systems and a framework for understanding the physician's relationship to the family. The following questions relate to a number of family interaction patterns that an alert family physician can observe in the course of routine medical care:

1. *Who is the family's primary health authority and health agent?* This is the individual through whom the patient gains access to health care and the physician's services; this is the key person in the therapeutic triangle. In practice, the wife/mother frequently holds this position, although a grandmother or another family member believed to possess special expertise may also fill the role. In Minuchin's terms, a family can only be "joined" if the physician acknowledges the family's health authority. One way to observe this family role is to ask patients routinely whom they have talked to about their health problem, and what advice that person gave.

2. *Which family members overutilize medical services?* The individual patient who comes to the office too frequently for minor complaints is bearing a message about the family. Often the family is supporting a habit of physician overuse by one of its members. This family probably lacks—or is not effectively using—its own coping resources. Therefore, it tries to incorporate the family physician into the family to do the family's job of supporting its members. For example, when a wife does not receive emotional support from her husband, she finds a way to get it from the doctor. When a mother feels unsupported by her husband and by her own mother in caring for small children, she may make an anxious pit stop at the doctor's office each time a child develops symptoms. The physician becomes the surrogate father and grandmother for the family—not without mixed feelings from being used in this way. Physicians have several options here: (a) trying to extricate themselves quickly from this burdensome role by avoiding or dropping such patients; (b) trying to educate such patients about appropriate use of medical care (often a fruitless endeavor, because the problem does not stem from lack of knowledge); (c) counseling the patients about underlying psychological insecurities (a sometimes helpful approach that unfortunately tends to pull the physician more deeply into the family system by creating more dependency in the patient); and (d) involving families in a way that creates the possibility for changing the underlying dynamics of the overutilization.

3. *Who is the family's chief underutilizer of medical services?* Often this is the husband/father of the family. The family physician may discover the underutilizer through conversations with family members who are more active patients. The wife, for example, may ask what her husband can do for

his month-long sore throat and cold. When the physician suggests that the husband come in for an examination, the wife says that her husband does not listen to her and never goes to doctors unless he cannot stand up any more. What might this husband's role in the therapeutic triangle suggest about the family's interaction patterns? It is quite possible that the husband fills the strong, inexpressive role in the family system. He is the "rock" whose denial of vulnerability may stem not only from a long-standing personality disposition but also from the dynamics of the marital relationship. His "strength" may allow his wife to be "weak." This marital balance may be somewhat precarious, however, because he may disdain his wife's vulnerability as much as she resents his inexpressive *machismo*. Patterns of help seeking during illness may be viewed as metaphors of the family members' general willingness to offer emotional support to and accept it from one another. A family with a blatant underutilizer may be a family at risk for dysfunction if it is placed under significant stress. One approach that the family physician can take to an underutilization problem is to strongly urge the wife (in this example) to insist that her husband visit the doctor. Her willingness to *insist firmly* that he see a doctor may signal to her husband that she is not so weak and therefore may not need him to be so strong; if she acts strong, he may be freed to act weak enough to accept emotional and medical support when he needs it. Such a subtle shift in a couple's complementary roles can produce benefits for both parties.

4. *Who visits the patient in the hospital—and for how long?* One of the best ways to observe the patient's *functional* family is to notice who responds to the patient's hospitalization by frequent visits. These people constitute for the patient a primary support system that can be marshaled by the physician. Routine questions to the floor nurses can yield the important information, for example, that a woman's husband is hardly ever present at her bedside. This may suggest a degree of disengagement in the marital relationship. (Of course, there may be benign reasons as well, and the physician should always ask rather than assume.) Not only is family disengagement observable in the hospital, but family enmeshment can be seen as well. Doherty observed a marital dyad in which the wife literally did not leave her husband's room for more than 5 minutes over a 3-day period. He was in the hospital for routine diagnostic tests related to abdominal pain. Their clinging behavior suggested an interaction pattern consistent with an enmeshed, overprotective relationship. It turned out that the husband was an alcoholic. In this case, the first family diagnostic sign was the hospital visitation behavior of the wife. In another case, a 10-year-old boy recovering from surgery for a ruptured appendix was never sure, during our daily hospital rounds, whether his parents would be visiting that day. He was not complaining; he did not seem to expect much attention in his large and rather poor family. The physician would be wise in this situation to entertain the hypothesis that this family is on the disengaged end of the cohesion continuum. If so, the family physician

might want to assemble the family at the boy's bedside and attempt to reinvolve the parents in their child's recovery.

5. *How does the family respond to the patient's disabling illness?* Serious acute illness taxes a family's ability to cope with high levels of short-term stress. The adjustment to a disabling chronic illness, however, makes perhaps even more demands on a family's resources, since there is no way to return to the old stable patterns. The physician can observe the extent to which family members over time are able to take over some roles abandoned by the disabled member while still permitting this member to feel useful in the family. A common example in family practice is that of the family crisis occurring when an elderly parent becomes disabled to the point of not being able to live independently. This situation challenges the family's ability to assemble its leaders and make a family decision. Some families will splinter at this point and try to leave the decision to the physician. Other families will hold together and adjust to the new reality. The family physician is observing here the family's adaptability under stress. Family physicians can be of enormous help to families at these times by serving as the "convener" of the family—the outsider who calls the family together and confronts the family with its need to make a decision about the welfare of one of its members. A family that shows little flexibility and cohesion during health-related crises is ripe for dysfunction down the road. The family physician can anticipate the appearance of physical or psychosocial complaints in this family's most vulnerable members.

6. *How do parents share responsibility for the children's health needs?* The family physician can learn about the parental subsystem in a family by observing how parents deal with their children's medical problems and health care. Is the mother fully responsible for this area? Does she seem to shoulder all the decision making about when to visit the doctor and when to keep the children home from school? Does the father get involved at all? Does she ask him to get involved? The totally responsible parent may be enmeshed with the children, while the uninvolved parent may be disengaged from both the children and the other spouse. On the other hand, a pattern of mutual support between the parents for their children's health care suggests a well-functioning family. This mutual support may be evidenced in both parents' participation in preventive health maintenance, screening children's symptoms, deciding on at-home treatment and visits to the doctor, and bringing the children to the doctor. When the mother is overly responsible in this area, she is likely to feel unsupported or even undermined by her husband, while at the same time she reaps less obvious rewards from her status as the children's primary caretaker. Unfortunately, many physicians reinforce this dysfunctional pattern by relating to the mother as if she were the only responsible agent. Such physician behavior in the therapeutic triangle may serve to prop up a dysfunctional parental alliance, often with unfortunate results.

7. *How do parents discipline their children?* Children's behavior in the physician's office is sometimes a source of stress for both the parents and the physician. (The children do not always enjoy themselves, either.) The family physician can gain valuable insight into a family by observing and interacting with a parent–child pair in the office. When the child is uncooperative, how does the parent respond? Some parents abdicate their authority to the staff by allowing the child free rein. If this occurs, it is likely that this parent is out of control of the child in other situations as well. When a child, say, is opening drawers in the examining room, a good way for the physician to learn about the parent–child relationship is to ask the parent to prevent the child from misusing the office equipment, rather than telling the child directly. This communicates to the parent that the physician believes that parents are responsible for children's behavior, and that the physician is not going to do the parent's job. The parent and child's interaction should be observed: Does the parent plead with the child, bribe the child, scream at the child, or resort quickly to spanking? Or does the parent speak firmly and lay down consequences for noncooperation? Does the child ignore the parent, yell back, escalate the conflict—or settle down when firmly reprimanded? The physician is witnessing a family interaction pattern; the fuller pattern can be witnessed only with both parents present. But before one parent is blamed for being "inadequate," the influence of the whole parental subsystem should be considered: Often when one parent is out of control, the other parent (or some other family member) is undermining the parent's authority. Allowing the drama of the parent–child interaction pattern to unfold in the office opens the door to asking the parent about difficulties in controlling the child at home and about whether the parents would like help in dealing with the problems. (We hasten to add that if the parent cannot or will not control the child's destructive behavior in the office, the physician should then step in and model an authoritative parent in action. Protecting the office property will provide the incentive.)

8. *Do family secrets block communication in the family?* Family therapist Murray Bowen (1978) uses the term "triangulation" to describe the process whereby two family members in conflict try to ease the strain by involving a third party in the conflict. A wife who is in ongoing conflict with her husband over sexual issues may unconsciously seek leverage on him by revealing their sexual problem to the family physician, all the while knowing that the husband is opposed to such a revelation of their "secret." When a patient discloses a family problem to the physician with the accompanying admonition not to let other family members know about the revelation, the physician should hypothesize the presence of rigid family interaction patterns that block communication among members. A mother brings her adolescent daughter for an abortion referral and asks the physician not to say anything to the father. A middle-aged man prefers to keep his wife somewhat in the dark about the nature of his heart problem; he does not want to "worry" her.

These family secrets represent powerful communication barriers in families. The family physician may sometimes be caught in a confidentiality bind that does prevent any revelation to other family members. At the minimum, however, the physician can use the presence of family secrets as useful background information about the family in case the family seeks help in the future. A more active posture on family secrets would be to urge the holder of a secret to bring in the other family member for a conference aimed at helping the family work more closely on its problems.

The answers to the above eight questions can help the family physician develop background information and valuable perspectives on families. This information comes primarily from interacting with patients and families in the therapeutic triangle. People wear their families on their sleeves for the ready observation of family physicians who know how to observe. Sometimes the physician does not have to *do* anything immediately with these observations, but the information can be quite valuable later if a fuller family assessment is needed.

CLINICAL "RED FLAGS" SUGGESTING FAMILY DYSFUNCTION

Some common clinical presentations in family practice may be related to significantly disturbed family functioning. The physician, of course, must evaluate each symptom individually, because biomedical and psychological factors may also be prominent in these symptoms. Our point, however, is that family dysfunction should be considered early in the differential diagnosis of the following symptoms (the list is based on our clinical experiences):

1. *"Atypical migraine" headaches of long-standing duration*, accompanied by a list of previous specialists who have evaluated and unsuccessfully treated the problem. It is not uncommon to have a young to middle-aged female patient who has intermittent but fairly severe headaches that have not quite fit the classic descriptions of migraine or muscle tension headaches. Frequently a careful history will reveal that the patient herself (or himself) has a clear association of family stress as a trigger point for the headaches, but has never discussed this with physicians. We find it useful to incorporate the spouse and/or other family members in the office management of this problem. Rarely have we met resistance to this approach, probably because of the chronic severe discomfort stemming from this problem.

2. *Persons with chronic depression, unmanageable by any long-term therapy, either medical or electroconvulsive.* It is not uncommon to have a history of depression for several decades with rather poor results from any management technique. Chronic family stress may be the root cause of poor recovery. In the history, the physician must look for interactive medications,

especially antianxiety agents that can aggravate the depression. These anti-anxiety agents may have been prescribed for many years by family physicians when the patient and family would become frustrated with side effects from antidepressants prescribed by a psychiatrist. In this situation, it is not unusual for the physician to have become incorporated into the dysfunctional family pattern and thereby to be perpetuating the problem. Treatment requires not only family intervention but also discontinuation of the aggravating medication and, if possible, incorporation of the prior physician in the treatment program.

3. *The patient presenting with "chronic anxiety" who has had many office visits over several years for multiple and diffuse complaints without significant diagnostic evidence of "organic" disease.* Long-term antianxiety medication is a frequent common denominator. In this setting, it is nearly universal that family functioning has deteriorated, even if it had been healthy early in the course of this set of symptoms. After years or decades the family interaction patterns have become distortedly organized around the anxiety symptoms. In these situations it is always helpful to have a family interview. Commonly, the primary patient has become psychologically dependent on the antianxiety medications; if so, the physician should move the patient and family into chemical dependency treatment.

4. *Patients presenting with a primary complaint of chronic fatigue.* Obviously a thorough medical evaluation is a fundamental responsibility of the physician. However, early in the review of symptoms, the physician must be sure to assess family relationships and to gather as much information as possible about how the family system functions. When initiating the medical evaluation, the physician can raise the possibility that life stress can cause fatigue, so that if laboratory evaluation proves negative, the physician and patient can move more smoothly to a family-centered evaluation and treatment. *Depression is a common denominator in these patients.* The patient may have assumed a chronically dissatisfying and dysfunctional role within the family and may recently have begun thinking of changing that role. The stimulus for this rethinking may have come from a friend who has found new meaning in life or from a book about seeking more satisfying family relationships or life styles. A family interview after the medical evaluation is often well received by these patients; indeed, the patient may be covertly requesting such help in presenting at this time with these long-standing symptoms.

5. *A number of pediatric complaints for which educating the parents has not been effective.* Classically these complaints are presented by the parents as serious medical problems, and no amount of explanation from the physician will change their minds. Medical evaluation makes the seriousness of the symptoms seem doubtful, unless that evaluation considers the possibility that the *family system* is dysfunctional rather than the physical health of the child. Common among these "red flag" complaints are the following:

a. Poor appetite in the first year of life is reported by the family, despite a healthy-appearing child.

b. Enuresis is reported by the parent for a child below age 2 who may not have the physical capabilities for bladder control.

c. Fussiness and poor sleep patterns are reported in children in the first year of life, where it is common that parenting responsibilities have become so overwhelming that the simple task of deciding as a parental team on a bedtime routine is more than young parents can agree upon. (It is not uncommon for this to be the first signal for serious maladjustment in an early marriage, but it might also be a simple case of young parents with no experience with young children.)

d. A parent presents a child with the primary complaint of hyperactivity, but the child behaves extremely well in the office. (The family system may have found a scapegoat in the "hyperactive" child. This complaint deserves serious attention, but is easily put aside by a busy physician, who may simply pass these symptoms off to the parent as insignificant and thereby deny the family access to any further consultation or referral.)

6. *Insomnia in certain patients.* Although insomnia is a very common symptom and often is not the primary complaint of patients in the family physician's office, in some situations it may suggest a more serious family dysfunction. Insomnia in middle-aged men may be an indicator of underlying depression and/or dissatisfaction with close relationships or occupational roles. A careful alcohol history may uncover inappropriate alcohol use as an aid to sleep. We have found it common that males with complaints of insomnia have developed over many years a habit of significant alcohol use every working day. Serious chemical dependency should be evaluated in these cases. Patients who are not significantly involved in inappropriate use of alcohol quickly respond to the suggestion to change their alcohol consumption pattern, and they seem to tolerate the 4 to 6 weeks of uncomfortable and unimproved sleep patterns required until their sleep cycle is reestablished. However, those who have developed a significant psychological or physical dependency on alcohol will not respond well to this approach and will need a family interview to assess the impact of the insomnia and the alcohol on their close relationships.

Generally, any consistent complaint that defies medical explanation after repeated examinations and perhaps previous consultation may be a clue to family dysfunction. The physician must always remain alert for subtle serious illnesses that often have obscure diagnoses early in their course but that become more noticeable or identifiable later in their progression of symptoms. While evaluating these complaints within a family systems context, the physician can safely leave the door open for further medical evaluation at any point, should symptoms change or become more recognizable as a clinical entity. Moreover, when the complaints are vague but persistent, a family interview is helpful, if only as a demonstration of the physician's sincere interest in the complaints and willingness to support the patient and family. These family conferences are much appreciated by most families.

ASSESSING FAMILY DYSFUNCTION
IN FAMILY PRACTICE

The previous sections have outlined a number of preliminary indicators of family functioning. This section discusses more specific assessment categories that the family physician can use to gain a clearer picture of the family. Generally, a confident assessment of a family's level of functioning requires sitting down with the whole family, but preliminary hypotheses can be formed from interviewing individual family members.

The field of family therapy unfortunately lacks the refined diagnostic categories and procedures available in biomedicine. There are no widely accepted and clinically practical diagnostic tests or instruments for family dysfunction, although quite a large number of instruments have been written up in the research literature (Cromwell, Olson, & Fournier, 1976). Two measurement procedures developed in the family medicine tradition are discussed later in this chapter.

Our conviction is that there is no substitute for careful analysis of the family's life situation and interaction patterns, and that this analysis can be done only through interacting with the family in the therapeutic triangle. The assessment categories and indicators described here are derived largely from the work of Salvador Minuchin (1974), although almost all family therapists would also use at least our four core dimensions: stress, adaptability, cohesion, and interaction patterns. Olson, Sprenkle, and Russell (1979) have documented the universality among family therapy theories of the concepts of *adaptability* and *cohesion. Interaction patterns,* as we have noted, are a core element in all systems approaches to the family. Finally, *stress* must be included in a family assessment to locate the trigger for much family dysfunction.

The family physician's assessment of family dysfunction, then, can be derived from the answers to four basic questions:

1. What are the sources of stress on this family?
2. How adaptable or how rigid is the family?
3. How cohesive is the family?
4. What are the family's repeating interaction patterns related to the problem?

WHAT ARE THE SOURCES OF STRESS ON THIS FAMILY?

Stress occurs when events or situations strain the family's resources. Minuchin divides the sources of family stress (or "stressors") into "internal" and "external" categories. Prominent among internal sources are family life cycle changes and the illness and disability or death of family members. External sources include stressful contact of one member with extrafamilial forces such as school and work, and stressful contact of the whole family with extrafamilial forces such as the welfare system or a depressed economy. Of course, families often are suffering from both internal and external sources of stress. McCubbin, Joy, Cauble, Comeau, Patterson, and Needle (1980) have discussed how stressors "pile up" in families: Some families can handle the main stressor, such as illness or unemployment, but fall apart under the added strain of adolescents' leaving home or elderly parents' becoming more dependent.

THE FAMILY LIFE CYCLE AS A STRESSOR

Families move through a common (though not universal) sequence of transitions and transformations, just as the individual human organism goes through predictable changes from infancy to old age. A prominent and universal source of stress for families lies in the challenge of adjusting to a new stage in the family's career. One way to demarcate stages in the family life cycle is as follows: (1) the newly married couple, (2) the family with young children, (3) the family with adolescent children, (4) the launching phase, and (5) the older family. An increasingly common variation on this "typical" sequence is a divorce, a period of single parenthood, and remarriage into a "reconstituted family." The main point is that any significant transition can strain the family's resources for reorganizing itself. *The presence of stress in a family may suggest "growth pains" more than serious family dysfunction.* Minuchin criticizes some family therapists for being too ready to label a family as a dysfunctional when it is merely reacting to a temporary dislocation:

> To focus on the family as a social system in transformation, however, highlights the transitional nature of certain family processes. It demands an exploration of the changing situation of the family and its members and of their stresses of accommodation. With this orientation, many more families who enter therapy would be seen and treated as average families in transitional situations, suffering the pains of accommodating to new circumstances. (Minuchin, 1974, p. 61)

Any of the clinical "red flags" discussed earlier, then, may stem from the stress of a transitional process in the family's career. The complaint may be related to the shakedown process of a new marriage, the new burden of a dependent infant, the addition of a second child, the challenge of an emerging adolescent, concern about the physical decline of one's parents, or the fear of being dependent on one's children in old age. Equally or more stressful are adjustments to being divorced and restarting a family. Carter and McGold-rick (1980) have developed an interesting table outlining the emotional processes and the systems changes required at each stage of the family's life cycle. These authors begin their stages with the "unattached young adult" (see Table 4-1).

ILLNESS AND DISABILITY AS STRESSORS

The threat of reality of the loss of a family member or of that member's normal role in the family is tremendously unsettling for the family. In one family we have worked with, the adolescent's acting-out behavior intensified after the mother was diagnosed with multiple sclerosis. In another family, the husband never resigned himself to his wife's multiple sclerosis, and their relationship began a slow decline toward eventual divorce. In neither case did the illness *cause* the family dysfunction, but it did tax the family system beyond its strength. Both families may have remained functional under less severe stress. In the face of a chronic illness or disability, some families reorganize satisfactorily and continue to support their members; some families never reorganize and suffer severe hardship; and other families adjust in such a way that the family needs the individual to remain sick and dependent. It is especially difficult diagnostically to differentiate families that are appropriately supporting their disabled member (such as retarded children) from families that are oversupporting the members by keeping these persons dependent.

EXTRAFAMILIAL STRESSORS

The physician may determine that the family is basically healthy but suffering from externally caused stresses affecting either individual members or the family as a unit. Job-related stress, for example, is reported to be widespread. According to Gunby (1981), the National Center for Health Statistics found that about one in four Americans report that they experience a "great deal of emotional stress on the job." In some cases, the physician may want to call upon community resources. Where such resources are inadequate, then the physician may want to take the plunge into "community therapy" by trying to bring new resources to the community. In any case, it is important to support the family, to help it adapt if necessary, and not to imply that the family itself is the locus of the problem.

How Adaptable or How Rigid Is the Family?

In the face of normal and abnormal stress, some families do quite well, and other families break apart or develop a dysfunctional stability. According to Minuchin and many other family therapists, *the key to family coping is*

TABLE 4-1. THE STAGES OF THE FAMILY LIFE CYCLE

Family life cycle stage	Emotional process of transition: Key principles	Changes in family status required to proceed developmentally
Between families—the unattached young adult	Accepting parent–offspring separation	a. Differentiation of self in relation to family of origin b. Development of intimate peer relationships c. Establishment of self in work
The joining of families through marriage—the newly married couple	Commitment to new system	a. Formation of marital system b. Realignment of relationships with extended families and friends to include spouse
The family with young children	Accepting new members into the system	a. Adjusting marital system to make space for child(ren) b. Taking on parenting roles c. Realignment of relationship with extended family to include parenting and grandparenting roles
The family with adolescents	Increasing flexibility of family boundaries to include children's independence	a. Shifting of parent–child relationships to permit adolescent to move in and out of system b. Refocus on midlife marital and career issues c. Beginning shift toward concerns for older generation
Launching children and moving on	Accepting a multitude of exits from and entries into the family system	a. Renegotiation of marital system as a dyad b. Development of adult to adult relationships between grown children and their parents c. Realignment of relationships to include in-laws and grandchildren d. Dealing with disabilities and death of parents (grandparents)
The family in later life	Accepting the shifting of generational roles	a. Maintaining own and/or couple functioning and interests in face of physiological decline, exploration of new familial and social role options b. Support for a more central role for middle generation c. Making room in the system for the wisdom and experience of the elderly, supporting the older generation without overfunctioning for them d. Dealing with loss of spouse, siblings, and other peers and preparation for own death; life review and integration

Note. Adapted by permission from E. A. Carter and M. McGoldrick, "The Family Life Cycle and Family Therapy: An Overview," in E. A. Carter and M. McGoldrick (Eds.), *The Family Life Cycle: A Framework for Family Therapy* (New York: Gardner Press, 1980). Copyright 1980 by Gardner Press.

family adaptability. Adaptability is the family's ability to respond flexibly—particularly to modify its interaction patterns if necessary—in the face of stress. Poor adaptabililty or rigidity is the sure indicator that the family will need specialized therapy instead of primary care counseling.

After discussing the misdiagnosis of dysfunction ascribed to some families who are experiencing the normal strains of adapting to change, Minuchin discusses the core family dimension of adaptability:

> The label of pathology would be reserved for families who in the face of stress increase the rigidity of their transactional patterns and boundaries, and avoid or resist any exploration of alternatives. In average families, the therapist relies on the motivation of family resources as a pathway to transformation. In pathological families, the therapist needs to become an actor in the family drama, entering into transitional coalitions in order to skew the system and develop a different level of homeostasis. (Minuchin, 1974, p. 60)

How can family physicians assess the family's level of adaptability? We propose two ways: first, through the family's history (as taken verbally from family members and as observed by the family physician), and second, through "nudging" the family in family counseling and seeing whether it changes. The history approach yields crucial information on precipitating events and on the chronicity of the problems. The longer the family has lived with the problem, the more rigid the family system is apt to be when faced with the task of changing its interaction patterns. For example, alcohol abuse of long duration clearly suggests a family with a low level of adaptability. A more flexible family would have either solved the problem or split apart. The same holds for dependency on prescription drugs, except that here physicians may be active participants in the family dysfunction. *We believe that dependency on prescription drugs generally indicates dysfunction in the therapeutic triangle.* In fact, rigid and dependent families frequently draw kindly but unwary physicians into rigid and enmeshed relationships with themselves. This dynamic renders the family more difficult to treat for an outside therapist unless the therapist can change the rigid family–physician interaction pattern (Selvini-Palazzoli, Boscolo, Cecchin, & Prata, 1980).

A second way to assess family adaptability is to engage the family in a counseling relationship to see whether change occurs. This approach is akin to the way physicians handle some medical problems of uncertain etiology. Sometimes it is worth beginning treatment with a low-risk therapy whose success or failure will yield diagnostic information, such as antibiotic therapy for infections of undetermined etiology. In assessing family functioning, the physician may be uncertain from the history about the extent of the family's rigidity. In such cases, primary care family counseling (with an agreed-upon limit of sessions before a referral) will give the physician a much clearer picture of the family's functioning. For example, if the physician helps a couple agree to spend a few hours together without the children during the next week, the spouses' success in carrying out the task will give the physician information about their flexibility, as well as about the likelihood that they will need therapy as opposed to primary care counseling.

HOW COHESIVE IS THE FAMILY?

Some families allow members to support one another emotionally and physically while holding on to an adequate degree of autonomy or separateness. Maintaining the balance between "family" and "self" is a continual challenge for all families. Too much cohesiveness ("diffuse boundaries," in Minuchin's terms) creates a situation in which family members are "inside one another's skins"; they are overprotective, overreactive to one another's pain. Diagnostic signs of enmeshment in a family include the following:

1. Members speaking for one another.
2. Continual interruptions while someone is speaking.
3. High levels of emotionality, such as tears in one member "spreading" quickly to others in the family.
4. Overprotective responses.
5. Either unwillingness to discuss conflicts and negative feelings for fear of hurting someone, or reactive conflict where family members flare up angrily at apparently small provocations.

Disengaged boundaries are synonymous with the noncohesive family. Family members go their own way, do not respond quickly to emergencies, and are emotionally unreactive to one another. The latter point is crucial to the diagnosis of disengagement, since avoidance behavior in a family can also be the temporary result of enmeshed relationships that have gotten too painful. The key difference is that enmeshed relationships will still be highly volatile emotionally even when members are trying to avoid one another, whereas people in disengaged relationships are generally emotionally "clicked off" from one another, although they will engage in conflict if one member provokes the other.

It should be noted that often in dysfunctional families, one subsystem or relationship (e.g., a mother with an adolescent child) may be enmeshed, while another (e.g., the father with the same adolescent child) may be disengaged. Secondly, terms such as "enmeshment" and "disengagement" are not precise diagnostic categories with unmistakable behavior indicators. They are among the best concepts we have in the field, but the dimensions of boundary clarity themselves still need more clarity.

WHAT ARE THE FAMILY'S REPEATING INTERACTION PATTERNS
RELATED TO THE PROBLEM?

The answer to this question provides the dynamic quality of family assessment. According to Watzlawick and Weakland (1977), leaders of the "interactional" school of family therapy, the heart of family assessment is the analysis of the interactional context of dysfunctional behavior (i.e., the problem can be understood as emerging from the ebb and flow of family behavior within the overall interactional "dance"). A fine-grained analysis of this interactional context can provide the key to solving the problem by changing its family context. Watzlawick gives the following example of an interactional diagnosis:

> For a relationship to be viable, there has to be a minimum of that kind of mutual understanding which is colloquially referred to as "knowing where one stands with the partner." What constitutes that minimum may vary greatly from one individual to another; for whatever reasons in their individual past, some people get along with very little of it, while others need a lot. Assuming now that a husband belongs to the former class of people and his wife the latter, a typical conflict will very probably arise in their marriage. Since the wife does not get enough information from her husband to know "where she stands" with him, what he thinks and feels about her and their shared life, etc., she is likely to try to get this information by asking him pertinent questions, watching his behavior, searching for further clues, and the like. In all probability he will find these behaviors excessively curious and intrusive. Notice that up to this point there is nothing even remotely "pathological" about their relationship. They simply operate with two different ideas about what their degree of understanding and closeness should be, and neither of these ideas is wrong *per se*—they are simply different. But the situation is unstable and unless they manage to decrease the discrepancy of their views, their interaction is bound to escalate. The more she seeks the missing information, the less likely he is to give it, and the more he withdraws and keeps her at a distance, the harder she will try to establish closeness. Both are thus caught in a "more-of-the-same" interaction in which, typically, a solution is sought through increased effort that precludes the solution. The rest of this fictitious, yet everyday story is easy to imagine. By the time professional help becomes necessary, her behavior satisfies the established clinical criteria of pathological jealousy. (Watzlawick, 1977, pp. xiii–xiv)

Minuchin (1974) and Haley (1980) emphasize those interaction patterns that maintain clear boundaries (optimal cohesion) across family subsystems, so that members can have both the support and the autonomy appropriate to their age and position in the family. Stated simply, Minuchin and Haley believe that parents should cooperate with each other, that the parents should give each other more emotional support than either gets from the children, and that parents should be in charge of their children. When this family hierarchy is firmly in place, then parents are not likely either to undercontrol or to overcontrol their children, and adults are free to work out their problems between themselves. Common dysfunctional interaction patterns that undermine this hierarchical arrangement include the following:

1. One parent repeatedly allies with a child against the other parent.
2. The oldest child is thrust into the "parental child" role with inappropriate responsibilities for the other children.
3. One parent develops a closer allegiance with a grandparent than with the coparent.
4. An unsatisfying marriage leads one parent to derive too much emotional support from a child.
5. The children continually play one parent off against another.
6. The family physician or other outside professional gets incorporated into a coalition with one family member against another.

Communication in families can be viewed as an aspect of family interaction patterns. As Watzlawick, Beavin, and Jackson (1967) maintain, *all* behavior—both verbal and nonverbal—in an interactional situation has message value (i.e., is communication). Two basic categories for assessing communication in families are (1) the directness of the communication and (2) the congruence of the communication. "Directness" refers to whether family members communicate through intermediaries—for example, a son tells his mother when he is angry at his father—or can deal in straightforward fashion with one another as individuals. In some families, the members speak for one another: For instance, if someone asks Sara a question, her mother will answer for her. The implicit interactional rule is that no one can have a direct relationship (communicate) with Sara except through the mother. "Congruence," which is closely linked to directness in communication, refers to whether the verbal and nonverbal channels of communication are sending the same message. When family members are angry with one another, do they laugh or give long speeches or avoid contact? Or do they more congruently express this anger by both words and tone of voice? Families develop implicit rules for what can be communicated about and what cannot; certain feelings or wants are acceptable, and others are negatively sanctioned. Since feelings tend to "leak out" whether they are sanctioned or not, families in which open expression of negative feelings is not permitted will experience high levels of incongruent—and confusing—communication.

Despite the importance of communication in families, however, we do not list it as a separate assessment category, because we believe that much "poor communication" stems from larger structural and interactional issues (such as ongoing coalitions) that make effective communication nearly impossible. For example, if a father and a daughter are aligned against the mother, then communication between the mother and the daughter is bound to be skewed. If a husband continues to have an affair against his wife's wishes, their communication will doubtless take a nosedive in quality. We note these points because newcomers to family counseling sometimes assume that all family problems stem from "poor communication" and can be solved by getting people to talk more directly with one another. Although it is often helpful to get family members to be more direct and congruent, communication patterns in our view flow inexorably from the underlying dynamics of the family system and therefore must be evaluated and dealt with in the context of wider family assessment and treatment issues.

TWO FAMILY MEDICINE CONTRIBUTIONS TO FAMILY ASSESSMENT

Academic family physicians have begun to direct more attention to biopsychosocial assessment (Medalie, Kitson, & Zyzanski, 1981; Smilkstein, 1980). From this promising early work, two techniques have emerged as potentially useful family assessment tools. These are the family tree (or family pedigree) and the Family APGAR.

The Family Tree

One way to get a handle on a complex family system, especially a three-generational family or a "blended" family created by the merger of two divorced people, is to diagram the family. This family diagramming is used extensively by the Bowen school of family therapy (Bowen, 1978) and has been used in a limited form by genetic counselors for years. Family medicine has borrowed the approach and expanded it by including both biomedical information and psychosocial information. Depending on the family physician's purposes and available time, the family tree can serve as (1) a quick overview of family members and their interrelationships, (2) a way to overlay biomedical and psychosocial information visually, or (3) a study tool for gaining a comprehensive understanding of multigenerational family systems. In his textbook *Principles of Family Medicine,* Rakel (1977) provides clear instructions for and illustrations of how to construct a family tree. Basically, he suggests including all members of at least three generations of the family, including both spouses' families. Ages or birthdates of family members can be added, dead members can be indicated with a slash, and known chronic diseases can be indicated by an appropriate symbol in the box for each member. A key for the symbols should be stored in the physician's head or at the bottom of the tree. Conflict can be symbolized by jagged lines between certain family members. Enmeshment can be marked by extra-heavy lines between two or more members; coalitions can be indicated by lines separating two members from a third. Divorce can be documented with a disconnected line and the year of the divorce, with the noncustodial parent's new family penciled in. The family tree, then, can be used to store almost any information the physician wishes.

Figure 4-1 contains the simplest form of a family tree, designed to provide the physician with a quick overview of the three-generational family. Figure 4-2 presents a more complex family tree for the same family, with biomedical and family systems data. This family has an alcoholic father and is characterized by a coalition of the mother and children against the father, a conflicted relationship between the father and the oldest son, and an enmeshed relationship between the mother and the asthmatic daughter. The father's side of the family contributes risks for depression and alcoholism, the mother's side for asthma, hypertension, and cancer.

The complexity of the family tree constructed should depend on the physician's purposes. Family physicians in busy office practices will probably confine themselves to a rapid sketch of the family tree when they are dealing

FIG. 4-1. A SIMPLE FAMILY TREE. ADAPTED BY PERMISSION FROM R. E. RAKEL, *Principles of Family Medicine* (PHILADELPHIA: W. B. SAUNDERS, 1977). COPYRIGHT 1977 BY W. B. SAUNDERS.

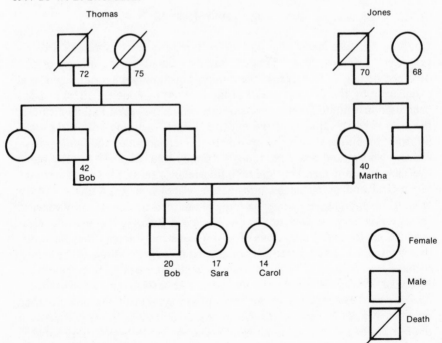

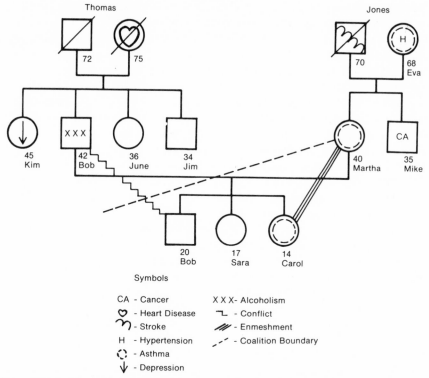

Symbols

CA - Cancer   X X X - Alcoholism
♡ - Heart Disease   ⌐ - Conflict
〜 - Stroke   /// - Enmeshment
H - Hypertension   ⟋⟍ - Coalition Boundary
◌ - Asthma
↓ - Depression

Fig. 4-2. A More Complex Version of the Same Family Tree. Adapted by Permission from R. E. Rakel, *Principles of Family Medicine* (Philadelphia: W. B. Saunders, 1977). Copyright 1977 by W. B. Saunders.

with large family systems. In other cases, when such information can be stored mentally or does not seem especially relevant to the presenting problem, many family physicians will not use a family tree at all. Generally, however, the family tree can be a useful tool for bringing order out of chaos. Its chief limitations are the time it takes to construct and the fact that it provides only "static" data and not interactional data about the ebb and flow of the family's interactional waters.

The Family APGAR

Although some would dispute the point, we believe that the family therapy field does not yet possess reliable, valid, and clinically practical assessment instruments. In other words, there are no simple tests for family functioning that lead to clear treatment decisions. Many of the best assessment instruments in the family field are either too long for use in family practice offices or require video equipment and trained observers (Cromwell *et al.*, 1976). One instrument out of the family medicine field, however, deserves consideration as a rapid screening instrument for family dysfunction—Smilkstein's (1978) Family APGAR scale.

The Family APGAR is a five-item paper-and-pencil test designed to elicit the patient's perceptions of the current state of his or her family relationships. The acronym APGAR stands for Adaptation, Partnership, Growth, Affection, and Resolve—core elements of family functioning that are purported to be tapped by the instrument. The Family APGAR seems to have adequate reliability and validity as a brief measurement of an individual's level of satisfaction about family relationships, although it cannot substitute for a more comprehensive assessment of the family as a unit. The scale and relevant instructions are included in Table 4-2.

How might the Family APGAR be used in family physicians' offices? Although we are generally skeptical of the ability of paper-and-pencil instruments to reveal more than could be learned in a brief interview with the patient, we think that the Family APGAR can be useful as part of a battery of tests conducted to determine the etiology of functional complaints and disorders that may be stress-related. Following is a possible scenario: The patient has presented with abdominal pain. The physician may choose to order diagnostic tests for the organic disorder and also may ask the patient to fill out the Family APGAR so that "I can get a better idea of what's happening in the rest of your life that might be causing your stomach to act up." By this patient's next visit, the physician will have the results of the lab tests and also an indication from the patient about the patient's level of dissatisfaction at home. If the patient has signaled in the Family APGAR the presence of distress at home, then these issues can be explored. However, this scenario depends on a trusting relationship between the patient and physician, since the scale will show only what the patient is willing to reveal. Generally, we favor discussions with patients rather than paper-and-pencil instruments, but the Family APGAR is a minimally disruptive and time-consuming instrument that can serve in some situations as a door opener to further assessment of psychosocial problems.

STORING FAMILY ASSESSMENT AND
TREATMENT INFORMATION

Anyone who has reviewed medical charts can testify to how little psychosocial information is generally recorded. One reason may be that traditionally only biomedical data have been considered worth documenting. But an additional reason is that physicians' medical records constitute a confidentiality risk for patients who report psychosocial problems. Almost everyone in the office can have access to the most sensitive information recorded

TABLE 4-2. FAMILY APGAR QUESTIONNAIRE

The following questions have been designed to help us better understand you and your family. You should feel free to ask questions about any item in the questionnaire.

The space for comments should be used when you wish to give additional information or if you wish to discuss the way the question is applied to your family. Please try to answer all questions.

Family is defined as the individual(s) with whom you usually live. If you live alone, your "family" consists of persons with whom you now have the strongest emotional ties.

For each question, check only one box.

	Almost always	Some of the time	Hardly ever
I am satisfied that I can turn to my family for help when something is troubling me.	☐	☐	☐
Comments: _____			
I am satisfied with the way my family talks over things with me and shares problems with me.	☐	☐	☐
Comments: _____			
I am satisfied that my family accepts and supports my wishes to take on new activities or directions.	☐	☐	☐
Comments: _____			
I am satisfied with the way my family expresses affection and responds to my emotions, such as anger, sorrow, and love.	☐	☐	☐
Comments: _____			
I am satisfied with the way my family and I share time together.	☐	☐	☐
Comments: _____			

Note. From G. Smilkstein, "The Family APGAR: A Proposal for a Family Function Test and Its Use by Physicians," *Journal of Family Practice,* 1978, 6, 1231–1239. Copyright 1978 by Appleton-Century-Crofts. Reprinted by permission.

Note. Scoring: The patient checks one of three choices, which are scored as follows: "Almost always" (2 points), "Some of the time" (1 point), or "Hardly ever" (0). The scores for each of the five questions are then totaled. A score of 7 to 10 suggests a highly functional family; a score of 4 to 6 suggests a moderately dysfunctional family; a score of 0 to 3 suggests a severely dysfunctional family. We think that a low score more accurately reflects a high level of current dissatisfaction in one family member than unmistakable evidence of severe family dysfunction. The latter diagnosis will require more evidence about the family system.

Note. According to which member of the family is being interviewed, the physician may substitute for the word "family" either "spouse," "significant other," "parents," or "children."

on the charts. This is especially problematic in small communities where the members of the office staff know the patients socially. Without adequate records, however, the physician is apt to forget important information. Based on Baird's efforts to deal with this problem, we suggest the following data storage procedure:

1. Keep a simple family tree in the chart to provide information at a glance about the family's composition. If you have used the Family APGAR scale, that information should be in the chart.
2. Record the main issues or problems either by symbols on the tree or by technical words such as "boundary problem" or "enmeshment issue."
3. Use cryptic symbols for sensitive issues such as alcoholism (e.g., "ethyl"), sexual dysfunction (♂ or ♀), or extramarital sex (EMS).
4. Record briefly any treatment agreements you have made with the family. Again, you can abbreviate or use technical terms where appropriate—for example, "agreed to 1 year abs." for a therapeutic agreement that an alcoholic family member would refrain from using alcohol for 1 year; "sens. focus" for a sensate focus exercise to treat sexual dysfunction.
5. When you have an unconfirmed report from one family member about another's behavior, put a question mark or some other notation in the chart to indicate that you do not yet have the whole story.
6. Baird sometimes tells the patient(s) or family member(s) that he may need their help remembering all the details of what they discussed during the last visit, especially when that visit was a month or more ago. The moral: When you have not recorded something and do not remember, ask for help.

CONCLUSION

In family treatment as well as in the rest of medicine, what you see is what you treat. The converse is probably also true: What you can treat is what you will see. This chapter has offered a set of "eyeglasses" to family physicians so that they can focus more clearly on family functioning. The family observation and clinical "red flags" have been based on our experience in family practice settings. Staying fairly close to Minuchin, we also propose four primary assessment categories: stress, adaptability, cohesion, and interaction patterns. Family physicians have so much information to carry around in their heads already that we think reducing family assessment categories to four has its benefits. Other important issues have been included under these four: the family life cycle becomes relevant as a stressor, family communication as an aspect of family interactional patterns. Family physicians need to know enough about families to detect and refer serious problems and to provide primary care counseling for less serious problems. If their family assessment framework is too simplistic, family physicians will miss serious issues and will handle less serious ones inadequately. If the framework is too complex, family physicians will hang back and leave all family assessment to the specialists, thereby depriving families of primary care services. The assessment approach in this chapter reflects our own training and preferences; other approaches may be equally valid and useful for family practice. But all primary care assessment frameworks must sustain the difficult balance between comprehensiveness and simplicity, between too many data and too few data.

5 FORMING A THERAPEUTIC CONTRACT THAT INVOLVES THE FAMILY

The therapeutic contract stage is the point at which observation and preliminary assessment turn into action. Forming a therapeutic contract is the process by which the physician and the patient come to an understanding that the patient has a problem that requires attention. This chapter focuses on the psychosocial aspects of the therapeutic contract, although many of these agreements will involve biomedical treatment as well. The physician skills required for this process of contracting constitute a *terra incognita*. Articles for family physicians on family counseling usually skip from assessment to treatment—or from assessment to referral. We believe that *the unique contribution of family physicians to psychosocial treatment occurs when they help patients view their somatic problems in a broader biopsychosocial context*. Without this agreement on the larger context of the presenting problem, assessment will be sterile, referral will be fruitless, and the offer of treatment will be rejected.

There are two main steps for the physician in facilitating family-related therapeutic contracts: (1) redefining somatic symptoms in biopsychosocial terms, and (2) convincing the patient to involve the family in further assessment or treatment. In some cases, the first phase is not necessary because the patient has already made the connection between the somatic and the psychosocial (e.g., between a headache and personal stress), or because the patient visits the physician for personal counseling unrelated to a physical complaint. More often, however, patients will need help in examining the context of the physical symptoms and in mobilizing the family to come to a family conference.

REDEFINING SOMATIC SYMPTOMS
IN BIOPSYCHOSOCIAL TERMS

A family physician with good observational and assessment skills will have little difficulty spotting symptoms that may be stress-related. The clinical "red flags" discussed in Chapter 4 are common examples. In these situations, the physician's responsibility is to pursue possible organic causes for the symptoms while at the same time setting the stage for the patient to accept the psychosocial dimensions of the problem. This is no easy task. The practical challenge consists of shifting back and forth between the biomedical and the psychosocial. These two domains should be blended during the interview rather than placed back to back—medical, then psychosocial. The following reconstructed interview conducted by Baird with a 23-year-old male patient exemplifies how the physician can gather both biomedical and psychosocial information in back-and-forth fashion, while at the same time moving toward both biomedical and psychosocial diagnoses.

PHYSICIAN: How can I help you today, Mr. J?

PATIENT: I've had this pain in my stomach for a while.

PHYSICIAN: I see. How long have you had this pain?

PATIENT: For about three or four months, I guess.

PHYSICIAN: Could you show me where the pain is? Tell me what the pain is like.

PATIENT: I don't know. It's this burning sensation in this area, mostly in the mornings. I thought it would go away, but it hasn't.

PHYSICIAN: It sure sounds uncomfortable. What happens in the morning?

PATIENT: It burns a lot as soon as I wake up. I feel like I want to vomit. My wife gets pretty alarmed.

PHYSICIAN: Are you married?

PATIENT: Yeah, I got married about four months ago.

PHYSICIAN: Congratulations.

PATIENT: Thanks, we're very happy.

PHYSICIAN: Great. You know, sometimes getting married can be a pretty stressful thing.

PATIENT: No, I don't think that's bothering me. My wife and I get along great.

PHYSICIAN: I'm glad. How did the rest of your family feel about your getting married?

PATIENT: My family got pretty upset because she belongs to a different religion. They won't come and see us.

PHYSICIAN: That must hurt a bit.

PATIENT: Yeah, it does. But I've accepted Jesus as my personal savior and I've never been happier. My wife is a Christian, too.

PHYSICIAN: Were you a churchgoer before?

PATIENT: No, I was into drugs and running around. But I've changed my ways completely now. So has my wife.

PHYSICIAN: But your parents are having trouble adjusting to their new son.

PATIENT: Yeah, but they'll come around.

PHYSICIAN: Let me ask you something about your stomach pain. What do *you* think is causing it?

PATIENT: I think I may have an ulcer. But I don't know.

PHYSICIAN: What does your wife think?

PATIENT: She doesn't know, but she has been after me to see a doctor about it.

PHYSICIAN: She must be pretty concerned about you. Let's have a look at you over on the table here. [Physician conducts exam, during which time he talks with the patient about his job and the local community.] Mr. J, I think we should have some tests run at the hospital to see if you have an ulcer. I don't think you have an ulcer, but you might have one in the early stages.

PATIENT: What if it's not an ulcer?

PHYSICIAN: Let's wait until after the tests before we do much speculating. But sometimes people's stomachs act up when they've been through some stressful changes in their lives. You've told me about several important changes in the past few months: You've gotten married, you've become a born-again Christian, and you've had an upsetting change in your relationship with your parents.

PATIENT: Yeah, but I've never been happier in my life. My wife and I get along great, and I'm a committed Christian.

PHYSICIAN: I can see that your life has changed in positive directions for you. But sometimes even positive changes, when they come one right on top of another, can cause enough stress to cause a stomach to act up.

PATIENT: Maybe.

PHYSICIAN: And what's happened between you and your parents is not so happy a change, is it?

PATIENT: No, but I'm not letting it bother me.

PHYSICIAN: Here's what I suggest. I suggest you make an appointment at the hospital to have some tests to determine if you have an ulcer. [Physician explains the tests and the patient agrees to undergo them.] If we find something wrong on the tests—like an ulcer—we'll start treatment right away. Whether you have an ulcer or not, I'd like to sit down with you and your wife and see if we can put our heads together to figure out if there are some stresses in your life that you might be able to change—with your wife's help. Even if we don't come up with anything, it might help your wife to get the chance to express her concerns and ask questions about your stomach problem. I'm sure she's worried about you. Would you be willing to bring her back with you after we get the X-ray report back?

PATIENT: Yeah, I want to get rid of this problem and I'll do whatever you think will help.

PHYSICIAN: Let's do first things first, however. And the first thing is to get a look at what's happening inside your stomach. If you have the tests done tomorrow morning, I'll be able to get back to you late tomorrow afternoon or early the next day at the latest. Then we'll proceed from there.

The young man in this interchange was resistive to viewing his symptoms in psychosocial terms. His image of himself was that of a happy, unstressed young man who had finally gotten his life straight. The physician, although suspecting stress-related problems in this patient, kept the somatic complaints in primary focus: The majority of time during the entire, unedited session was devoted to exploring the organic source of the pain, and the primary action taken was aimed at assessing organic damage. However, the physician laid the groundwork for a biopsychosocial perspective on the problem by suggesting the possibility of a stress-related stomach disorder. *Never did the physician imply that the discomfort was imaginary.* In addition, the physician set the stage for family involvement by announcing his intention to invite the wife to the next interview. Note that the physician did not suggest that the patient's marriage was a negative source of stress or that the patient had marital problems. Rather, the wife was cast as a potential source of information and assistance to help the physician and the patient understand what might be causing the stomach disorder. In addition, the physician mentioned the importance of involving the wife for her own benefit as well, since she was affected by her husband's illness.

We have found a number of strategies useful in helping patients see the psychosocial context of their physical symptoms:

1. *Allow time for nonfocused, open-ended questions.* Examples include the following: "What brings you to the office today?" "How do you feel when that happens?" "What does your spouse say or do when that occurs?" "How does this symptom affect you? Your family? Friends? Work?" If the physician asks open-ended questions, then the patient may spontaneously provide information about psychosocial stresses. In the foregoing interview with the man with stomach pain, for example, the question "What happens in the morning?" gave the patient enough latitude in his answer to bring up his wife's worry about his nausea. A more narrow question focusing only on the abdominal discomfort in the morning would not have yielded the same information. Furthermore, if the physician asks open-ended questions about family and other psychosocial areas, the patient will sense that these areas are acceptable for discussion. If given permission in this way for discussion of family, personal, or emotional topics, many patients will quickly dismiss a

vague medical symptom such as fatigue and seek help directly in the psycho-social area. When this occurs, it transforms the discussion from physical to family issues *at the patient's initiative* and thereby greatly reduces the burden on the physician in attempting to force such a redefinition.

2. *Introduce psychosocial issues while evaluating medical symptoms.* The physician can go back and forth between the biomedical and the psychosocial domains during the same interview. Not asking questions about personal or family stress until after an exhaustive assessment of somatic symptoms may communicate to the patient that such issues are either unimportant or uncomfortable for the physician. The ability to shift routinely from lower back pain to an unhappy marriage and then return to the lower back—this is the fine art of comprehensive medical interviewing. It also gradually prepares the patient to look at a psychosocial problem instead of "springing" the issue on the patient after a strictly medical interview.

3. *Assure the patient that you are conducting an appropriately thorough medical evaluation.* Patients must feel confident that the physician is ade-quately assessing the physical symptoms before they are likely to accept the role of psychosocial factors. The physician, too, must be confident about the nature of the symptom and its biological implications in order to feel comfortable incorporating the role of the family or other psychosocial factors into the treatment equation.

4. *Avoid premature reassurances about benign complaints.* If a vague, nonserious symptom serves as the patient's ticket to receive help for a family problem, then the physician could block this help seeking by offering happy reassurances that "nothing serious is wrong." Something serious in fact may be wrong in the patient's life, and the patient will not feel as optimistic as the doctor. In some cases, the patient will push for more and more tests until either the physician acknowledges the presence of psychosocial problems or the patient gives up and tries another specialist.

5. *When complaints are serious, do not lose sight of the family implica-tions.* Problems in the real world often do not neatly divide themselves into biological or psychosocial domains. Patients with serious illnesses may also have serious family problems, which can worsen during the course of the illness. In the same way, illness can create problems for families who other-wise have been functioning well. It is tempting for the biomedically trained family physician to latch onto the serious medical problem exclusively, as if "real" medical problems have no family overlay.

6. *Stay involved with the patient after a referral.* When the symptoms are complex or the seriousness of the illness requires consultations outside the family physician's office, it is important to arrange specific ongoing care plans that involve the family physician. This allows the possibility of further assessment and handling of the psychosocial context by the family physician, as well as better medical care in the long run. Such continued contact also

avoids the problem of the patient and family's feeling rejected by the family physician. Family counseling may need to be postponed until after the assessment of the consultant or until after medical treatment has been initiated, but continued contact between the patient and the family physician will keep the door open to dealing later with psychosocial issues. Ideally, the physician should be able to insure that the outside consultant will not prescribe tranquilizers to pacify a patient when a family interaction pattern is closely linked to the symptom. Even more ideal would be the situation in which the consultant would identify the family problems and refer the patient back to the family physician for further assessment and treatment.

7. *Bide your time if your first attempt does not work.* Sometimes patients are not yet ready to hear that they have stress-related symptoms or psychosocial problems. A woman who has headaches after arguing with her husband may prefer to postpone the day of reckoning with her marital problems. Here the family physician's best tool may be *persistence over time.* If the patient's headaches continue, she will be back in the office again. Some physicians who are unsure of their counseling skills choose to back away from psychosocial issues after one failure to convince the patient. Continuity of patient care gives the family physician and the patient a number of opportunities to form a therapeutic contract. Of course some patients never will deal with their personal or family problems, despite your best efforts. But there are plenty of patients who will respond to their family physician's low-key but persistent attention to these stresses in their lives. The challenge in a busy medical practice is to be ready when the patients are.

8. *Make a strong confrontation of patients who are in serious psychosocial difficulty.* If biding your time is not getting the patient anywhere and if the problem is serious, you should consider decisively confronting the patient about the problem. One strategy we have found useful is to declare our impotence to help the patient further unless we take a different tack (i.e., work on family or other psychosocial problems). This approach has the advantage of keeping the physician out of the role of directly demanding that the patient start "shaping up." A second strategy is to confront the patient's spouse or other family members about the problem, rather than just confronting the patient. An alcoholic patient, for instance, is probably quite accustomed to ignoring physicians' suggestions about drinking but may be more responsive to the insistence of a spouse and children.

9. *What not to say.* In addition to the above strategies for effectively confronting patients about their problems, we offer a number of things *not to say* to patients in the confrontation process. Unfortunately, we have overheard these remarks more than once in medical interviews.

- "How's the marriage?" is a perfunctory question that usually elicits a perfunctory "Fine" from the patient. Be more specific. For example, if a woman who has recently returned to work is complaining about back pain, you might ask, "How does your husband feel about your returning to work?" Asking the more general question "How's your marriage?" is like asking someone "How's your body?"—hardly an astute diagnostic inquiry.

• "I can find no physical cause for your pain, so it must be mental." This kind of statement stirs up both the patient's fears of mental illness and the patient's concerns that the physician does not take the pain seriously. Sensitive family physicians know how to communicate to the patient an appreciation for stress-related physical pain as a normal human experience. Generally, a term like "stress" is more helpful than terms like "psychosomatic" or "in your head," because the latter suggest that the pain is not real. Furthermore, the "stress" image leads naturally to an exploration of the sources of stress in the patient's life, including family relationships.

• "I think your family is part of this problem." Having discovered the importance of family issues in patients' problems, it is tempting for some family physicians to be too fast and too blunt in approaching these issues. Many patients will deny family difficulties if confronted directly in this fashion, out of feelings of family loyalty or personal threat. The same patients, however, will often respond to gentle probing and to reflective statements about what the physician hears the patient to be saying. The physician must be careful not to get too far ahead of the patient in suggesting family involvement in the problem. In fact, some patients rankle at the word "problem" but will readily accept the idea that certain stressors are affecting them and their families. Generally, it is wise to make verbal assessments of family problems in a tentative fashion at first so that the resistive patient will not slam the door on the issue.

One of the most debilitating aspects of medical practice is the ongoing treatment of psychosocially stressed patients who will not admit or work on their problems. These are the patients whom the physician dreads seeing but who are among the most needy in the practice. A physician who develops good psychosocial assessment and therapeutic contract skills will be spared some of this bloodletting—and will help more patients in the process.

STRATEGIES FOR INVOLVING THE FAMILY

We suggest that family physicians routinely conduct family conferences for a variety of patient problems. Since the family is the principal context of illness and health care, it makes sense to meet with the family to explain the illness and its treatment, to elicit members' support for the patient, to support them when they are distressed by the patient's illness, and to help them change when change is needed. Generally, any serious, chronic, or recurring problem merits at least one conference with the spouses or the family. Stated differently, whenever the physician must engage the patient in ongoing treatment of health problems, the family should routinely be assembled in the office or hospital. In addition, informal supportive and educational conferences can be held with couples during premarriage visits, routine Pap smears and pelvic exams, prenatal visits, and routine child health care visits.

Families will seldom decline the invitation to meet with a physician who has established the precedent that there is nothing unusual or threatening about assembling the family. Figure 5-1 outlines a continuum of urgency about assembling families in the office or hospital, ranging from generally not important to essential. Generally, the more serious or chronic the problem or the greater the preventive care opportunity, the more important it is to assemble the family. In some cases the family conference will be the starting point for continued family counseling, while in many cases only one or two meetings will be needed.

Even if the physician decides to refer the patient and family for therapy, we recommend that a family conference be held first, for the following reasons: First, the physician can make a firmer assessment of the patient's and family's problems; second, direct referrals for family therapy are notoriously ineffective when the physician talks to only one family member; third, assembling the family may begin the process of constructive change in the family, whether or not the physician continues to work with the family; fourth, a family that has been assembled in the physician's office may see benefits in holding family meetings on their own. Except in unusually volatile situations, there is little to be lost and much to be gained by assembling a family in the primary care setting in order to facilitate a referral for specialized therapy.

Although family members are usually willing to comply with request for family conferences concerning a physical illness, often members—particularly husbands—are wary about this sort of family meeting to discuss such psychosocial problems as marital distress and chemical dependency. From our experiences in family practice offices and in mental health settings, we have developed a number of strategies for involving reluctant family members in family sessions (Doherty, 1981c).

1. *Confidently indicate that other family members are simply expected to come.* Be matter of fact about this (e.g., "I'd like to meet with both you and your husband next week. What would be a good time for your work schedules?"). Of course you cannot coerce a patient into bringing in a spouse, but you can communicate your clear expectation that this will occur. Avoid tentative questions such as "Do you think your husband would be willing to come back with you?" In fact, the reluctant family member may not be the husband but the wife. You may be giving her a way to hide behind her husband's imagined reluctance. Furthermore, to be most effective, a confident expectation for family involvement must be expressed not only by the physician but also by the entire supportive staff. If the physician has asked a mother to bring in her whole family, including children, and the

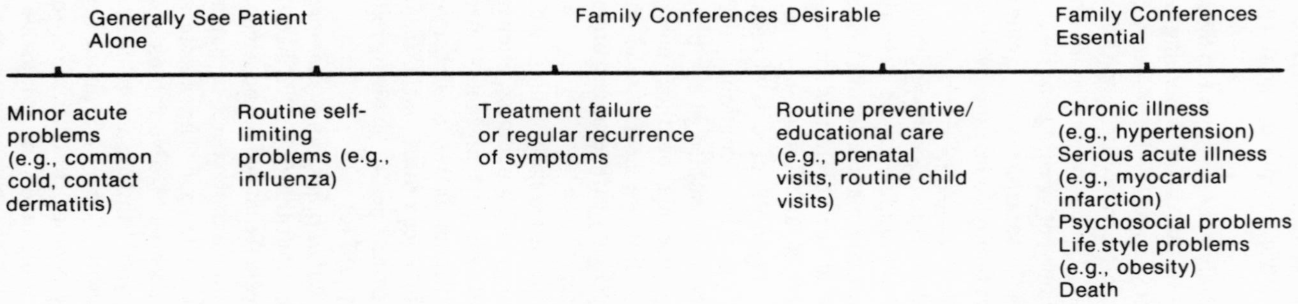

Generally See Patient Alone | Family Conferences Desirable | Family Conferences Essential

Minor acute problems (e.g., common cold, contact dermatitis)

Routine self-limiting problems (e.g., influenza)

Treatment failure or regular recurrence of symptoms

Routine preventive/ educational care (e.g., prenatal visits, routine child visits)

Chronic illness (e.g., hypertension)
Serious acute illness (e.g., myocardial infarction)
Psychosocial problems
Life style problems (e.g., obesity)
Death

FIG. 5-1. WHEN TO ASSEMBLE THE FAMILY.

mother calls on the day of the appointment to ask whether the physician meant *all* the children (including the baby or the "perfect" child), the receptionist should be prepared to assure her that if the physician said "the whole family," then everyone should come to the session.

2. *Communicate a sense of urgency to the patient about assembling the family.* A patient who believes that family involvement is an optional procedure—desirable but not necessary—will be less likely to take the risk of mobilizing the family. You may be asking the patient to overcome obstacles at home in order to hold a family session. A sense of urgency and seriousness will help the patient deal with the obstacles. Assembling the family may be as important for the patient's well-being as diagnostic X-rays or antibiotic therapy. Physicians who believe in family involvement should convey the same sense of urgency about assembling the family as they would about these biomedical tests and treatments. When trying to persuade the spouse of an alcoholic, for example, to bring in the whole family, we have found it useful to remind the spouse that alcoholism is a chronic, progressive, and sometimes fatal disease—and that family involvement is the only way we know how to help a poorly motivated alcoholic patient.

3. *Ask for a spouse's help in order for you to understand the patient's problem fully.* As exemplified in the interview earlier in this chapter, the physician's safest route to family involvement is to take the role of an information gatherer who needs input from all important sources. Once again, if the husband has medical information you need, you would find a way to get the information from him. Appealing to the spouse's helpfulness in the area of psychosocial stress often meets with the same success—if the physician is not timid about asking. This approach has the advantage of not raising the spouse's defensiveness unnecessarily and of not asking for an early commitment from the spouse for counseling or therapy.

4. *Use the hospital as a setting for assembling families.* If the patient with psychosocial problems is in the hospital, the family physician is in a powerful position for calling a meeting with the family. Most families hold strong cultural beliefs about the importance of any hospitalization. Family members who have not spoken to each other for years will rally to the hospital bedside. The physician's imputed authority is never so great as in the hospital. In our experience, families of a hospitalized patient rarely decline the physician's request for a family meeting. If the patient is ambulatory, this meeting should be held in a conference room with the patient in street clothes, in order to deemphasize the patient's sick role in the family temporarily. If this is not possible, then privacy in the patient's room must be insured for the family conference; the hospital staff should be notified to stay away. We have found in-hospital family sessions quite effective in mobilizing families to confront alcoholic members who had been unwilling to come to

the office. Faced with temporary sobriety, physical illness, and an empowered family, an alcoholic is more likely to agree to treatment. And since the meeting involves the whole family, the family is more apt to continue collaborating with the treatment. When efforts to reach a therapeutic contract with an individual patient have not been effective, then sometimes this agreement can be reached by assembling the whole family in the hospital.

5. *Contact other family members to reassure them that you are not looking for villains.* Family members may be understandably concerned that they will be blamed or scapegoated for the patient's problems. This fear is especially acute if the family members believe that the index patient has a special relationship with the family physician. Since the patient with the special relationship is often the wife, the husband may believe that the family meeting has been called to tell him to stop causing his wife so much difficulty. One way to avoid this misperception is to stress to the patient that the first meeting will be for information gathering. Another approach is for the family physician to telephone the reluctant family member with (a) a request for help, and (b) an explicit statement that the physician does not believe in family villains—that everyone in a family is hurting if one member is hurting. Of course you must *believe* this in order to persuade anyone! A family systems perspective can help you resist searching for villains or scapegoats for family problems. Another way to avoid blaming other family members is to keep out of long-term individual counseling relationships with patients prior to trying to involve the family. The family will know whose side you are on—everyone's or your special patient's.

6. *Be patient and persistent.* Sometimes the "guests" take a long time deciding to come to "dinner." Some patients need time to assimilate the idea of asking their family to come to the doctor with them. Other patients are willing immediately, but their family members resist. While waiting patiently, however, you should keep the pressure on the patient and family to get involved together in handling the problem. If you ask once but fail to repeat the request each time you see the patient, then the patient and the family may suspect that you are willing to drop the matter and leave the family out of treatment.

7. *Declare the limits of your ability to help unless the family gets involved.* The family physician can "declare impotence" in being able to help a patient with family problems unless family members get involved. In fact, such impotence is a reality. It is like a patient's requesting treatment for chest pain but not permitting the physician to conduct X-rays, electrocardiograms, or blood tests. The patient who is motivated to work on a family-related problem will usually respond to the physician's *minimum requirement* for helping with the problem—namely, a family meeting. The more common obstacle is that the physician does not realize the probable futility of treating family problems without the family.

If the patient accepts the importance of a family meeting, then the physician and patient can work on strategies to persuade other members to come. If the patient expresses firm expectations to other family members, *and* if the physician makes personal contact with reluctant members, *and* if both the patient and the physician persist in these efforts—then the whole family will usually appear in the office for a family session. The chief exception to this generalization occurs when a reluctant spouse is no longer committed to a marriage. In this case, the physician can help the patient understand the possible implications of the partner's refusal to cooperate. Another exception arises when a spouse distrusts the family physician's bond with the patient and is unwilling to accept the physician's reassurances of impartiality. In such cases, if the spouse is truly interested in helping, then the physician can make a referral to another physician or to a family therapist who knows neither partner.

CONCLUSION

This chapter proposes strategies for redefining somatic symptoms in bio-psychosocial terms and for involving the family in therapeutic contracts. The chief difficulty in both tasks lies not with the techniques of persuading patients, but with the family physician's practical commitment to biopsychosocial and family perspectives. Patients generally will cooperate with a physician who believes strongly in the importance of family involvement in assessing and treating a wide range of problems. With time, family-oriented therapeutic contracts can become routine for a family physician. Eventually, patients come to expect that their doctor is inclined to ask them about their families and to call family meetings in the hospital and office. At the risk of sounding pretentious about the importance of our advice, we note that a century ago most physicians did not pay much attention to sterile procedures, and that the first physicians to insist on sterilizing and quarantining were preceived as overconcerned with small matters. Family-oriented physicians have an equally large educational task with professionals and lay people alike.

6 GUIDELINES FOR REFERRING OR TREATING

The daily nemesis of the generalist is the decision to treat the problem oneself or to refer to a specialist. Referring too readily makes the primary care physician merely a conduit for patients into subspecialty medical treatment; referring too stingily brings the risk of inadequate treatment and malpractice suits. Sometimes the referral decision is straightforward because the family physician has limited training in the area—for example, in cancer, neurological disorders, and serious eye problems. At other times the grounds for the decision are murkier, especially when the physician has been trained to treat relatively uncomplicated presentations of diseases, such as diabetes, hypertension, and gastrointestinal disorders. Often the disease presents in such an early, undifferentiated form that the family physician must treat the symptoms while waiting for the real animal to show itself—at which point diagnosis by the specialist is straightforward.

When faced with psychosocial problems, family physicians face similar dilemmas. Most family physicians will never be trained as experts in psychotherapy. Knowing one's limits is as important in the psychosocial area as in the biomedical area; some psychosocial problems require treatment from specialists. However, family physicians have an essential role in the diagnosis and treatment of psychosocial problems. We term this role the "primary care" of psychosocial problems. Unfortunately, family physicians generally are less well trained for primary psychosocial care than they are for primary biomedical care. This lack of training creates the danger that the family physician either will ineffectively treat psychosocial problems that should be referred, or will fail to offer immediate help to patients and families by making inappropriate or premature referrals to the specialized mental health sector. Our model attempts to avoid these pitfalls by involving the family physician in the early assessment and treatment decisions regarding the problem—thereby setting the stage for an immediate referral—and by proposing the ground rule that a referral should be made if the problem is not ameliorated through primary care counseling. Optimally, a referral attempt should be made only after the patient and the physician agree about the presence and urgency of the problem and after the physician has had contact with the family. We believe that a referral made after assembling the family is more likely to succeed—especially a referral of a couple or family as a unit—than one made after dealing only with the individual patient. *Referring a family is best accomplished at a family meeting.* The family physician may also choose to counsel the family in primary care modes in order to discover whether the psychosocial problems are amenable to a supportive and educational intervention or appear to require more specialized treatment.

This chapter is intended to help the family physician with the decision about attempting counseling with a patient and family versus referring to a therapist. The chapter's second purpose is to help the family physician handle the process of making referrals.

CRITERIA FOR DECIDING TO TREAT OR REFER

Based on our experience in family practice and family therapy settings, we propose three criteria for deciding to treat (counsel) or refer patients and families with psychosocial problems: (1) the nature of the problem, (2) the family physician's knowledge of and ability to treat the problem, and (3) the family physician's time and outside resources.

THE NATURE OF THE PROBLEM

Integrating the disciplines of family therapy and family medicine requires an effort to demarcate the kinds of problems that are best treated initially in the primary care arena of the family physician, as opposed to those problems best assigned from the outset of treatment to family therapists. Although generalizations are always hazardous, we believe that the average family physician should refer patients and families who present with *serious, chronic psychosocial problems.* The following are leading candidates for referral:

1. *Chronic depression and anxiety* that have not responded to previous biomedical or psychotherapeutic treatment. In these cases there is a high likelihood that the family interaction patterns have become rigidly stabilized around the patient's dysfunction. A powerful therapeutic intervention is needed, particularly if the patient and family have become expert at deflecting professionals' attempts to "rescue" them.

2. *Chemical dependency.* Like individually oriented psychotherapists, family physicians are notoriously ineffective in treating alcoholics and other

chemically dependent persons. One of the reasons for this failure is that chemical dependency generally is accompanied by a rigid family system. The combination of a manipulative, chemically dependent patient and a rigid family is too much for an isolated family physician to handle effectively. Specialized treatment—especially when it combines AA and family therapy —holds greater opportunity for success (Barnard, 1981; Kaufman & Kaufmann, 1979). In the treatment of chemical dependency, the family physician's greatest contributions occur in assessing and confronting the problem in both the patient and the family, in vigorously using community resources, and in providing posttreatment care.

3. *Chronic family dysfunctional patterns.* When the family history indicates long-standing dysfunctional interaction patterns, the family will probably need intensive family therapy. When a wife complains that she and her husband have been battling for 7 years about their sexual relationship, the problem probaby is rooted much more deeply than if she complains that their sexual relationship has declined since the birth of their first child last year. Similarly, a family that has been organized for years around a problem child and mutually undermining parents is going to be difficult to help in a primary care counseling mode. The key notion here is that *chronicity suggests low family adaptability.* The lower the adaptability, the more the family will require therapy as opposed to counseling.

4. *Serious, acute family symptoms, particularly child abuse, spouse abuse, and incest.* The family physician's important role in these crises lies in the early assessment and referral of families with these problems. Indeed, the physician may be mandated by law to engage outside agencies to assist the child and the family. Part of the family physician's challenge here is to make a referral without alienating a family that will need all possible social and medical support in the coming months.

We want to reemphasize that the above-mentioned problems are part of the family physician's health care responsibility, since these are among the most serious and even life-threatening disorders experienced by patients. Many distressed patients and families will never obtain treatment unless family physicians involve themselves more deeply in the assessment and referral of serious psychosocial problems. To say that chronic marital distress should not ordinarily be *treated* by primary care physicians is not equivalent to saying that these physicians should keep their "hands off" such difficult problems. In fact, unless a family physician puts his or her "hands on" marital problems in the form of assessing and initiating therapeutic decisions about these issues, many of the walking wounded among married couples will never receive the specialized treatment they need.

What kinds of problems are most appropriate for primary care counseling by a family physician? We suggest three categories:

1. *Family transition problems.* These are the adjustment difficulties experienced by families as they undergo the stresses associated with life cycle

changes. A common example we have encountered is fatigue and dysphoric mood in a young mother who recently has had her second baby. She regularly brings in one of the children for minor illnesses as a way to ask for help herself. By offering supportive counseling for this woman and her husband, the family physician may relieve distress now and forestall more serious problems later. At the other end of the family life cycle are family transition problems related to the increased dependence of older family members—problems that upset normal families and that can respond to supportive counseling.

2. *Other problems of recent origin.* A first-time depression, a sudden increase in alcoholic consumption, an upsetting new behavior by a child, an uncharacteristic attack of nervousness—these may be symptoms of new stresses for the patient and the patient's family. A family member presenting to the physician with nonspecific complaints may serve as the emissary for a family suffering an acute, situational crisis. When psychosocial problems are of recent origin, the family probably has not yet become rooted in rigid interaction patterns based on the symptoms. Such families may respond well to primary care family counseling.

3. *Many illness-related problems.* The family physician is uniquely positioned to provide counseling to patients and families suffering from the emotional and social implications of illness. Such counseling can help families from the point of diagnosis through the treatment and recovery processes, and especially during adjustments to life style changes and the death of a family member. We underline the value of sitting down with the family to work on these issues—thereby letting family members help one another in the physician's presence—as opposed to the more traditional approach of talking to one or two family members separately. The family physician can serve as the catalyst for the family's recovery from a health crisis.

Sometimes mild psychosocial symptoms, like their medical counterparts, mask greater underlying pathology. In both cases, a reliable indicator of a more serious problem is that primary care treatment is not working. Referring apparently mild psychosocial problems that do not respond to primary care help will keep the physician and family out of a frustrating and unproductive long-term counseling relationship.

THE PHYSICIAN'S KNOWLEDGE AND ABILITY

Family physicians differ rather widely in their training and skills in various aspects of medicine. Some family physicians, for example, do no obstetrics, while others perform Caesarean sections. Similarly, in the psychosocial area some family physicians have received a modicum of training in family counseling during their residencies, while others have received practically none. A few have received extensive training, including Balint-type seminars aimed at helping residents understand their personal reactions to patients and families (Balint, 1964). Hence, an important criterion for deciding whether to counsel a family is the physician's knowledge and ability in the area of family counseling—in other words, the physician's competence.

This competence is difficult to measure, even for a family therapist with academic coursework and supervised clinical experience. Family medicine has even fewer standards for evaluating competence in family counseling. Ultimately the individual family physician must set personal standards for judging which kinds of psychosocial problems to handle personally and which to refer immediately. These standards presumably will change over time—at least if experience and consultation enhance the physician's skills. Some problems, moreover, will stir up so many personal or family issues for the physician that it may be best to avoid counseling patients in these areas. Some issues are literally too close to home—and should be referred to someone else.

THE PHYSICIAN'S TIME AND RESOURCES

You are a physician who has determined that a patient and family need counseling. The problems appear to be within your competence as a family physician to treat. But flu season is reaching its peak, your partner is heading for Bermuda for 3 weeks, you have three OBs in the wings, you are already counseling four families, and you are beginning to think that the biomedical model was not so bad after all. One option would be to begin counseling the family anyway. (See Chapter 16 for an antidote for the affliction known as "super doc.") Another option would be to postpone seeing the family until you have more time. A third option would be to refer the family to a family therapist if one is available.

The point is that the decision to counsel or not to counsel should be based in part on the availability of the physician's two greatest resources—time and outside consultants. The most important issue is that the patient and family receive help from a qualified source and in a reasonable amount of time. Problems that are serious and urgent generally should be referred anyway—after appropriate assessment and therapeutic contracting—while problems that are less serious probably can be placed on a short waiting list before the physician begins counseling. Problems in the middle range might be tackled if the family physician has a therapist or other consultant with whom to discuss the case. Finally, busy family physicians should consider limiting the number of families they will see each week. Protecting one's own time and carefully cultivating consultants and referral resources will serve the needs of patients and physicians.

THE ART OF REFERRING

A family physician skilled at assessing, assembling the family, and referring patients with psychosocial problems could keep a family therapist quite busy. Although no data are available on the success of referrals to family therapists, the corresponding data on general mental health referrals are discouraging. In a study of the referral process between primary care physicians and a community mental health center, France, Weddington, and Houpt (1978) found that only 10% of patients referred for the first time completed the referral.

While referrals to therapists will never achieve a perfect success rate, we believe that physician-caused barriers are part of the problem. (For a study of physician resistance to psychiatric consultations, see Steinberg, Torem, & Saravay, 1980.) Specifically, the lack of medical school and residency exposure to psychotherapy and family therapy leaves many physicians unfamiliar with these treatment modalities and doubtful about their efficacy. Familiarity breeds better referrals. Since family physicians generally have taken surgery rotations, they can make convincing referrals to surgeons by saying, for example, "The surgeon will make a small incision in this area; you'll have some pain for a while, but in a few weeks you'll be back to doing most of your normal activities." Patients know when the physician is speaking from first-hand knowledge. This surgery example may be contrasted with a referral for marital therapy when the physician has little idea of what goes on during the treatment. Patients are reluctant to sign a blank check for therapy when they sense that their doctor is unfamiliar or even dubious about it. In addition to physician barriers, other important difficulties is making successful referrals derive from the complexity of relationships in the referral triangle.

THE REFERRAL TRIANGLE

If the physician, the patient, and the family constitute one important therapeutic triangle, the physician, the patient or family, and the therapist–consultant constitute a second.[1] Figure 6-1 presents this referral triangle. This configuration assumes that the physician has assembled the family and has a relationship with the index patient and the family as a unit. The referral social system becomes much more complex and difficult if the physician has not successfully engaged the family—in other words, if the

---

[1]We acknowledge the contributions of Paul Williamson, MD, to the notion of the referral triangle.

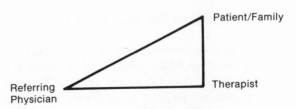

FIG. 6-1. THE REFERRAL TRIANGLE.

family is not the patient. This situation creates a rectangle, a social system consisting of four different combinations of triangles (see Fig. 6-2)!

In the referral triangle, the family physician must be concerned with three relationships, all of which must function well for the referral and subsequent treatment to be successful. These are the physician's relationship with the patient and family, the physician's relationship with the therapist, and the patient and family's relationship with the therapist. (For simplicity, we truncate the expression "patient and family" to simply "patient.")

THE PHYSICIAN–PATIENT RELATIONSHIP

In Minuchin's terms, a successful referral requires "clear boundaries" in the physician–patient relationship. The twin pitfalls are "disengaged" and "enmeshed" boundaries. If the physician has not adequately engaged the patient interpersonally in the process of assessing the problem—if the physician–patient relationship is not close enough—the patient may experience a referral attempt as a brush-off. ("My doctor doesn't want to be bothered with me and my troubled family.") *The physician has to earn the right to ask the patient to expose personal and family problems to a mental health professional.* A disengaged physician–patient dyad is unlikely to give birth to a triad. In the same way, an *enmeshed* physician–patient relationship will be wound too tightly to permit the threat of an outsider. This occurs when the

FIG. 6-2. THE REFERRAL RECTANGLE WHEN THE FAMILY IS NOT THE PATIENT.

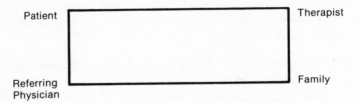

physician has labored mightily in a counseling relationship with a patient or family, only to feel frustrated at the lack of progress. The physician feels caught in a desire to rescue the patient or family. The patient, who has become quite attached to the physician, interprets the referral request as a rejection. In an enmeshed relationship, distance feels like loss and rejection. Characteristically, the patient sabotages the referral by not liking the therapist or by doing poorly in treatment. The enmeshed physician may sabotage the therapy by communicating inaccurate expectations. In contrast to these twin dangers of disengaged and enmeshed relationships, clear boundaries in the physician–patient relationships allow the patient to accept a referral while still maintaining a trusting relationship with the family physician.

THE PHYSICIAN–THERAPIST RELATIONSHIP

Arranging a referral is like setting up a blind date: The arranger had better be able to vouch for both parties. Unfortunately, many family physicians do not have personal knowledge of the skills and personalities of the therapists to whom they refer patients. In the biomedical area, family physicians carefully develop working relationships with consultants; even here communication is tricky, and competition over patients is common. In the psychosocial realm, the gap between the referring physician and the consultant is widened by ignorance on both sides: physicians do not understand therapists and therapists, most of whom are not MDs, do not understand physicians. Hence, there tends to be little communication between the two about their common patients. The patient gets caught in the middle—or at least fails to obtain all possible help for the problem. Some patients learn to use the tenuous physician–therapist relationship to manipulate the treatment—for example, by obtaining Valium from the physician but not telling the therapist. Dealing collaboratively with such patients is the litmus test of the physician–therapist relationship.

THE PATIENT–THERAPIST RELATIONSHIP

The main goal of the referral is to establish a helpful relationship between the patient and the therapist. Some of the burden for success or failure of this relationship rests with the referring physician, who communicates a number of expectations to each party about the other. Perhaps most important are the expectations about the nature of the therapy. Physicians who are not clear about what the patient should anticipate (e.g., about fees, length of treatment, or involvement of family members) will be less convincing about the referral, and at worst may undermine the new therapeutic relationship by setting up false expectations. After the patient–therapist relationship is established, the physician continues to serve as a supporter or an underminer of this newest relationship in the referral triangle. Sometimes the "blind date" leads to a "love affair"—with many thanks to the friend who made the introduction—while other times recriminations are heaped upon the "matchmaker's" head.

SELECTING THERAPISTS FOR REFERRAL

We offer two basic prescriptions here: First, spend enough time to meet and get to know the mental health referral sources at your disposal; and, second, opt where possible for therapists who involve families in the treatment. Referring to an anonymous mental health center will not be as successful as mentioning the names of colleagues who work at the mental health center will be. In biomedical referrals, the family physician generally sends the patient to a specific trusted consultant—or to a prestigious tertiary care center —rather than to "the surgery group across town." The physician must get to know the local therapists in order to make intelligent referrals. Unfortunately, we have never found the therapist's academic degree—MA, MSW, PHD, or MD—particularly helpful in sifting out skilled therapists. Good ones and bad ones come with all kinds of sheepskins.

Even if you do not feel competent to evaluate therapists' academic training, philosophy, or treatment approaches, you can get a sense of which therapists appear interpersonally competent. Talk with them about patients you are treating and evaluate the helpfulness of their reactions; also try asking yourself if you would send a member of your own family to this or that therapist. Once you have found a trusted therapist colleague or two, you can ask them for advice about the merits of other local mental health professionals. Such colleagues will probably be willing to offer you consultation about your own office counseling and help you enhance your primary care counseling skills. Eventually, you may arrange to have an in-office family therapist for easy referral and consultation.

Why refer to family-oriented therapists? We believe that a family physician with an appreciation of the therapeutic triangle should refer where possible to a therapist who shares this systems orientation. We are not suggesting that the therapist must function exclusively as a family therapist, but rather that family therapy be an integral part of the therapist's treatment repertoire. (A useful guideline for judging whether the therapist has been trained in family therapy is membership in the American Association for Marriage and Family Therapy, the only national accrediting body for family therapists, or the American Family Therapy Association, an organization for leading teachers and researchers in family therapy.) This recommendation to refer to family-oriented therapists holds for so-called "individual" problems such as depression and anxiety, as well as for the more classical "family" problems such as marital conflict and parent–child conflict. *When the patient lives with or interacts closely with relatives, there is no good reason to exclude the family from the mental health treatment, except in unusual cases.* We ourselves do individual therapy only when the family is inaccessible, since individual therapy, in our experience, tends to be slower and more difficult than family therapy. In sum, family therapists are natural allies of family physicians.

GETTING THE PATIENT AND THE THERAPIST TOGETHER

The road from the doctor's office to the therapist's office is paved with good intentions. Although ultimately it is the patient's own responsibility to follow through on the referral, the family physician can add weight to the referral process by attending to a number of practical matters.

1. Have the names and phone numbers of your referral sources immediately available. Baird keeps this information in a date book he always carries with him.
2. Give patients realistic notions about the therapy: time and travel commitments, inpatient versus outpatient setting, short-term versus long-term treatment, requirements that other family members be involved in treatment.
3. Ask the patient to make the appointment with the therapist before leaving your office. Some family physicians have discovered a highly effective tool for making a referral: The physician places the call for the patient and hands the phone to the patient to work out the details. Such personal involvement communicates that the physician is serious about this referral. Of course, this procedure requres prior consent by the patient. The therapist or agency should also be acquainted with the procedure.
4. Ask the patient to let you know when the referral has been successfully completed. Again, this request suggests that you are taking the matter seriously. It also gives you the chance to regroup if the referral appointment is not kept.
5. Check with the patient on how the therapy is progressing. During the patient's or other family member's next office visit, inquire about the therapy. Is the patient pleased? Is the therapy helping with the problems? Patient satisfaction with therapy is one of your best criteria for judging the effectiveness of the therapist, although you must be alert against becoming triangulated into a conflict between the patient and the therapist.
6. Ask the therapist to keep you informed about the main therapeutic strategies and about the progress of the therapy. This will allow you to support the therapist–patient relationship. Sometimes a family must become disorganized temporarily before it can reorganize itself. Dur-

ing this period of family stress, a member may present to the family physician with physical symptoms and a complaint that the family has been worse since going to therapy. If the therapist has informed the physician about the likelihood of disruption during the early treatment stages, then the physician will not assume that the therapy is ineffective or harmful.

7. Work out a continuing care program after the therapy. The therapist will probably be a temporary figure in the life of the family, whereas the family physician may be involved for the long haul. The lasting effectiveness of the treatment may be enhanced by periodic follow-up counseling from the family physician, or at least by continued monitoring of the patient's and family's functioning.

8. In some circumstances, join the patient and family in the therapy. If the physician is enmeshed with the patient and family, then a referral may be doomed: The family feels forced to choose between their "good old doc" and a strange "shrink." This is no contest. If you sense this kind of entanglement, consider referring yourself with the family in order to hand over the treatment responsibility to the therapist in question. Your involvement in the therapy may be short-term, but it is nevertheless essential.

These suggestions presuppose that the therapeutic contract process has been successfully negotiated. If careful referral mechanisms have been established, most referral failures can be traced to the therapeutic contract stage: The physician and the patient have not agreed about the importance of treatment. The physician may then choose to renegotiate treatment options with the patient at that time or to wait until another crisis provides the opportunity.

CONCLUSION

The appropriate treatment of psychosocial problems in family practice consists of providing direct physician services to patients and families who can benefit from primary care counseling—and of referring problems that appear to require therapy. As in primary biomedical care, the guidelines for treating or referring are sometimes clear and sometimes blurred. In practice, the critical variables may be the skill and interests of the family physician, as well as the physician's support systems and referral options. Since counseling training has been accorded the lowest priority in medical education, many family physicians—especially those without a trusted consultant—will feel inadequate to treat any but the simplest psychosocial problems. We think the best place to start for such uncertain novices is to emphasize the stages of assessment, therapeutic contract, and assembling the family in the treatment process—followed by referral for most problems. Learning that many families can rally their resources to cope with difficulties may encourage timid physicians to try their hand at more counseling, particularly for the kinds of biopsychosocial problems (such as heart attacks) that only primary care physicians are situated to treat in a family context. With time and experience in a primary care family counseling, each family physician ideally will achieve a "comfort zone" for handling psychosocial problems and will find it easier to determine which problems are in the "referral zone." Neither simply a friendly next-door neighbor nor a trained therapist, the family physician has a role somewhere in between—in that fertile but poorly mapped landscape of primary care family treatment.

7 COUNSELING FAMILIES

Willing or unwilling, trained or not, family physicians are family counselors. Patients expect it and demand it. The philosophical underpinnings of family medicine require it. But there is perhaps no area of practice in which family physicians feel more unprepared, inadequate, and vulnerable. No one likes to feel submerged in the turbulent waves of a major family conflict—one's own or another family's. Small wonder that when faced with threatening family storms, physicians often seek shelter by hospitalizing or tranquilizing the most symptomatic family members, by making a hasty and ineffective referral, or by avoiding a family altogether.

Along with the personal risks involved in family counseling, however, come the rewards. Physicians who get seriously involved in family counseling may find it an enlivening experience. They are enriched by their exposure to the deep emotional experiences of family life. They are stimulated to rework their own family relationships, both with their family of origin and their current family. It is uncanny how families in one's professional practice bring up issues not successfully resolved in one's own personal life. Such a professional confrontation carries the opportunity for personal development for the counselor.

The general point we are making is that family counseling demands more personal investment from the physician than perhaps any other aspect of medical practice does. Assessment tools help reduce the uncertainty, and counseling techniques help reduce the anxiety, but ultimately family counseling is a human encounter between the counselor and the family. Of course this is true for individual counseling as well, but the physician is more apt to feel in control of a one-to-one counseling session than of a family session. Spouses may bicker or refuse to talk, children may tear up the office, and the family may gang up on the doctor.

What does a family physician need in order to get seriously involved in family counseling? ("Seriously" refers to a planned and thoughtful approach to developing one's skills in this area.) The first requirement is a basic knowledge of family dynamics and family assessment. Second come reasonably well-developed individual interviewing skills: Family counseling builds on the foundation of the physician's ability to engage and help patients at the individual level. The third requirement is support in the form of more experienced counselors or therapists. The family counseling techniques presented in this chapter are not meant to be used in isolation from professional feedback and consultation; family counselors at all levels of experience—especially novices—need colleagues to talk with about what goes on in family work.

To reiterate distinctions made earlier, this chapter presents skills in primary care family *counseling* as opposed to family *therapy*. Therapy interventions differ from counseling interventions in that the former are more intrusive, more suited to dealing with resistance, more potentially destabilizing, and more far-reaching in intent. In other words, family therapy is aimed at major family system overhaul or at least at a decisive breakthrough in serious family dysfunction. Therefore, although Minuchin's *assessment* model is stressed in this book, many of his *therapy* techniques are not suitable for the kind of counseling most family physicians will do.

The second point to be reiterated is that we consider family counseling an appropriate part of the treatment of most psychosocial problems—those traditionally considered "individual" problems, such as depression and anxiety, as well as those typically considered "family" problems, such as marital or parent–child conflict. Depending on the presenting issue, primary care family counseling may be used in conjunction with individual counseling or psychopharmacological treatment, or it may serve as the primary treatment for the psychosocial problem. Hence, we are not fostering family counseling as a panacea, but rather as a useful and potentially powerful treatment approach in the family physician's repertoire. This chapter introduces the general functions and processes of family counseling in family practice. Subsequent chapters apply the general approach to specific problems.

FUNCTIONS OF PRIMARY CARE FAMILY COUNSELING

We propose that family counseling in the context of family medicine has four distinct functions or purposes: education, prevention, support, and challenge.

EDUCATION

Sometimes families get themselves into trouble because they are faced with unfamiliar situations. The new parents argue heatedly over getting up with their baby daughter when she cries at night. The wife of a man depressed over the loss of his job grows progessively more agitated when he does not "snap out" of his depressive symptoms. A husband is upset over his wife's diminished sexual interest during pregnancy. A recently divorced woman believes that she must be going crazy because of her mood swings, and fears her children will inevitably be damaged by the divorce. If these individuals and families are functioning reasonably well, the above situations lend themselves to a family counseling intervention by the family physician in the role of teacher. Physicians of course have been filling this role for centuries, but generally the teaching has been done mainly with individual patients (usually the wife/mother) rather than with a couple or family. *It is far better to educate all the involved parties as a group.* This way the physician can maintain a relationship with the whole therapeutic triangle. Many a brilliant educational move has come to naught when translated by a patient who wants to make a point—for example, "The doctor says to let the kid cry, just like I told you," or "The doctor says you're making things worse by nagging me." In one of our favorites, the mother of three small children told her husband, "The doctor said my stress comes from being cooped up with little kids, so I'm going back to bartending in the evenings." This husband, by the way, tended to be jealous of his wife, and she tended to be flirtatious with men.

Educating the whole couple or family gives each member access to the same knowledge and the same opportunity to ask questions. With the physician's help, the family can then apply this information or advice to their own situation; for example, clear expectations about the course of an illness can help the family decide to reassign family responsibilities. If education is to lead to action, the commitment of all the involved family members will be required; sometimes this means bringing grandparents into the family counseling, especially if the doctor's ideas are quite different from the family's traditional notions.

Family sessions also give the physician the opportunity to teach in one of the most effective ways—by modeling. A physician can deal with the depressed, unemployed husband in a way similar to that in which the wife could deal with her husband—that is, with sympathy for his suffering, with understanding that depression cannot usually be "willed" away, but with firm expectations that he participate in his own recovery and that he refrain from manipulating others into catering to him unnecessarily. The same kind of modeling can be quite helpful for families trying to cope with the physical illness of a member: The physician can show the family how to combine strong support with clear expectations for the patient's independence. Opportunities for such family life education occur every day in family medicine.

To summarize, the educational function of family counseling brings the family physician's knowledge to bear in such areas as family dynamics, child development, stress during the life cycle, and mental and physical illness. By assembling family members to discuss their current difficulty, the physician can more effectively educate, can avoid disturbances in the therapeutic triangle, and can model the behavior being taught.

PREVENTION

Prevention in family counseling may be viewed as a special kind of education concerned with avoiding common problems encountered by families during their life cycles. If education to ameliorate problems is more desirable than waiting until therapy is needed, then *preventive* family counseling is better still. Since people have routine medical needs throughout their lives, family physicians are uniquely situated to deliver preventive family counseling. Any of the transition points in the family life cycle is appropriate for such an intervention, but perhaps the most well-documented need is for prophylactic treatment of couples who are expecting their first child. One of the most consistent findings in family sociology is that the average couple experiences an enduring decline in marital satisfaction following the birth of the first child, a decline not experienced by couples who do not have children (Rollins & Cannon, 1974). Clinically, the move from a dyad to a triad can be seen as leaving someone feeling outside. The father may feel jealous of his wife's preoccupation with the baby; she may feel pulled between husband and baby. The wife may experience diminished power and self-identity in the marriage if for the first time she is without employment and her own source of income. The husband/father may experience stronger needs to earn money and be successful in his job; thus at a time when she needs him more, he may be more preoccupied with the outside world.

What are the other predictable stresses during the first year with a first baby? Russell (1974) assembled the following "bothersome issues" most often cited by a randomly selected group of 200 Midwest urban couples who had had their first child within the past year. Notice the differences between the husbands' and wives' lists:

Wives	*Husbands*
Worry about my personal appearance since the baby	Baby interrupted sleeping and rest
	Suggestions from in-laws about our baby
Physical tiredness and fatigue	Baby increased money problems
Baby interrupted sleeping and rest	Baby's birth made it necessary to change some plans
Worry about my "loss of figure"	
Feeling "edgy" or emotionally upset	Additional amount of work required by baby

The family physician can try to prepare couples for these transitional stresses through preventive marital counseling. Prospective parents tend to be focused on the childbirth to the exclusion of considering their future life as parents. Seeds can be planted during prenatal visits, and then more intensive preventive counseling can begin after the birth. Issues the physician can bring up include the partners' expectations of each other for child care; their employment plans; their plans to spend time alone as a couple; use of relatives and babysitters for relief from child care burdens; whether and how soon to have another baby; birth control; and child-rearing values and techniques, including those learned in their families of origin. One research finding that can be stressed is that couples who maintain a high level of companionship activities may not experience a decline in marital satisfaction after the baby comes.

The transition to the first child is just one of many examples that could be developed to suggest the place for preventive family counseling. Some other family life cycle stress points include the birth of the second child, the challenges of adolescent children, and the increasing dependency of elderly family members on their adult children. Preparing families for these expectable stresses can allow them to cope more successfully.

In addition to preventing problems associated with life cycle transitions, preventive family counseling can help avoid dysfunctional coping with medical problems. A common illustration is a husband's first myocardial infarction. Here a preventive intervention with the couple should be considered part of the standard treatment protocol. The danger these couples face, of course, is that their marital roles will quickly come to resemble a nonsexual nurse–invalid relationship. The preventive counseling should be done with both spouses present, even if one or both appear uncomfortable (and even if the physician is uncomfortable). If the spouses are counseled separately, neither will be certain about what the doctor told the other one. Together they can both hear the good news that the husband is still a man and that the wife can still be a woman.

SUPPORT

Providing support for individuals and families is the foundation of all counseling. Hence, support is involved in the other three functions of family counseling. It is singled out here because sometimes support is all the family physician needs to provide a family. The supportive function of family counseling is aimed at helping the family through a difficult time by being available, by listening attentively, by helping family members express their feelings, by showing one's concern, and by letting the family take responsibility for its own resolution of the difficulty. In a primarily supportive family counseling session, then, the physician would do little in the way of education or problem solving. This relatively passive counseling role may be quite difficult for activist physicians.

Supportive family counseling is most clearly indicated when a family has suffered the death of one of its members. Trained to view death as a personal failure, the physician may be reluctant to give the family the time and attention required for supportive grief counseling. The emotional force field that families create is nowhere more keenly felt than when a member has died, particularly if the death was unexpected or ill-timed. The death of the family patriarch or matriarch, the death of a spouse/parent in the child-rearing years, and the death of a child are examples of particularly trouble-some losses for families. What a family needs is support through the process of grieving, healing, and recovery. Family members must learn to accept the loss and to reorganize themselves without the missing person. If not handled carefully, the wound opened by a significant loss may become infected—leading to the impairment of one or more members—or may scar over, resulting in a diminished quality of personal and family life. Following is an example of such a situation.

A colleague, Stanley Greenwald, MD, has observed that the torment following the death of the older son in the book and movie *Ordinary People* could have been allayed by a supportive primary care physician working with the whole family. In the plot line, the older boy is killed in a boating accident; the younger boy is involved in the accident but survives. The parents are not able to talk with each other or their son about the loss. The mother never cries. The mother and the son become antagonists, with the father in the middle. The son eventually is admitted to a psychiatric hospital. As Greenwald asks, "Where is their family doctor? Why doesn't their doctor notice the unresolved grief and bring the family together for supportive counseling?" The family's communication and healing channels are blocked; an early supportive intervention might have prevented serious personal and family dysfunction. Once the damage is done, however, supportive counseling would not be enough for this family. They need therapy as a family, but unfortunately only the son is singled out for treatment—a quite common event. While the individual psychotherapy in the story is a fine illustration of that treatment modality—the therapist is empathic, confrontive, and insight-ful—other equally needy family members, particularly the mother, are not involved in the treatment. By the time the therapist invites the parents to participate, the therapeutic triangle is dysfunctional: The mother distrusts the therapist and will not meet with him. The patient survives and the family dies—an outcome that could have been avoided, in our judgment, by a more family-oriented treatment. To recap, *Ordinary People* depicts missed op-portunities—first, for primary supportive counseling from a family physician, and then, failing such counseling, for therapy that involves all the hurting parties.

CHALLENGE

There is an old statement of purpose among pastoral counselors that applies to family physician counselors as well: to comfort the disturbed and to disturb the comfortable. "Comforting the disturbed" refers to the supportive function of counseling. "Disturbing the comfortable"—shaking up those with an illusory sense of good health or with rigid ways of viewing problems—this is the goal of *challenging* the family. One of the most effective ways of constructively challenging a family is to offer a family systems perspective on the problem and then to stress the urgency of a collaborative solution. The physician can point out a couple's troublesome interactional dance and challenge them gently but firmly to work together at changing it. Or parents can be challenged to collaborate in disciplining their children instead of arguing about who is responsible for the family troublemaker. A test of the family's adaptability is how it responds and whether it changes after the counselor makes a challenging observation about the family's interaction patterns. Some adaptable families will have an "Ah ha!" experience and begin to change their interaction patterns. Other families will reject alternative solutions or be unable to implement them.

Challenging or confronting families about serious problems is a risky but sometimes necessary part of the primary care of families. It is risky because the family may resist, disagree with, or verbally attack the physician who is bearing bad news about the family. Why is it sometimes necessary? Since families often become stabilized around the major dysfunctions of their members, a major jolt may be needed to create the possibility of change and healing. Chemical dependency is a classic illustration in primary medical care of the symptom that the family protects as in a cocoon. The husband may say, "I have a few beers every evening." The wife may add, "Yes, he doesn't pass out like he used to. Now my uncle, *there* was an alcoholic."

Sometimes the family physician may initiate supportive or educational counseling with a family and subsequently discover that the family is more dysfunctional than anticipated. The physician can then switch from a supportive or educational mode to a challenging mode. The family of *Ordinary People* could have provided such a scenario. Let us assume that when the family physician assembles the family to help them verbalize their grief and regrets, the parents bicker and the son refuses to talk. The physician tries valiantly to help them open up, but meets with continued resistance. This is the time for challenge and referral: The physician observes to the family members that they have been having some serious difficulties in getting along with each other since the death, that this loss has brought problems to the surface that they have needed to work on for a number of years, and that they could benefit greatly from working together with a family therapist. Once having made this challenge and referral attempt, the physician/counselor should express reluctance to continue with business-as-usual supportive or educational counseling, since all the participants in such an enterprise will feel pessimistic about success. While pulling back from the primary counseling role, however, the physician can assure the family of his or her ongoing concern and involvement. One way to accomplish this reassurance is to attend the first family therapy session with the family. Sometimes the physician needs help too, especially when a family's loss is also the physician's loss or stirs up feelings of failure.

One outcome of a successful challenge concerning a serious family problem, then, can be a referral for therapy. All the guidelines discussed in Chapter 6 apply: Referral should be made to a known and trusted source; it should be rapid; and it should be followed up to make sure that the family has kept the appointment and is progressing in treatment. Successful use of challenge and referral during the process of family counseling can keep the physician out of long-term unproductive counseling relationships and can mobilize the family to accept the more intensive help it needs.

GUIDELINES FOR PRIMARY CARE FAMILY COUNSELING

Family counseling is more an art than a science, more a fluid series of exchanges than a set of discrete behavioral techniques. Counselors and therapists with widely different styles may get very similar results: Some counselors are more "feeling"-oriented and some more "task"-oriented; some are quite active in the session, others relatively more passive. Despite these differences, we think there are a number of fundamental guidelines for family counseling by family physicians—guidelines that cut across the personality types of counselors and, to some extent, the kinds of family problems being treated. Table 7-1 outlines the basic family counseling processes that we think are important in primary care work.

ENGAGING THE FAMILY

The first step in any helping effort is to engage the patient—in this case, the family. "Engaging" refers to the process of meeting and establishing the

TABLE 7-1. BASIC FAMILY COUNSELING TECHNIQUES

1. Engaging the family
2. Initiating discussion of the problem
3. Structuring the session
4. Defining the problem
5. History taking
6. Remaining neutral
7. Encouraging a collaborative set
8. Facilitating family discussion
9. Giving support
10. Teaching
11. Challenging
12. Dealing with resistance
13. Helping families make behavioral contracts
14. Assigning homework

beginning of a trusting relationship with family members. Engaging a couple or family is more difficult than is engaging an individual patient. Accustomed to one-to-one relationships, physicians are apt to relate to a couple as "a patient plus one," and to a family as "a mother plus others." Making personal contact with a family requires making personal contact with each family member. This is the first guideline for engaging a family: Talk to each member separately at the beginning of the session. The conversation can be casual and informative: "How old are you?" "Where do you work?" "What do you do for fun?" "How do you like school?" You might want to begin with the spouse/parent who is less familiar—for example, the husband whose wife is the primary patient. In other words, it is often useful right away to begin building a bridge to the person who is farthest out on the therapeutic triangle. When there is an identified patient, such as an acting-out child, you should probably *not* begin by asking that child any questions. A child on the hot seat will not communicate if you move in too quickly. Generally, a good rule of thumb is to start interacting with the adult family member who is least familiar or with the child who seems furthest removed from the problem.

This warm-up period is intended to put the family at greater ease and to give them a sense of who you are. Social time also helps the counselor begin to get a feel for the family—its mood, activity level, authority structure, and language patterns. The counselor is then able to adapt to the family's unique style, a process Minuchin calls "joining the family." Some families are "hot" and some are "cool"; some use intellectual language ("We don't communicate") while others talk concretely ("He watches TV instead of talking to me"). The counselor can best engage a family initially by employing the language of the family. Similarly, families tend to have a member whose opinion counts most on matters of importance (such as whether to return to family counseling). The family counselor can sense this role and make a special point to honor this member's authority. The underlying goal here is that the counselor communicate to the family members an acceptance of them as a family.

Engaging the family, in summary, involves two steps: (1) making social conversation with each family member, and (2) adapting the counselor's style to the family's style.

INITIATING DISCUSSION OF THE PROBLEM

After the initial social time of engaging the family comes the business at hand. Since the physician/counselor usually has talked with one family member about the problem, it is a good idea to begin with the other adult member—usually the husband—who has been invited to participate by the original patient.

Here is one discussion opener: "Mr. J, would tell me how it came about that you and your wife decided to meet with me today?" This can give you an idea about the process whereby his spouse got him to come to counseling and about his willingness to participate. Responses may range from "I've known there was a problem and when she mentioned talking to you, I was glad to do it," to "She said if I didn't show up today she'd divorce me," to "I don't know what this is about; she just asked me to show up."

Or you can begin with the wife: "Mrs. J, the last time we talked you said you were going to ask your husband to return here with you. Tell me about how you asked him to get counseling with you and how he responded." Here you can begin with the primary patient's viewpoint on the discussions leading up to the marital counseling.

Where there is an obvious presenting problem (such as an alcoholic husband) that everyone in the family believes is the *only* problem, we have found it useful to avoid a direct opening question such as "What problem can I help you with?" The automatic response will be to implicate Mr. J's drinking: "If he stopped drinking, everyone would get along fine." In such cases, we prefer to begin the family counseling with a question that keeps the focus on the way the family members relate and the way drinking affects those relationships: "Tell me what it's like being in this family these days. Johnny [the youngest child], would you begin?" The youngest children will often state the unvarnished truth.

When the family presents child-related problems, begin the discussion with the parents rather than the child. Not only may the child feel dumped on by all the adults, but the parents may sit back to let you handle their child. Alternatively, if the child is especially quick and verbal, the parents may feel put on the defensive immediately. For example, if you engage an adolescent in an extended first-session discussion of his or her parents' shortcomings, the confidence of the parents in the counseling process may be inadvertently undermined. Generally, it is best to work through the parents to help them help their children.

One way to initiate the discussion of parent–child problems is as follows: "Mrs. J, we've talked a bit about the problems you've been having with your children. Mr. J, would you fill me in on what you see as the problems your family needs to work on?" Even if the initial discussion repeats what you already know, or if you are dealing with a single parent who has discussed the problems with you privately, it is important that the whole family hear and participate in a calm airing of the problems. After initiating the problem-oriented discussion, you can then systematically solicit everyone's perspective on the difficulties that brought the family to the office. These opening remarks from family members should be relatively brief, a kind of getting-the-feet-wet exercise.

The above guidelines are designed for problem-focused discussion. In preventive or supportive counseling for life transitions, illness, or grief—

when there may be no concrete "problem"—the discussion of the family's major issue can be initiated with an acknowledgment such as this: "I know you are going through an important change in your lives [or have gone through a painful loss] and I'd like to help you in any way I can." Or this: "When someone in a family has been very ill, I like to sit down with the family to answer questions and find out how everyone is doing." First, address the family member who appears to be the neediest: "How are you holding up today, Joe?" Then check in on the others.

STRUCTURING THE SESSION

Just as a successful artist must be in control of the artistic medium, a successful counselor or therapist must have control over the counseling session. The counselor must be able to decide on the structure of the session and adhere to it within reasonable limits. For example, the time to socialize with each family member may have to be protected from a family member who wants to monopolize the physician's attention. The following is a structuring statement: "Mrs. J, I'd like to come back to that point after I've had a chance to get to know the rest of your family."

Family counseling presents greater control difficulties than does individual counseling. Family members may collude unconsciously with one another to stay away from topics the counselor wants them to discuss. Members may vie for "air time" in the session, or they may struggle to stay as far away from the action as possible. The counselor is apt to be swept away by the family's well-rehearsed interaction patterns. When family meets counselor there is always an underground power struggle; failure to gain control over the counseling sessions after repeated tries indicates that the physician/counselor should seek consultation or refer this family for therapy.

"Structuring the session" means being able to enforce your rules when they conflict with the family's. We suggest several core family counseling rules:

1. *Each person has the right to speak without being interrupted.* Some families are chronic interrupters; no one finishes an important thought. If you permit interruptions, you perpetuate this dysfunctional interaction pattern. With an interrupting family, you can make the rule explicit: "I would like everyone to get a chance to speak without being interrupted." Then you must enforce the rule.

2. *When you have announced a procedure or plan of action, do not let yourself become sidetracked.* If you say you want to ask *everyone's* opinion, an argument between two family members must not prevent you from checking with every member. The family will know that you did not follow through on your intention, and the two combatants may have unconsciously wanted to avoid hearing someone else's response.

3. *Steer the family back to the issues at hand when the discussion strays.* One of the best ways to avoid confronting a problem is to keep changing the subject, as anyone who has ever served on a committee can attest. An effective counselor has a homing sense for staying with important issues. A common family escape is to complain about people not present in the session, such as in-laws, school teachers, or other physicians. In the presence of one's wife, it may be easier to complain about one's mother than about one's wife. A simple way of getting back on the track is to say, "I'd like to return to what you were talking about earlier." After repeated failures to retrack the family, the counselor can confront them about their pattern of jumping away from certain issues. This confrontation can be done with a supportive acknowledgment of the family's fear: "I've noticed that when I ask you to talk about your relationship as a couple, you end up talking about Mr. J's mother. She must be an important person in your marriage. And I think it may be hard for the two of you to just talk about your own relationship. Is that true for you, Mr. J?"

4. *Resist requests for solutions if such requests seem premature or inappropriate.* Some patients and families want to jump from a hasty identification of a problem to an immediate solution, preferably one proposed by the physician. To spend enough time exploring the problems and getting family members to talk with one another honestly, you may have to sidestep family members' requests for definitive advice. They may be expecting you to write a family prescription after 20 minutes. A "What shall we do?" question can be handed back to the family in a number of ways:

• "I think we need to understand more about what's going on first."

• "The solution is going to have to come from all of you as a family. I will have some ideas to offer, but only *you* know what kind of family you want to have."

The point here is that you should take responsibility for the timing of the counseling process, and therefore must resist being pulled into the role of expert advisor for a family that has not squarely confronted either its problems or its own resources for change.

5. *Take charge of the physical arrangements of the session.* We prefer to have family members sit in a circle, with the counselor reserving a favorite chair. It is diagnostically useful to see how family members place themselves within the space you provide (e.g., do the spouses sit far apart?). If you want people to change seats during the session so that, for example, a married couple can talk more directly with each other, ask them to move. In other words, you should be in control of the physical environment of the counseling.

6. *Take charge of who attends the counseling sessions.* If the children are asked to be present, insist that they should be there. If a child or spouse feels free to show up one time and not the next, the counseling cannot work. You must be in charge of the membership of the sessions.

In Carl Whitaker's approach to family therapy, the first significant phase of therapy is the "battle for structure" (Whitaker & Keith, 1981). This issue is just as important for primary care family counseling. It is only when the family perceives the physician as able to lead the session that the family will feel secure enough to delve into painful material. Family counseling can begin with an authoritarian flavor and move toward democracy: The counselor controls the sessions at the outset like a parent or teacher, then later— when this leadership is clearly established—the counselor can let the strings of power return gradually to the family.

DEFINING THE PROBLEM

After each family member has had the opportunity to give an initial statement about the problems that have brought the family to counseling, the counselor can move to define these issues more clearly. A common approach used by family therapists is to ask family members to specify the *changes* they would like to see in the family. This puts the issue in positive form—changes they would like—as opposed to a negative form of complaints about others' behavior. Often this reversal of direction requires coaching from the counselor.

PHYSICIAN: Mrs. J, what changes would you like to see in your relationship with your husband so you could be happier in your marriage?

MRS. J: I just want him to stop avoiding me so much.

PHYSICIAN: Rather than putting it as what he should *stop* doing, would you say what you would like him to do more often, or something you would like to see him start doing?

MRS. J: I would like him to stay home with me in the evenings and pay some attention to me.

A start has been made toward defining this marital problem. The problem is constructively described as the wife's wanting more time and affection than the husband is giving her. "I want to be around you more" is a more positive beginning for problem solving than "You go out too much; you just want to avoid me."

Thus, the first guideline for defining the problem is to specify what changes family members would like to see. Preferably, these requests for change should be concrete rather than global:

MRS. J: I wish he would be more attentive to me.

PHYSICIAN: How could he show that he was attentive?

MRS. J: By staying home with me once in a while and talking to me instead of watching TV.

By asking the wife to specify what sort of specific behavior change she wants from her husband, the counselor has begun the process of helping them find solutions to their problems.

When one person has made a clear statement about goals, move on to another. It is very important, especially in marital counseling, that *both partners* state some change they would like to see occur in the relationship. If Mr. J gets off the hook by claiming to be perfectly content, then Mrs. J falls into the role of the complaining shrew. Both partners must own the need for change if change is to occur. An exception is in the area of child discipline problems: Sometimes the parents must force a reluctant child to change.

As each problem gets clarified, the counselor can summarize the issue for the family. By the end of the first session, the family can be presented with an agenda of changes they have said they want to work on. Further problem definition will continue during subsequent counseling sessions.

HISTORY TAKING

Minuchin recommends taking only a brief history of the presenting problem during the first session. We agree with this procedure for family physicians. It is important to learn about the origins of the family problem and how it developed to its present level; however, this need not encompass more than a third of the initial interview. *Onset* of the problem and *previous efforts to cope* with the problem are two essential pieces of historical information. Tracing the start of the problem may suggest that the family is suffering a life cycle adjustment difficulty, as in the case of a couple whose dissatisfaction begins after the birth of a first child or after their last child has left home. Similarly, it is useful to know whether a patient's depression or anxiety began after a particular family event (such as an affair) or has pervaded the patient's life since childhood.

In addition to questions about the origins of the presenting problem, the second important piece of history concerns the family's attempts to solve the problem. The Palo Alto school of family therapy (Weakland, Fisch, Watzlawick, & Bodin, 1974) has proposed that families get into trouble not because of the "problem" itself (e.g., depression, acting-out behavior), but because of how the family attempts to solve the problem. Thus the physician/counselor should inquire about the family's coping attempts. How did family members try to help Mr. J when he got depressed? How did he respond to their gestures? Often people will tell a depressed individual to "cheer up," thereby making that person feel worse. Or parents may try to crush their son's incipient rebellion by controlling him more and more closely until the family explodes. The "problem" may have begun as relatively normal behavior from an adolescent or as a normal reaction to situational stress, but the "treatment" may have made the patient seriously ill.

We suggest a problem-focused approach to family counseling, which deemphasizes extensive history taking and elaborate assessment of all areas of family functioning. The problem with such data gathering is that you end up with more information than you know what to do with. Data constipation may result: You know a lot about these people, but may not be able to help them any better. Families that can only be helped with the assistance of comprehensive three-generational biopsychosocial family assessment ought to be referred to a therapist in any case. Family physicians, as primary family counselors, do not have the time or the training for such analysis. And many families do not need it anyway. Minuchin's here-and-now approach to assessment is taxing and complicated enough for the training level of most family physicians. Furthermore, we think the biggest payoff in successful interventions comes from the physician's understanding of the interaction patterns that maintain the problem and that influence the physician–family therapeutic relationship. These dynamics can only be assessed by face-to-face interaction with the family.

REMAINING NEUTRAL

The therapeutic triangle is like an electromagnetic field that pulls the counselor in one direction or another. Counseling a family requires an overall stance of neutrality, or, stated more positively, an alignment with each member and with the family as a unit. The therapeutic triangle can remain functional in the face of brief coalitions of the counselor with one member against another—as when the counselor supports a wife to confront her husband's drinking behavior—but the counselor's support must on balance be perceived by family members as flowing equally to all members. This is difficult to achieve for a physician who has already formed a bond with a primary patient. In such cases, during the first counseling session with the family, the physician should work especially hard at communicating to other family members that you understand and appreciate their positions and feelings. In other words, you can draw on the "savings account" accumulated with the primary patient by temporarily paying more attention to others.

Neutrality flows from an internal state in the counselor rather than from a body of techniques. In other words, you have to *believe* that there are no villains in the family—and no faultless victims—in order to refrain from casting family members in these roles. A husband will know if you regard him as an irresponsible bum; a wife will detect your judgment that she is lucky her husband has put up with her all these years. If you feel this way—and often such judgments are involuntary—then do not try to counsel the family. Refer the case to a therapist or to one of your family physician colleagues.

If you can avoid internally taking sides and scapegoating individuals in the family, the following techniques may be helpful in communicating this neutral support to the family:

1. *Paraphrase each person's major complaint or proposed solution in terms that sound as reasonable as possible.* This communicates to family members that you think that their feelings are understandable and not stupid or bad.

MRS. J: I want him home more in the evening. I can't stand being a single parent. But when I ask him to stay home, he gets mad at me. Am I expecting too much?

PHYSICIAN: You're saying that he's your husband and you need his support at home with the kids. But when you bring up this problem, you feel like it just leads to a fight. Mr. J, what's your side of this?

MR. J: I'd be willing to stay at home more in the evenings, but I can't stand it when she nags at me. She doesn't appreciate that I work hard all day.

PHYSICIAN: If I understand you correctly, the problem for you is not that you don't *want* to stay home with your wife but that things get so bad between the two of you that you tend to stay away. Is that right?

MR. J: Yeah, that's right.

The counselor has attempted to communicate to each spouse that each is understood.

2. *Juxtapose each person's position on the problem and point out any similarities you see.* One of the best ways to remain neutral in a conflict is to articulate both sides' positions in back and forth fashion, therefore implicitly saying that neither side has cornered the market on truth and righteousness.

PHYSICIAN: Both of you are saying that you would like to feel more appreciated by the other. Mrs. J, you feel like your husband doesn't think housework and child care are difficult burdens. Mr. J, you've said that your wife doesn't seem to appreciate your need for relaxation after working outside the home all day. What I hear are two people who very much want support from each other but who are ending up driving each other farther apart. Does that sound like what's going on?

Such interventions serve notice to the couple that you see them as in the same marriage boat, albeit rowing in opposite directions. You are saying that they both have legitimate needs and claims on each other, and you have identified the problem as stemming from their ineffective efforts to give and receive support. Even if one member is an alcoholic whose drinking you want to see stopped—and on this issue you may be allying with the other spouse— you can openly acknowledge the unhappiness this person feels in the family and the changes he or she wants to see occur. There is a good chance, for example, that the nonalcoholic spouse has denied any personal contribution to family problems by placing all the blame on the partner's drinking. While not supporting an alcoholic husband's self-deceptions about the drinking, you can support his effort to escape the scapegoat role in the family.

ENCOURAGING A COLLABORATIVE SET

Family members need help in seeing that they got into the mess together and must get out together. In Benjamin Franklin's phrase, "If we do not hang together, we will surely hang separately." When family alliances are fragile, the family physician can help by communicating the expectation that the family will work together on the problem.

One way to encourage the family to take a collaborative set is to help them see the dance they have been doing to create or sustain the problem.

PHYSICIAN: Mr. and Mrs. J, it's not very surprising to me that you've been having trouble controlling Jimmy's behavior. He's a pretty clever thirteen-year-old who knows how to take advantage of his parents when they're at odds with each other. You each have some pretty good ideas about disciplining him, but you don't have your act together as a parental *team.*

It is not enough, of course, to point out the mutual participation in the problem formation; you must also help them *change* their interactional dance. Generally, resolving family problems requires complementary changes by all the participants. A brilliant solution that requires changes in only one member is probably doomed from the start. That person will feel unfairly burdened. In the case of the J family, it would be a mistake to settle for Mr. J's promise to stay home more in the evenings. Unless his wife also behaves differently toward him, he will not stay home long. Cave-ins do not contribute to family growth.

When helping families negotiate change or when offering suggestions for handling common family problems, therefore, you should look for tasks or solutions that involve two or more people. When new parents are fighting over how to handle their baby's crying, it is better to give them a suggestion that they can implement together than it is to give one that involves only one partner (typically the mother). A couple whom Doherty counseled agreed to alternate getting up each night to feed and change their fussy baby. This was their first collaborative parenting venture. They eventually got to the point where they let the baby cry and go back to sleep, but at the beginning it was important that they learn to share the nightly burden.

In encouraging a collaborative set in these ways, the family physician is calling upon the family's *esprit de corps*—their sense of belonging to each other in bad times and good. Fairly well-functioning families will respond positively to being approached this way. More debilitated families will probably not get worse, but they will not get much better without specialized treatment.

FACILITATING FAMILY DISCUSSION

Generally it is best for the counselor to begin the first session by talking individually with family members. This procedure helps build rapport with each member and helps establish the counselor's control of the session. At some later point, however, it is often helpful to have family members speak directly with one another. Inducing the family to have such a discussion can be difficult for the novice counselor.

Several moments in family counseling lend themselves to family discussions. When the family is approaching a joint decision, the counselor can step back and ask them to talk with each other about what they want to do. A second appropriate time is when a family member tells the counselor something positive about another member:

HUSBAND: I guess I don't tell her very often that I think she is a good wife.

PHYSICIAN: Why don't you tell her now?

A third case is when someone speaks of poor communication with someone else. If a wife says that her husband will not listen when she tells him something, the counselor can ask her to talk with him in the session. *A good rule of thumb for family counseling is that people must first change in the office if you expect them to act differently at home.* If they cannot communicate in front of the counselor, then they will not do any better at home.

Sometimes family members are reluctant to speak directly with one another in front of the counselor. Common expressions of this resistance are "I've already told this to her," "I feel silly," and continuing to speak directly to the counselor instead of the family member. If you decide to ask spouses or other family members to talk with each other, you must firmly insist that they do so. Gently but persistently repeat your request:

PHYSICIAN: I know you feel a little strange talking with your husband in front of me, but I'd like you to try it anyway.

WIFE: He already knows how I feel about it.

PHYSICIAN: Tell him again anyway. I'd like to just listen while the two of you talk together.

Sometimes getting two people to interact requires changing the seating arrangement. You can ask the spouses to turn their chairs so they can face each other more directly; and you can also move your own chair back so that its position is less central to the family system. One technique we have used when spouses continue to look our way instead of at each other is to refrain momentarily from looking at either one of them as they begin talking. Thus they have only each other to look at. Like all counseling techniques, this one has its limits: After Doherty suggested to a resident that he look away from the couple in order to encourage them to keep talking with each other, the resident proceeded to stare out the window for 10 minutes while the couple made befuddled, furtive glances in his direction.

When family members engage in serious conversation in your presence, you can learn much about their communication patterns and can coach them in more effective communication and/or more constructive problem solving. The trick is to move into their conversation to make an observation or suggestion, but then to get back out again so they can continue talking. This is the essence of coaching as opposed to playing the game oneself.

WIFE: When I am depressed, you seem to avoid me all the time.

HUSBAND: No, I don't.

PHYSICIAN: Would you tell your husband what he does that makes you think he is avoiding you?

WIFE: Well, he . . .

PHYSICIAN: (pointing to husband) Tell him directly.

WIFE: You listen to me for a while and then go putter around your shop or watch baseball or something. You always have something else to do when I'm feeling down.

HUSBAND: (to wife) I don't know how to help you. I just feel awful for you but I don't know what to say after a while, so I just get up and leave.

WIFE: It would help if you stayed and listened to me.

The physician in this vignette is helping this couple deal directly with each other around the issue of how the wife gets support during her depressed moods. Since this couple apparently uses physical distance as a way to handle difficult communication episodes, the physician can help them best by coaching them to talk openly with each other in the counseling sessions. The wife can be helped to tell her husband more directly what she wants from him when she is depressed, and the husband can teach his wife about the limits of his tolerance of her discussions about how badly she feels. If he offers more brief supportive gestures to her, she may feel less inclined to talk about her troubles at great length. At any rate, their best chance of progress lies in their face-to-face interactions in marital counseling.

Giving Support

At the risk of stating the obvious, we note that in order to give support to a family, you must *want* to support them. You must *feel* supportive if you want to communicate genuine support. Counseling techniques are empty without the underlying disposition. Furthermore, some counselors can break all the counseling "rules" about how to express concern and helpfulness, but they still leave the patient or family feeling supported. In this spirit of caution about techniques when they are not in harmony with the intentions of the counselor, we offer some guidelines for communicating support to families:

1. *Be willing to be quiet and let people express their feelings.* When families are experiencing great stress or grief, one of the best ways to help is to listen much and talk little. This can be difficult for active physicians.

2. *To let people know you are with them emotionally, reflect back to them from time to time the feelings you hear them expressing.*

PATIENT: I should be over his death by now, but I still think about him all the time.

PHYSICIAN: You still miss him a lot.

Feeding back to patients what you hear them saying is an alternative to the persistent habit of asking questions. The above physician's statement, "You still miss him a lot," may be contrasted with the probably less empathic question, "Do you still miss him a lot?"

3. *Stay with the patient's and family's feelings rather than trying to push their feelings along toward resolution.* Your own discomfort may lead you to premature efforts to make everyone feel better. Certain wounds take time and patience to heal. Statements like "You'll feel better soon," or the more contemporary "You will someday see this as a growing experience," serve only to communicate impatience and disapproval to the patient and family. *In supportive counseling, you must trust the family members to heal in their own time.* If you think that the healing is being blocked by psychological or family forces, then switch to a different counseling mode—for example, educational or challenging. But avoid trying to support the family too emphatically into moving faster! In the following example, the physician supportively confirms both the fears and the confidence of a man whose wife has just left him.

PATIENT: These next two weeks are going to be the hardest. It's going to be hell.

PHYSICIAN: I agree that you're in for some real pain over the next couple of weeks.

PATIENT: But I can handle it. I've been through hard times before.

PHYSICIAN: I think you can handle it. And I'd like to be available to you over the next couple of weeks if you need me.

A family practice resident observing this exchange said later that he would have been tempted to say something like "It may not be so bad as you think; you can handle it," when the patient first expressed fears about the immediate future. In so doing, the resident might have moved ahead of where the patient was emotionally—leading to patient resistance—rather than following the patient's movement from fear to confidence.

4. *One of the best ways to support a patient and family is to help them mobilize the supportive people in their social environment.* The physician is only one person and has enormous time demands. As soon as possible, try to share the burden of support with others—extended family, other health care professionals, clergy. For example, if a couple has given birth to a handicapped child, the physician's first task is to support the partners personally but then to connect them rapidly with the network of self-help groups and professional services. Continued intermittent follow-up support from the physician may then be sufficient.

Supportive counseling is best suited for helping families through temporary stress, grief, and dislocation. The counselor helps by listening, by communicating an empathic understanding of their difficulty, by patiently respecting the family's own pace of recovery, and by helping them contact others who can offer support. A chief limitation of supportive counseling is faced when the family does not progress toward healing, when it does not reorganize after a loss, or when it becomes more rigid in the face of adversity. This is what happens in *Ordinary People.* Such a "stuck" family may require therapy.

TEACHING

All counseling is in some way an educational activity. However, some situations call for explicit instruction from the counselor. Physicians are accustomed to the role of expert teacher, but they tend to have difficulty moving out of that role once in it. The art of teaching in family counseling involves moving in and out of a teaching role with the family: *in* when information is needed, and *out* when the family needs to make decisions on the basis of the information; *in* when facts can clear up confusion, and *out* when people need to express feelings.

PHYSICIAN: One thing we know about teenagers is that they try to test the limits their parents set. Jimmy in that way is acting like a normal kid, although he can be infuriating. And it's also normal in his development that he is so concerned with his appearance.

MRS. J: I'm glad to hear he is normal. But how can we handle him?
PHYSICIAN: That's for you and Mr. J to decide. All I can do is talk about some general principles of discipline. It's clear to me that you and your husband must agree first, then let Jimmy know what you expect, and then follow through with consequences if he does not cooperate. That's the general principle, but only you two can decide what is best for your child. Why don't you talk right now with your husband about how you can work together more in handling your son?

The physician here has done some explicit teaching about adolescent development and discipline, but then has moved out of the expert role by tossing the problem back to the parents. Similarly, in sexual issues, the physician can communicate accurate information about the risks of sexual intercourse after a myocardial infarction without telling the couple how they should relate sexually.

Like all good teaching, the art of instructing families should be tailored to the specific issues faced by each family. Discourses on psychology, philosophy—or even family systems!—are almost always inappropriate. Families in crisis need only enough information to cope more effectively with their presenting problem. Later they may be interested in the fuller picture. Especially to be avoided are attempts to convince the family that things will get better, such as "He will certainly grow out of this nasty streak," or "First you'll feel shock at your loss, then denial, then anger . . . then you'll come to accept it." Teaching from physicians can be the best of experiences, and when it sounds like these two statements, the worst of experiences.

CHALLENGING

The best way to challenge a family is to get someone in the family to do it. At least one family member must be feeling pain and wanting change in order for a family confrontation to be successful. In other words, you generally must have some leverage within the family in order to challenge the family's status quo. If the wife of an alcoholic man is ready to push for change in the family and in herself, then the physician can challenge the family as a group to confront the problem. If no one in the family is prepared to go out on a limb—to take a risk—over a serious dysfunctional pattern, then you should be leery of rushing in to save them. An exception to this principle is family violence, where a physician can mobilize community authorities to disturb an unhealthy family balance.

Before you challenge a couple or family to work on a serious problem, you should have already done preliminary counseling with the family member who most wants change. This person may need strengthening in order to lead the family in a different direction. The most common example in our experience is the wife/mother who is concerned about her husband's drinking behavior. Another example is the single-parent mother who is involved in a power struggle with her ex-husband over disciplining the children: The children are out of control and will not get back in control unless the parents work collaboratively instead of competitively. In the latter case, the family physician can ask the mother to bring in her ex-husband for a discussion about the children.

As suggested above, most of the actual challenging—or pushing for change—should be done by family members themselves, not by the physician/counselor. You are serving here as a catalyst for the chemical reaction rather than as a prime mover:

WIFE: Our family is so miserable I can't stand it any more. We're always fighting.

PHYSICIAN: Would you talk with your husband about what you want changed?

WIFE: (to husband) We're going to have to do something to stop this fighting all the time. And I don't think I can take you getting drunk any more on the weekends. You get so mean to me after you've been drinking.

HUSBAND: I don't think I have a drinking problem.

PHYSICIAN: (to wife) Would you tell him what it's like for you when he drinks?

WIFE: You become a different person, not the man I married. You either leave the house and don't pay any attention to me, or you yell and pick on me terribly.

PHYSICIAN: (to husband) I think what your wife is telling you is that your drinking is causing a problem between the two of you. You may think you are in control of your drinking, but your wife is saying she is never sure how you're going to treat her when you come home. Even if you've only had one beer, she is going to suspect that it's the alcohol that's talking to her and not her husband. (to both spouses) I think the two of you have a serious problem in your relationship. You're arguing a lot and not sharing much affection with each other. And alcohol keeps you from getting to first base in dealing with your problems.

In this exchange, note the advantage of piggybacking one's challenge of the husband's drinking on the wife's confrontation. The wife opens the door for the physician. At the same time, the physician ends the interchange by challenging them as a couple to work on their full range of problems, including the drinking problem. In challenging a family member, it is important to refrain from moralizing; others have undoubtedly tried and failed with this approach ("You owe it to your family . . ."). Instead, the family member can be confronted with the family problems that others in the family are articulating and with the personal problems this individual has faced (such as loss of job or poor health). If necessary, you can speak frankly and ominously about your *concerns* for the long-term consequences of not dealing with the problem. There is an important distinction between saying "I am concerned about . . ." and saying "I think you should. . . ." The former respects the patient's right to choose a course of action; the latter puts the physician in a godlike position almost certain to turn off the patient.

A challenge should always be accompanied by a treatment plan. For serious psychosocial problems, this treatment plan will probably involve a referral for therapy. The details of the referral should be carefully worked out before the family counseling session. If the treatment plan for alcoholism involves family therapy and AA, then these sources should be prepared for the referral and should be ready to accept the patient or family into care. If the referral is first to inpatient treatment, then the bed should be ready at the treatment center. Finally, as the family's physician you should promise to continue supporting the family throughout the treatment process. The skill of challenging in family counseling, in sum, consists of delivering both bad news—"You've got a serious problem, as some of you already know"—and good news—"Effective help is available for you."

DEALING WITH RESISTANCE

Major family resistance to change or to the counseling process should signal the need for a referral to a therapist, but some forms of resistance are inevitable in every counseling relationship. A skilled primary care counselor must know how to deal with at least two forms of resistance: failure to cooperate with the structure of the counseling (no-shows, lateness, unreasonable time demands), and the tendency to argue with the counselor ("Yes, but . . ."). The structuring issue requires an assertive posture from the physician/counselor. Families that miss appointments or come late to sessions should be confronted about this. One way to use this resistance therapeutically is to ask what the family members are trying to tell you by their behavior. If everyone denies any deeper meaning in the uncooperativeness, then you can deal with it straightforwardly by saying, "My time is important to me, and I would like you to respect it." You can also confront the family about how high a priority they are placing on the counseling, particularly if other activities become excuses to skip a family session. Unreasonable time demands can be dealt with in a similar straightforward way: "I realize you would like to meet weekly (instead of biweekly) or in the evenings, but my schedule cannot accommodate that." There are two other options: Try to deal directly with the family's doubts about their internal resources for getting through the week by themselves, or refer a particularly demanding family to a therapist who has more time for family sessions.

Arguing with resistive patients and family members is a common pitfall for beginning counselors:

PATIENT: I don't think I will ever get over this divorce.
COUNSELOR: You will probably be feeling better soon.
PATIENT: I don't think so. I don't know how you can say that.
COUNSELOR: I've worked with other people in your situation, and I'm sure you'll be feeling better.
PATIENT: Huh.

It is quite frustrating to have a family member—or a whole family—disagree with one of your most brilliant biopsychosocial observations. The counselor's art generally requires bending with such disagreement rather than meeting it head on. People often need time to assimilate new information about themselves and their families. There are two ways to deal with disagreement: (1) Suggest that family members think about what you have said; or (2) encourage them to say more about how they see the issues and how they would like to change things. Their disagreement with you may not be a sign of resistance at all; they may be closer to the truth and to the best solutions. Therefore, one of your options is to follow where they lead and to see if you can find an area of common agreement. The worst option is to try repeatedly to persuade the family of the wisdom of your position.

Generally, the best approaches to dealing with a family's resistance are to be assertive with family members when they are uncooperative with the structure of treatment, and to follow their thoughts and feelings when they disagree with your assessment of their situation—and then to seek a blending of the two views.

HELPING FAMILIES MAKE BEHAVIORAL CONTRACTS

Behavioral marital therapists such as Jacobson and Margolin (1979) and Stuart (1980) have demonstrated the usefulness of helping spouses make clear agreements with each other for changing their interaction patterns. It is often not enough to help couples or families understand their problems better and communicate more honestly with each other; solutions may require agreements or contracts about what each person will do differently in the future. The counselor's role here is that of teacher and mediator—stressing the importance of each person making a commitment to change and facilitating the working out of a complementary decision about what behaviors each is willing to change. Some families never move to this stage of decision making about their problems, and other families handle it with unilateral calls for everyone else to change ("If you would pay more attention to me, stop drinking, etc., we wouldn't be having this problem"), or with unilateral confessions of guilt and promises to change ("I know my temper is the problem; I'll try to control it better"). *Complementary* change offers better promise of success.

Other important ingredients in effective behavioral contracts include the following:

1. *A positive emotional environment during the negotiations.* The quality of the outcome depends heavily on the quality of the process. If the family members are speaking angrily or resentfully, then the agreement is unlikely to be implemented successfully: "All right. I'll start cleaning the house more often. You'll be able to eat off the floor by the time I get finished! You'll see!" It is better to wait until negative feelings have subsided and you have helped the partners see the benefits of collaboration. Behavioral contracts should be made with calm voices and positive feelings.

2. *Clear and specific behavior changes agreed to by all parties.* It is not enough for the husband to promise to be "more attentive" and the wife to be "more supportive of his work." They need to nail down the particular behaviors that make each other feel good.

3. *Good-faith commitment by all parties to carry through with the new behaviors.* Jacobson and Margolin (1979) and Stuart (1980) have discussed the value of "good-faith" contracts, where each party is unilaterally committed to following through, as opposed to "quid pro quo" contracts, where each party will change only if the other does. The good-faith approach builds positive feelings in problem solving: "I want to do something that will make you happier, and I will do it because I want to, not just because you will do something for me in return."

4. *Evaluation to see if the contract is working.* Family members should plan in advance to evaluate the success of their agreement at a later time. There does not have to be a "do or die" quality to the contract; the partners need to learn the importance of renegotiating agreements that are not working.

The following is a case illustration of behavioral contracting:

A young woman presented with an uncontrolled seizure disorder related to marital distress, which she said led her to not taking care of herself. Her biggest complaint about her husband was that he nagged her all the time about not taking care of herself (eating well, getting enough sleep) and made her feel stupid and incompetent. She was taking her Dilantin faithfully and demonstrated an adequate blood level of the medication. When the couple was seen together, the underlying interactional power struggle over her health became apparent. He was in the role of a stern parent in their relationship, and she was in the role of an admiring but uncooperative child. He felt frustrated and scared by her seizures and continually nagged her about taking better care of herself. She agreed with his criticisms but would get angry at him for putting her down. After they fought, she would apologize for acting irresponsibly, but nothing would change.

During the marital counseling session, the counselor pointed out some of these interaction patterns and empathized with the frustration that each partner felt. After these and other issues were explored, the counselor helped them negotiate a behavioral contract. The husband volunteered that one thing he could do would be to not nag her about her health; the wife agreed that she would remind him if she felt his comments sounded like nagging. By itself, this contract would have been insufficient and negative—an agreement to *stop* doing something. So the counselor asked the wife what kind of support she would like from her husband. She then asked him to listen to her more when she talked about her frustration at work. He promised to do this as long as he could stop her when she discussed the technical aspects of her job too much; she agreed to this, commenting that such technical talk was probably something she used to sound smarter than her husband. Thus, the final behavior contract called for diminishing a negative interaction pattern and enhancing a positive one. The wife could "own" her health behaviors but could still ask for support from her husband; he could support her without becoming a frustrated parent. Two follow-up sessions over the next 3 months revealed that the couple had followed through on their contract; the wife had experienced no further seizures, marital satisfaction had improved, and the husband was acknowledging that he was now more able to work on some of his own career decisions. Six months later this couple was continuing to do well.

In summary, helping families make behavioral contracts is a way to bring about collaborative arrangements for changing the daily context of family life. Success in carrying out the contract also gives the family members a sense of accomplishment and confidence in their ability to solve their problems.

ASSIGNING HOMEWORK

Since families spend at most 1 hour per week in family counseling, most of the important changes will have to occur at home. An effective way to extend the influence of the family counseling session throughout the week is to assign a task for the family to accomplish before the next session. The task should be designed to provide follow-through on some issue dealt with in the session. For example, spouses who have spent little time alone may be asked to go on a date during the next week. Or an uninvolved father might be assigned the task of supervising his son's homework every night. It is essential that the details of the task be worked out and agreed upon during the counseling session. The spouses assigned to go on the date should be asked to make specific plans during the counseling session; the father and son should decide what time homework will be done. Such clarity is particularly important early in the counseling relationship, when the family members may need a lot of structure from the counselor to change their ways of relating. Do not, however, assign tasks for behavior that the family has not managed to engage in during the counseling session. Spouses who have not communicated effectively about their household responsibilities with the counselor present should not be asked to continue their discussion at home. Save such issues for the next session. However, if they have made a breakthrough on this issue in counseling, then you might ask them to work out the details on their own and report back at the next session. Finally, the homework task should always be followed up on by the counselor. Failure to do the task suggests either that the family is resisting change or that the task was inappropriate or not agreed to by the family. In any case, the counselor should see failure to follow through on homework as an important issue for discussion with the family.

WHERE COUNSELING ENDS AND THERAPY BEGINS

All of the family counseling skills discussed in this chapter were developed by family therapists, who as a profession have pioneered the treatment of whole families. Family therapy involves everything that family counseling does—but more. Like family counseling, family therapy involves education, prevention, support, and challenge. But family therapy often proceeds to major restructuring of the family's interaction patterns. One important signal that primary care treatment should give way to therapy is a family's resistance to changing its interaction patterns. Some parents will have enough adaptability to follow their physician's educational approach in handling their child's temper tantrums. Such an educational approach is an appropriate way to begin treatment in either a primary care (family medicine) setting or in a secondary or tertiary (family therapy) setting. However, if the parents return the next week having sabotaged the plan for change and having fought extensively over other aspects of their relationship, then the helping process should probably be handed over to a therapist. The therapist may have to explore the ways in which the struggle over the child reflects, for instance, an entrenched power struggle in the marriage or deep-seated resentments about other issues. Therapy takes off, in other words, where education and support have reached a standstill.

There are many medical analogies to the distinction between counseling and therapy. Family physicians are trained to treat the relatively uncomplicated presentations of certain chronic diseases, such as diabetes. At some point when the basic treatment repertoire is not proving effective—when the disease process is resisting the first line of treatment—the family physician usually refers the patient to an internist. To refer all diabetics upon diagnosis would be as inappropriate as referring no diabetics no matter how the treatment is progressing. A similar situation holds for obstetrical treatment:

Most family physicians are trained to handle relatively uncomplicated pregnancies and deliveries personally, but to refer more complicated cases where further skills are required.

Family counseling in family medicine, then, is a vehicle for the primary care of families' biopsychosocial problems. Not all family-related problems require the specialized treatment of a family therapist, and family therapists—working at the secondary or tertiary level of health care—are not in the position to deliver widespread preventive care to families. The unfortunate limp in the analogy of family counseling to primary medical care is that family physicians are far better trained to treat uncomplicated disease than they are trained to treat uncomplicated family problems. To get the nation's family physicians to the point where they are delivering sound primary care of family-related problems would require a revolution in medical education. In the meantime, this book is aimed at those who have been working on their private revolutions in the primary care of families.

8 FAMILY COUNSELING AND STRESS-RELATED DISORDERS: TWO CASES

This chapter presents two case illustrations of family-oriented treatment of two stress-related disorders—headaches and lower back pain. The first case concerns a boy presenting with headaches that had no objective physical cause. The boy and his family were seen once for a family meeting by Doherty and Garold Moyer, MD, a third-year family practice resident and the family's primary physician. The case write-up begins with a grand-rounds presentation and a tape-recorded interview with the family during the grand rounds. This grand-rounds transcript gives the background of the problem. Next comes a reconstructed version of the one-session family counseling treatment and a final comment about the outcome of the treatment. Names and other identifying information have been changed.

The second case comes from Baird's practice. It concerns a middle-aged woman who presented with lower back pain. The case is written up in two-column format—the left column for description of the case and the right column for Baird's commentary. Unlike the first case of the boy with headaches, which was conducted as a primary care intervention, Baird's treatment shifted after the first few sessions into a family therapy mode. Specialized training in family therapy was required to carry out the treatment program that Baird used, whereas we believe the first case was of a type that can realistically be handled by family physicians who receive some basic training in family counseling. Thus the two case studies illustrate both the family-oriented treatment of stress-related disorders and the differences between primary care family counseling and specialized family therapy.

A BOY WITH HEADACHES

GRAND-ROUNDS PRESENTATION AND INTERVIEW WITH FAMILY

DOHERTY: This is a review and discussion of a headache problem of an eight-year-old boy and his family, the Lowes. We're going to have the presentation in three segments. First, we'll talk about the medical background that led to the point at which Dr. Moyer asked me to come and meet with him and the family. And then the Lowes and I and Dr. Moyer will form a circle and recreate a little bit of our interview and hear what they experienced in dealing with the problem. And then we'll thank them, and they'll be on their way, and we'll have some discussion.

MOYER: I'll briefly go over what has happened over the last couple of years with Ron and his family. I wrote a letter to the pediatric clinic here in October, so I'm just going to basically go over that letter, because it explains everything I have done. I said Ronald Lowe is an eight-year-old White male who was first seen in the Family Practice Clinic at Children's Hospital on January 4, 1979, with a complaint of frontal headaches. His mother said that at that time the child had had intermittent frontal headaches which showed no pattern and seemed to be related to nasal congestion; however, this was not definite. The patient was started on dimetapp elixir and aspirin for headaches. The child continued to have difficulty and in follow-up examinations was noted to have hypertropic mucuosa. He was referred to Dr. McFarland in Towncrest. He, indeed, did have hypertrophy of the right upper and middle turbinates and drainage. He was treated with erythromycin and Dimetapp. Two weeks later he showed total opacification of his maxillary sinuses bilaterally and underwent sinus irrigation. Ron was not seen again by Dr. McFarland until July 1980. He did not have a history of frontal headaches. Sinus X-rays at that time were within normal limits; he was felt to have headaches probably of tension origin, rather than sinus headaches. It is worthy to note that he was seen in our clinic during the interval there, and no problem was mentioned in the chart.

I first saw Ron October 1, 1980, when his mother said that he had had chronic frontal headaches for most of the summer and that he had had some difficulty in 1979. Ron described the headaches as feeling as if there was a rock behind his forehead. There were times during the days when it was worse and times when it was better. He said that he had the headaches when he woke up in the morning and when he went to bed at night. His mother stated that he seemed to complain about it more some days than others, but he had been able to maintain normal activity and only missed one day of school for the entire fall. He had been eating well and sleeping well at night, and his mother was unable to delineate any problems at home. In the summer Ron had had an eye examination and a trial of glasses for about two weeks, and these did not relieve his headaches. Because of the history of the physical examination, which I felt was completely normal for his age, I decided to do some laboratory work, which also came back normal. Because of this persistent problem I also had a CT scan, which was normal. Again, unable to give an answer for the headaches, we referred him to the pediatric clinic where he was evaluated and felt to have possible vascular headaches, and we attempted to reassure Mrs. Lowe that his headaches needed to be watched but there wasn't anything acutely wrong at this point that needed to be treated. At that point, there came the idea: Are these headaches psychogenic or is there something we're overlooking? This is where I decided to have Dr. Doherty come in and talk with the family.

DOHERTY: There aren't a lot of rooms to meet with families in this building, so we met right about here. I'd like to introduce the Lowes to you all, starting with Sarah and her father Bill and her mother Diane, and this is Ron. By the way, I'd like to thank them now, and I'll thank them before they leave for coming out. Mrs. Lowe had to get off work today and do some arranging to come in. I appreciate it. (to Ron) He said a lot of big words in describing what you had, didn't he?

RON: I don't know what they meant.

DOHERTY: Neither did most of them. (general laughter) I'd like to find out what it has been like to be a family with a boy with headaches. I'll be asking you what that has been like for you. I wonder if you could start, Mrs. Lowe, when you first began to get concerned.

MRS. LOWE: Well, it would probably be like in the middle of the summer. He kept complaining of the headaches. We wondered what was wrong. We figured there had to be some reason for them. Everybody we talked with said that he doesn't seem to be the type to get upset about things. So, we got the idea that something was wrong. When you keep going from one place to the next—"No, that's not it; no, that's not it"—it gets a little discouraging.

DOHERTY: Where did you start?

MRS. LOWE: In the summer, we started again with Dr. McFarland because I thought maybe it was his sinuses again. He said no, and then he went to the optometrist thinking maybe he needed glasses since John and I both wear glasses. He said no. So, we came here and started because we didn't know where to go after those couple of things were suggested.

DOHERTY: Were you getting frustrated during that time too?

MR. LOWE: Well, what bothered me the most was that when he got a headache, aspirin didn't seem to help him. Once he got to sleep it was fine, but there were times when the headache bothered him so much that he didn't want to eat, and times when he'd lay in bed that trying to get to sleep would bother him. When the aspirin doesn't help—that's when it really bothers you. Nothing seems to help, your common remedies such as aspirin and sleep, and that's when it bothers you. You keep on taking tests and they come up blank, so that's when it affects you. You start doing a lot of thinking and worrying.

DOHERTY: What kinds of things did you start to worry about?

MR. LOWE: Well, you think about things when they talk about the brain scan—tumors and on that order, something serious, since they didn't find anything from the eye test and the test prior to that.

DOHERTY: Did you two spend some time talking about all this?

MRS. LOWE: Yes.

MR. LOWE: What to do next?

DOHERTY: (to Ron) Did you know your folks were worried about you? (Ron shakes his head "no.") They did a good job of just taking care of you and doing their worrying on their own. What were you thinking about? You never used to get headaches? (Ron shakes his head "no.") So this was something pretty new for you. Did you think about what they might be— what they might be from? (Ron shakes his head "no.") Sarah, did you know your brother was having headaches?

SARAH: Yes.

DOHERTY: How did you know that?

SARAH: He'd tell me.

DOHERTY: You believed him when he told you?

SARAH: Yes.

DOHERTY: Would he tell you while he was having them? What would he say?

SARAH: I don't know.

DOHERTY: Would he say "My head's killing me"? You don't remember how he said it? (to parents) So, you went through the process of running down different explanations. Different doctors.

MR. LOWE: More or less what we were told. We went where we were told. When they said sinuses, we went to Dr. McFarland. We just kept going back and forth. Like the eye test.

DOHERTY: Now, Ron was scheduled to be seen by a psychiatrist once. Was he evaluated? Or did they decide not to do that?

MRS. LOWE: We went over to the university, we thought, for a neurology and psychology workup, only we didn't get that.

DOHERTY: So, you were expecting a psychological/psychiatric workup, and didn't get that.

MR. LOWE: Right.

DOHERTY: How did you feel about not getting that?

MRS. LOWE: Very upset.

DOHERTY: Why did they tell you that they were not going to do a psychiatric workup?

MRS. LOWE: That morning I went over and was in pediatrics, and as I was sitting there all these people were being sent off to all different parts and this place and that place. I thought, "Well, this is the place where we come and we get sent off to from here." And then we got put back in a little room and sat there for four-and-a-half hours and there's a doctor in and back out and I'm thinking all this time, I'm thinking, "He's going to have to send him now for what we came here for." And then he said, "You can go home and I will call you if they think he should be seen in neurology." Well, that's what we were here for, why were we going home without that? And after quite a few phone conversations we found out that basically they don't see you in neurology without being seen in pediatrics first. Because headaches are too common of a thing to just have everybody with headaches go to neurology. That's basically what I was told.

DOHERTY: Did they tell you why no psychiatric evaluation?

MRS. LOWE: No.

DOHERTY: So that must have been one of the most frustrating times. (*to Ron*) Do you remember that day, sitting over there? What did you do all that time?

RON: I just sat there while one of the doctors talked to my mom.

DOHERTY: Did you have a headache that day? A big one?

MR. LOWE: What number?

RON: One hundred.

DOHERTY: Ten is tough—but you had a big one. So, you went home that afternoon and told your husband about it?

MRS. LOWE: Right. Well, they wanted to send us back to the ophthalmology clinic. And I said that he had had a complete eye exam. And they said, "He probably didn't have this or that done," and I said, "I'm not going through it again if it's been done." Because of the cost, for one thing, and because I wasn't going to sit for another four hours over there in the clinic. I got hold of our optometrist and he wrote a letter stating everything that was done, and what they wanted done had been done. So, I canceled that appointment.

DOHERTY: So you were taking more things into your own hands at this point. You were not just going to follow along.

MRS. LOWE: I wasn't going to go through the same tests that I had gone through. Because they, as far as I could see, did the exact same thing over there that Dr. Moyer did here for the exam. And it's no fun sitting in an office with a kid for four hours waiting. So I just decided I was not going to go through a lot of repeats.

DOHERTY: Did you have to miss a lot of work for these appointments?

MRS. LOWE: No, because I just work part-time evenings and weekends.

DOHERTY: (*to Mr. Lowe*) So, you were getting these reports of frustrating times?

MR. LOWE: I called to talk to my wife that afternoon and it's something you just hear about once in a while, but once it happens to you, you realize it, and it's a different report you get and every now and then people running around and the waiting time and stuff like that.

DOHERTY: Do you remember what your reactions were when Dr. Moyer suggested that you sit down with a counselor and talk?

MRS. LOWE: I think it was "Anything."

DOHERTY: Even that, right?

MRS. LOWE: Right. I wasn't upset about the idea of it. We were just looking for answers. Just if someone can give us an answer.

DOHERTY: Okay, let's talk about our session for a bit. And then let some others ask some questions.

RECONSTRUCTED SEGMENTS OF THE FAMILY COUNSELING INTERVIEW

DOHERTY: What time of day seems to be the worst for your son's headaches?

MRS. LOWE: Bedtime is the worst. A lot of times he's fine after supper watching television, and then around bedtime he starts to complain about this pain in his head.

DOHERTY: Who's in charge of putting the kids to bed in your family?

MR. LOWE: I usually put them to bed.

DOHERTY: Tell me what happens at bedtime when your son has a headache.

MR. LOWE: Well, I didn't know what to do for him. That was the hardest part. He'd be complaining about this pain in his head, and I would take him some aspirins and I would talk to him and I would hope this would help, but it never seemed to. I just couldn't do anything for him. I used to ask him whether anything was bothering him, whether he was worried about something, tense about something. He never said there was anything wrong.

MRS. LOWE: We both talked to him about whether there was anything bothering him.

DOHERTY: How was Ron doing at school during this time?

MRS. LOWE: He was doing fine. His grades didn't suffer—he was second in his class. We thought he was doing fine, but he got headaches in school too.

DOHERTY: I would like to talk to your son for a while about all of this. Ron, what's your favorite part of school?

RON: Recess.

DOHERTY: What do you like most at recess?

RON: Oh, playing football, soccer, or any game that we play—that's my favorite.

DOHERTY: Are you any good at it?

RON: Yeah.

DOHERTY: How do you and your sister here get along?

RON: Rotten.

DOHERTY: Yeah, what does she do that gives you a headache?

RON: She knocks over my toys.

DOHERTY: Oh, really? (*to Sarah*) You don't really do that, do you?

SARAH: Sometimes.

RON: She does it all the time.

DOHERTY: Ron, I'd like to play a little game with you. I'd like you to give a number on how much the headache hurts. Zero would be that you don't feel anything at all, and ten would be just the worst humongous headache that you think you have ever had. Five would be right in the middle. You understand that?

RON: Yeah.

DOHERTY: Now, when your sister knocks your Legos over, what kind of headache do you get then?

RON: A twelve.

DOHERTY: A twelve—that bad? (*general laughter*) Does your mother ever give you a headache?

RON: Yeah.

DOHERTY: What does she do to give you a headache?

RON: She won't let me go and visit her when she's working at the store.

DOHERTY: So you like to go see her when she's working but she sometimes won't let you do that. Who's watching you at the time when she's at work?

RON: My daddy.

DOHERTY: So he tells you that you can't go visit her.

RON: That's right, because Mom says she's too busy sometimes. Sometimes we can go but sometimes she says she's too busy and we can't go.

DOHERTY: What number headache do you get when your mother won't let you go?

RON: Oh, about a seven.

DOHERTY: It's not as bad as when your sister knocks your Legos over?—Still not a nice one.

RON: Right.

DOHERTY: What does your father do that gives you a headache?

RON: When he puts me to bed when I really want to stay up and watch television.

DOHERTY: He makes you go to bed anyway, huh?

RON: Yeah.

DOHERTY: What number headache do you get when your father makes you go to bed?

RON: Oh, about a six.

DOHERTY: Not quite as bad as when your mother won't let you go to the store and visit her, and not nearly as bad as when your sister knocks your Legos over.

RON: That's right.

DOHERTY: You're coming up as the best guy in the family there, Dad.

MR. LOWE: Yeah, looks that way, doesn't it?

DOHERTY: Ron, do you ever get headaches at school?

RON: Yeah. Sometimes I get really bad ones in the afternoon.

DOHERTY: What time in the afternoon?

RON: Sometimes right after recess.

MRS. LOWE: That doctor thought maybe the exercises started up the headaches.

DOHERTY: Ron, what was the worst headache you ever had in school?

RON: A couple of weeks ago right after recess.

DOHERTY: What were you doing at recess?

RON: I was playing football with my team.

DOHERTY: How did you do in that game?

RON: Terrible. I fumbled in the end zone twice and the other team recovered it and went for a touchdown and won the game.

DOHERTY: That's terrible. I bet that gave you a real high-number headache.

RON: Yeah, that was a ten.

DOHERTY: Have you gotten other headaches when you haven't done real well at your games at recess?

RON: Yeah, sometimes I get headaches then.

DOHERTY: Do you have a headache now?

RON: Yeah.

DOHERTY: What number?

RON: Three.

DOHERTY: So just a little one right now. Are you just a little nervous being here?

RON: Yeah, but it's not so bad.

DOHERTY: (to parents) What are you thinking about what you've been hearing here?

MRS. LOWE: Well, it's real clear—when Ron gets upset with one of us or when he's at school he gives himself a headache.

MR. LOWE: Yeah, I've never seen it so plainly before.

DOHERTY: We all learn to handle angry feelings and frustrating feelings in different ways, and for Ron, instead of talking about them he's learned to give himself headaches. [Doherty asks to meet with the parents alone; after the children leave the room, the conversation continues.] You have enjoyable children.

MRS. LOWE: Thanks. I think they're pretty good kids. I think that's amazing to hear him talk about his headaches and what causes them.

MR. LOWE: And the things that he talked about at home that gave him headaches really made sense. He hates to go to bed.

MRS. LOWE: And he really doesn't talk about his feelings much. He hardly ever gets angry. What can we do to help him with this?

DOHERTY: A good start has been made by making everyone aware that Ron gives himself headaches when he gets upset. This is a good start. This is a problem that is not as serious as a brain tumor, and it is something that you can work with. He's a good kid. He's pretty well adjusted at home and at school and he's got friends. He's second in his class. He gets along with both of you. You're both involved with him. This has been going on for a number of months, but it's not like it's been going on for years. He's had pain and you've undergone some emotional stress about his health, but you seem to have held on to your sense of humor and your perspective. I have a few suggestions about what you can do.

The first thing is to downplay the importance of headaches when you're talking with Ron. If he says he has a headache, express sympathy and give him aspirin or do whatever you would normally, but try to treat the headaches matter-of-factly. What you can do—as I did a few minutes ago—is to ask him what sort of headache it is on a scale of 1 to 10. This is the way of giving you and him an idea of how badly it hurts; it can also help you play a little bit with the headaches. If you noticed, there's kind of a playful quality in the conversation I was having with Ron about his headaches. I take his pain seriously, but we can also be a little light-hearted about it—that light-hearted quality comes from having some perspective on it. So that when Ron tells you that he has a headache, you can ask him to put a number on it, you can ask him who gave it to him, or what gave it to him. He can give it a number and if he can say, "My sister gave me the headache"—then Ron can learn to talk about his headaches with you, and you can help to express the kinds of feelings of frustration and anger that give rise to his headaches. You might be able to help him prevent getting headaches by talking about those feelings.

The other thing is that he should not get out of any responsibilities, he should not get any extra desserts, he should not be able to stay up late at night—in other words, no extra rewards for having headaches. But now that you know that his headaches are coming from the way he deals with his feelings of anger and frustration and probably not some serious physical illness, I think it would be a good idea to let *him* bring up the topic of headaches and for you not to ask him if he has a headache. When you are concerned that your son may have something seriously wrong with him, then you naturally want to find out if he's having headaches at suppertime, or bedtime, or after school, and so it makes sense that you've asked him from time to time about his headaches. But now it would be a good idea for you to low-key it. In other words, if he doesn't bring up that he has headaches, then you don't ask him if he has a headache. The biggest danger with something like this is that Ron uses it as a way to control the family. You could end up falling all over yourselves asking him how he is doing, and he could end up using this as a way to gain some privileges and to gain leverage over the rest of the family. I think you've done a good job of keeping this from happening so far. I want to urge you to continue treating him like a normal eight-year-old boy, and so my suggestions are, first, that you not bring up the subject of headaches, not ask him whether he has a headache, let him bring it up. Second, when he tells you he has a headache, make a little game out of it by asking him to give it a number. This way you can also monitor his progress. If after his sister knocks over his Legos he says today he has a number seven headache, and three days ago he said it gave him a number nine, you can point out how much better he is doing. Third, you can ask him who or what is giving him the headache and encourage him to talk about his feelings. Then, in situations where you see him frustrated or angry, you can try to get him to talk about these things.

FINAL COMMENTS

The family left the session on a very optimistic and upbeat note. Since the Christmas holidays were coming up, no subsequent appointment was scheduled at that time. They were asked to phone the office after the first of January to report on Ron's progress. At that point a decision would be made about scheduling a follow-up session. The mother did phone approximately 3 weeks after this initial session, reporting that Ron's headaches had subsided substantially, that they were using the techniques suggested in the session, and that progress was impressive. The follow-up two months after the initial session indicated that Ron was rarely having headaches and that according to his parents he was talking about what was bothering him. The parents felt that the problem with the headaches had been resolved by the time of the grand-rounds presentation.

A WOMAN WITH LOWER BACK PAIN

Description	Comments by Baird
3/28/79—Mrs. A presented to the office with a complaint of back pain, "especially since exercising at the YMCA," and gas and a bloated feeling in her abdomen. The nurse's history revealed that she took an occasional Maalox as needed for heartburn, and Dalmane occasionally at bedtime for sleeping. As I greeted Mrs. A on her initial office visit, she seemed noticeably upset and appeared to be	The patient's demeanor in response to initial questions led me to pursue a rather thorough family and stress history early in this interview. She responded rather openly and seemed to be visibly relieved as she was allowed to reveal more and more stress that related to close relationships. My overall impression was that of a "super mom" who pleased everyone else at her own expense and was eager to have

in some discomfort with back pain. She repeated the history given to the nurse and described back pain that seemed to be rather constant, located in her lower sacral area and without radiation of the pain. She denied any history of previous back injuries or chronic low back pain. In her opinion, the pain had gotten worse over the past several months. This was her first office visit for this problem, although she had had previous office visits for urinary tract infections, minor respiratory problems, and complaints of stomach discomforts. Further review of systems revealed that she had been hospitalized only for childbirth and considered herself in good health except for being overweight. She had recently begun YMCA activities in order to lose weight. A brief family history revealed that her five children were apparently in good health. Two older sons and one older daughter were away from home, but none of them were married. A sixteen-year-old daughter and eight-year-old son were still at home. Mrs. A stated that her husband worked very long hours as a sales and service representative of a farming equipment firm.

Mrs. A stated that she really felt quite blue at this time. She was frustrated about being overweight and seemed to have very few friends outside her immediate family. She expressed frustration over lack of support and lack of meaningful contact time with her husband, a problem that seemed to have gotten worse over the past several years. She stated that she had a hard time making friends even in her new YMCA activities. She and her husband had never established a circle of friends within their rural community, and both of their families were some distance from them. She had never worked outside the home, but had recently become interested in some type of paid employment, partially to occupy her idle time. She denied any actual hobbies outside her exercise classes and denied having any close friend or family member with whom she could talk meaningfully. When asked about her family of origin, she described a history of abuse by her parents. She stated that her husband grew up in a family where abuse was also present. Her husband's father was an alcoholic, as was her own father. She volunteered that it was very difficult for both her and her husband to face conflicts; in fact,

her husband be the "villain." Her nonspecific symptoms were helpful in that they, also, suggested that I should review family and emotional stresses. At the end of the physical examination, I offered her the option of further objective evaluation through X-rays or laboratory testing, therefore shifting a part of the responsibility for her care plan to the patient. Without hesitation, she opted for pursuing her family stresses rather than going through an exhaustive laboratory evaluation. The door was left open for further testing; however, the decision relieved me of the entire responsibility for perhaps missing a serious organic lesion. The entire interview lasted for approximately twenty-five minutes.

All of the above history flowed rather easily and almost spontaneously in the initial interview. The patient definitely seemed relieved that I was probing in these rather personal areas of her life and stated that no one else had ever talked to her about these issues.

they avoided discussing any issue that created conflict.

Physical examination revealed that the pateint was, indeed, overweight. Her weight was one hundred ninety-five pounds; her height was five feet one inch. Blood pressure, pulse, and temperature were all normal. Except for obesity, her physical exam was unremarkable. There was mild tenderness in the low back. Neurological examination was normal, including deep tendon reflexes and sensation in the legs. Straight-leg raising test was mildly positive at eighty degrees.

After completing the physical exam, I asked the patient what she felt was the most significant contributing factor to her back pain. She quickly answered that her pain became much worse whenever she was angry with her husband. She felt that she would rather pursue conversations with her husband than proceed with X-ray or further laboratory evaluation. Therefore, a treatment plan was established in which she would continue with her exercising; specific back exercises were added to her daily exercise program. She was asked to return with her husband for conjoint marital therapy, perhaps to be followed by family therapy. She was quite pleased with this treatment plan and seemed noticeably more comfortable upon leaving the office. No medications were offered.

This question was open enough to allow any answer—picking up something, sleeping on a soft mattress, or going through emotional stresses.

4/5/79—Mr. and Mrs. A arrived for a conjoint interview. Mr. A was tense. He stated that he was here at the request of his wife "to help her." They were seated apart. Mrs. A was talking eagerly; Mr. A was quite reserved. Both families of origin were reviewed. Mr. A was the oldest of four children. He remembered a great deal of conflict within his family and still retreated from any area of open conflict in his own married family. His father had died as a result of alcohol-related problems. He rarely saw other members of his family, partially due to their distance from him and partially due to his own preference. Mrs. A again reviewed her family of origin. She briefly described mistreatment by her parents. She was the fourth of five children. In reviewing their own marriage of twenty-seven years, they described a major event in their lives approximately nine years ago when they declared

This initial interview revealed that neither marital partner had had satisfactory models for parenting or spouse roles. Their previous economic difficulties seemed to propel Mr. A into continual overinvestment in his work role and underinvestment in his family. His coming to the office seemed to be his way of complying with his wife's request in order to avoid further conflict. I learned very little about their children during this interview, but I felt that I had gained their trust.

bankruptcy and Mr. A changed his occupation. Since that time, he has been in constant fear of a second financial collapse, inspite of continued notable success in his occupation as a sales and service representative of a farming equipment firm. He described a lack of energy for family and home activities, due to his constant drive for continued economic security. His occupation demanded calling upon farmers six days a week. He had had very few vacations over the past nine years. When they did go they were usually company-related retreats designed to stimulate him to further heights of salesmanship. Each of those trips had resulted in continued frustration on the part of Mrs. A. Mr. A's primary support outside the family was a group of friends with whom he had breakfast each day in a small town near their home. They had no social friends mutually and could describe no common interest outside work and family business. Mrs. A described her life style now as understimulating, uninteresting, and lonely. She projected a great deal of anger toward her husband. Mr. A quietly accepted her criticism. During that initial joint interview, I seemed to gain their trust and respect but offered no short-term solution. I outlined the areas of major conflict that I had observed; these seemed to center around their continual avoidance of conflict, which prevented meaningful resolution of their problems. I asked that they continue to share their feelings as they had done today in the office, and said that I would see them again as soon as possible.

4/20/79—Mr. and Mrs. A again arrived in a somewhat angry state. They sat apart and continued to express frustrations about past events. In reviewing the impact of their style of communication, both realized that they seldom expressed their true feelings and had frequently misunderstood each other. Each of them would walk away in silence during past conflicts or would carry grudges for several days, frequently having misinterpreted the other's intention. When allowed to express their feelings more openly during this session, they appeared visibly relieved and did move physically closer toward the end of the interview. They agreed to return for continued work at more honest communications and more direct resolution of conflict. In the meantime, it had become apparent that Mrs. A's back pain had completely resolved.

5/10/79—Mr. and Mrs. A arrived and immediately became angry with each other over multiple frustrations. Now they felt free to discuss their lack of sexual intimacy, which had been a problem for many years. Mr. A described his physical exhaustion and lack of interest in physical closeness. Mrs. A expressed extreme frustration. Neither had openly discussed this topic at home nor with me, but now felt free to do so. After they vented their feelings I described a plan of gradually increasing sexual contact and intimacy, such as sensate focus therapy. They planned to return in one week.

5/18/79—The plan to carry through with sensate focus therapy had been stalled just as they had begun to practice this technique. They had had an upsetting event relating to their oldest son, who apparently had been in trouble many times over the past ten years while drinking. Both spouses described their opposing philosophies for controlling his behavior. Mr. A had decided years ago not to be involved in his son's life and had never confronted him about his irresponsible behavior. Mrs. A had talked to her son many times; she had often threatened him with withdrawing her level of support, but continued to offer him food, shelter, money, and rescues from various troubles. After a rather angry discussion, they agreed that they would try to protect themselves from his further manipulations and assaults upon the family's economic status and would try to work as a team in that regard. They were also confronted with the fact that this event had interrupted their work as a couple on becoming more intimate sexually.

8/12/79—Mrs. A presented for a medical visit alone. At this time she was complaining of dizziness and tingling in her fingers. She had gained approximately nine pounds since her initial visit and was feeling quite distraught. The description of her symptoms with tingling in the hands and fingers, respiratory anxiety and distress, and light-headedness—all associated with family stress—suggested a diag-

It was predictable that Mr. and Mrs. A would not be able to carry through with even the early stages of sexual intimacy training. They had not been emotionally or sexually close for many years, and I expected resistance. At this time I also became aware of my error in not initially including the entire family. At this point I offered family therapy, but did not want to neglect the spouse dyad just as they were approaching intimacy.

nosis of hyperventilation. Her physical examination was normal except for her obesity. I reviewed the history of her son's apparent chemical abuse and/or dependency. She then revealed that her second son had problems that had never been discussed at home or with me. He was now separated from his wife of two years. They had one child. He was using Mrs. A's home as a point of rendezvous with various female companions. I suggested that we continue to discuss that in conjoint therapy. She agreed to return with her husband. She understood that her new symptoms were apparently related to continued stress.

9/14/79—Mr. and Mrs. A again returned for conjoint therapy. We reviewed their oldest son's problems. Apparently the two older sons were using the family home as a staging area on Friday nights for weekend forays into a nearby city. They would return Sunday evening inebriated and without food or money, would receive both from the parents, and then would return to their nearby apartments. Mrs. A was nearing despair. Mr. A was reluctant to confront his sons about their behavior. But as the interview continued, it became more and more difficult for him to avoid the conflict, and Mrs. A became more effective in expressing her feelings. They finally agreed to a family interview with all of their children in order to assess the nature of their problems fully.

10/15/79—The entire A family was present. Terry, aged twenty-six, and Steven, aged twenty-four, were sitting together, noticeably separated from the remainder of the family. Lynn, aged twenty-three, sat between her mother and father. Lisa, aged sixteen, sat between the father and the two oldest boys. Michael, aged eight, sat next to his mother. The interview began with open-ended questions, such as "What is it like to be living in your family at this time?" The discussion quickly focused on the chaos that was caused late at night by Terry's arriving home while inebriated and awakening the entire family. This had been going on for many months, especially on weekends, but had not been openly discussed by the family. Terry initially denied that this was a problem, but then recog-

I did not wish to label or try to assess the oldest son's diagnosis or nature of problems without him being present. Therefore, during the interview I focused primarily on this couple's ability to face each other with conflict in order to proceed toward a resolution. One step toward resolution at this time was to agree to more complete family participation in therapy. It should be noted that Mrs. A's back pain had never returned, but that she was getting more upset as the nature of their conflicts became more openly expressed. Mr. A was now more fully involved in his family's conflicts, but the couple was still avoiding many of their own interpersonal conflicts and now was focused on the children. I was aware of this but felt a priority in dealing with what may have been a serious chemical dependency in their oldest son.

It appeared that there were relatively no rules of appropriate conduct established within this family. Mr. and Mrs. A had never been able to establish norms of behavior or to communicate their expectations to their children. My plan at this time was to strengthen the marital dyad but not to ignore what now appeared to be a significant chemical dependency problem for Terry. Formal chemical dependency treatment was offered to Terry as an alternative if his problems continued.

nized that his behavior was upsetting other
people in the family. Mr. and Mrs. A took
charge and stated that this was no longer
acceptable and that he would not be allowed
to return home unless he behaved responsibly.
Other areas of manipulation and financial distress caused by Terry's drinking were discussed
to reinforce the nature of the problem.

Steven remained quiet during the interview. When confronted by his mother and
father about his bringing female companions
home when he was not divorced, he shrugged
his shoulders. The older daughter, Lynn, intermittently defended her older brothers and
seemed somewhat resentful of the entire interview. She felt that she did not belong in the
office for this type of interview and stated that
she would continue to try to help Terry and
Steven by loaning money or her car or whatever they needed, whatever they asked for.
The younger daughter, Lisa, also felt that her
older brothers were unfairly maligned. The
only time she had become upset by either of
their behavior was when Terry literally broke
down the front door at 2 A.M. when he did not
have the key. She felt that this was a reason
for others to become upset; less serious occur-
rences were tolerable to her. The youngest
son, Michael became noticeably upset whenever Mrs. A became angry or tearful.

Near the end of the interview I asked if
there were well-understood rules of behavior
within this family. Mr. A stated that yes, there
were; and after our meeting he would continue
to have family meetings in order to emphasize
clearly what those rules really were. He did   In fact, there were no rules at all!
not feel comfortable in delineating basic family
rules now, but agreed to have them agreed
upon and discussed by our next meeting.

11/9/79—Mr. and Mrs. A and the three
younger children returned. The work that they
had done at home was apparent. Mr. and
Mrs. A were more comfortable. They said
they seem to be taking charge of their family
now and had established reasonable norms of
behavior which have now been communicated
to all children. The oldest two, Terry and
Steven, had decided that they could not comply and were no longer visiting the family.
This seemed most difficult to accept for Lynn,
who felt that the parental expectations were
too severe. Lisa denied that there were any

problems in the first place; however, Mr. and Mrs. A continued to stand together on this issue and appeared more confident in their parental role.

12/10/79—Mr. and Mrs. A returned for conjoint therapy without their children. Previous conflicts were discussed and progress was reviewed. Mrs. A now seemed to have an upset stomach when she felt upset about her older sons; however, it did not deter her from enforcing her newly established family rules with her husband. Both partners were more able to express disagreement openly. They also stated that they had become more comfortable with sexual intimacy, although we had not discussed that explicitly during the past several interviews. They had had relatively little contact with their sons, Steven and Terry, since our last session. I recommended a return with Steven and Terry explicitly to discuss their differences and to resolve their conflict more openly.

12/17/79—Mr. and Mrs. A and Steven and Terry returned. Mr. A expressed his feelings and expectations very openly. He outlined what all agreed were reasonable expectations for behavior. Mrs. A essentially agreed with her husband. She expressed herself openly and, this time, did so without shedding tears or being distraught. Steven discussed his life style more openly. He expressed some regrets about his past relationships. He did not plan to change his life style, but agreed not to upset his family by bringing guests home unannounced and uninvited. Terry seemed rather subdued. He discussed his life style in detail. He felt that he could be in control of his drinking and declined formal chemical dependency treatment. He agreed not to abuse his family privileges by returning late at night or otherwise disturbing the family. This was the first time these four had talked in many years. They now agreed that they understood one another's positions although they did not agree about one another's life style or expectations.

1/28/80—Mrs. A was seen in the office for evaluation of a painful mass in the right side of her neck. Laboratory data were normal. The physical exam revealed mild lymphadeni-

Mr. A had now taken charge of some of his family responsibilities. He and Mrs. A were aligned as a team and seemed to be more confident in their family tasks. I felt that it was still unlikely that Terry would avoid further problems with his drinking behavior, but at least the confrontation had begun and he understood his parents' expectations. Steven was free to continue with his own life style as long as he did not force his parents to participate in it. He was still welcomed home when he respected their wishes to be notified ahead of time and when he did not try to cohabitate with a new friend when he returned home.

tis. She was started on antibiotics and reassured. I briefly reviewed her family situation. She felt that she would like to return with her husband for further therapy with just the two of them.

3/17/80—Mr. and Mrs. A returned. They stated that for several months they had been doing quite well, having comfortable conversations and becoming more intimate. Now they felt worse again; Mrs. A was especially angry. As the conversation continued it became apparent that Mrs. A was blaming her husband for her own unhappiness. He was feeling pressure in being responsible for her and had avoided her contact for many years by remaining for long hours at work. Now that this probably central issue was opened, Mrs. A realized that she had been dependent upon her husband and not self-reliant. He realized more clearly that he had avoided family responsibilities by becoming overly involved in work. I requested that they continue this discussion at home and return in two months.

Now that parenting issues had been openly discussed and were progressing toward some type of resolution, the spouse issues were surfacing more clearly. I had tried to explore these issues several months earlier, but I had been unsuccessful. It seemed that now that they were more confident parents, they had greater willingness and ability to discuss more personal spouse issues. Mrs. A was finally able to become more responsible for her own well-being. Mr. A could now be more honest about his work role and his absence from his family. He seemed especially relieved after this session.

7/10/80—Mr. and Mrs. A returned for conjoint therapy. Mrs. A had lost thirty-two pounds with her exercise program combined with a dietary group. She presented herself in a proud and assertive manner and expressed increasing sexual frustration, which had resurfaced as a theme. Mr. A seemed unsettled and defensive. He felt "pushed" into sexual activity for which he had no interest or energy. After an open expression of their conflicted feelings, they agreed that we would once again resume a sensate focus plan, which would decrease sexual demands, especially for Mr. A.

More and more intimate spouse topics were surfacing. They seemed more appropriate to this couple now that they continued to be more comfortable with their parenting roles. In the background was the relative lack of conflict with their older children, who had much less contact with their parents now but whose behavior remained unchanged otherwise.

9/29/80—Conjoint therapy. Mrs. A had now lost a total of thirty-five pounds. Both partners appeared more self-confident. They were expressing some warmth for each other and were seated together for the entire interview. Mrs. A had accepted a more self-reliant role within her family. Mr. A seemed to have more energy for his family activities, partially because Mrs. A was now accompanying him for most days of the week on his rounds throughout the farming area that he served. This allowed him to resume family activities at approximately 6 P.M. rather than 8 P.M., which previously was the end of his work day. Weekends were more enjoyable because he was only working half a day instead of a full day on Saturday, again because of her helping him with his work-related tasks. They were able to enjoy more sexual intimacy and to feel confident of their success as a marital couple and parental team. No new issues were discussed. This was more of a reinforcing visit.

10/13/80—Mrs. A presented again with right-sided neck pain. She was referred for consultation at a large medical institution. At the time of presentation for the physical complaint, she expressed confidence in her continued ability to function at home in a satisfactory manner. Further details of family issues were not discussed. It was a rather quick office visit. (The consultant agreed that her neck problem was benign and required no treatment.)

11/24/80—Mr. and Mrs. A returned with their youngest children, Michael, aged eight, and Lisa, aged sixteen. Conflicts between both children were discussed. There were multiple areas of rivalry and what appeared to be unfairness from Lisa's perspective. All four members participated in the discussion. Lisa also expressed concern about peer pressure for alcohol use. She was supported by her parents and felt relieved to be able to discuss this with them. Both parents and children agreed that they could return on an as-needed basis, and all expressed confidence in their continued survival as a family.

This was a generally pleasant visit, which included all those living under one roof at this time. Lisa seemed reassured that she could discuss troublesome topics with her parents. She was especially pleased that her father participated in the discussion and that her mother did not become upset. None of them were troubled at this time by either Steven or Terry, although all assumed that their life styles had been unchanged by their family confrontations.

1/20/81—Conjoint therapy. This was Mr. A's busiest season; Mrs. A was no longer accompanying him on his work. They both felt that they had relapsed into some of their previous noncommunicative pattern. I confronted both of them quite forcefully about my inability to change any of their behavior; I could only challenge them. I emphasized that they were now responsible for their continued growth as a couple. If they had conflicts, they needed to resolve them together without my presence and encouragement. I offered them my continued support, but only if they continued working on their issues at home as ground work for our office visits.

It had become apparent that the couple would delay effective communication until they came to my office. Therefore, I felt compelled to confront them about this in order to motivate continued growth. Many of their conflicts had been at least partially resolved. They were now faced with their own marital conflicts, which required their continued open communication and honesty. The initial symptoms of back pain had long since resolved. Underlying issues of behavior problems in their children had changed in a manner that was satisfactory to them for the time being. The remaining conflict was their own intimacy and willingness to face their interpersonal conflicts. This issue would surface whenever they approached resolution of the other, slightly more distant problems. We had become quite good friends by the time; they seemed to accept my challenge as one of support rather than rejection.

2/9/81—Mrs. A returned for evaluation of a viral respiratory infection. After reassurance about that problem, I briefly reviewed her family situation. At this point, they were in the final stages of arranging their first family vacation in nine years. They planned to take two weeks' travel and get away from their current environment. They were beginning to establish some social friends, although this was still difficult for them. Mr. A had arranged for weekend coverage of his business, especially during the busy time of the year. Mrs. A had continued to maintain her weight loss and often accompanied her husband in his work. Their sexual relationship was now satisfactory most of the time, and they had occasional late-night discussions about events and life problems. She no longer had back pain, but still tended to get an upset stomach when she was confronted with conflicts with her older sons, Terry and Steven. Neither of the sons frequently visited their home except when invited or on special holiday occasions. Mrs. A had recently confronted the mother of one of Steven's new girlfriends about his usual life style. In doing this she was quite upset for some time, feeling that she had betrayed his motherly trust; however, she could not stand by and passively observe his manipulation of another young woman. She had discussed this with her husband and was now resolving this conflict satisfactorily. In this incident she also had support from her daughters, Lynn and Lisa. I congratulated her on her continued growth as a person, parent, and spouse. She asked if she and her husband could return from time to time—especially when Terry finally accepted help for his drinking problem. I agreed to this plan and offered my optimism about their ability to resolve problems as they arise.

9 A FAMILY APPROACH TO PATIENT COMPLIANCE

Despite advances in biomedical treatment technology, many patients remain ill because they do not adhere to prescribed therapeutic regimens. Hypertension provides a useful illustration of the problem. Over 50% of hypertensive patients have been found to discontinue therapy within 1 year of starting treatment (Caldwell, Cobb, Dowling, & Jongh, 1970; Wilber & Barrows, 1969, 1972). Among patients who persist in medical treatment, an estimated 40% fail to take enough of their medication to achieve the desired therapeutic benefits (McKenney, Slining, Henderson, Devins, & Barr, 1973; Sackett, Haynes, Gibson, Hackett, Taylor, Roberts, & Johnson, 1975). A commonly mentioned rule of thumb among researchers in this area is that only one-fourth of hypertensive individuals are under treatment and that only one-half of those under treatment are actually controlling their blood pressure (McKenney et al., 1973). Clearly, treatment technology has surpassed patient management in modern medicine.

In this chapter, we use the commonly accepted term "compliance," even though we do not like the term's connotation of a one-sided physician–patient relationship. Only in the fantasies of beginning medical students does the doctor simply diagnose and prescribe and the patient gratefully "comply." But despite attempts to substitute such terms as "adherence" and "concordance" (Rakel, 1977), "compliance" continues to serve as the common term to describe the extent to which the patient follows the treatment regimen prescribed by the physician. Aspects of the treatment regimen may include taking medication, changing diet or other aspects of one's life style, and telephoning the office or scheduling a return visit if the symptoms do not remit. The following section reviews some of the research support for a family approach to patient compliance. Then we present a family systems approach to compliance and describe practical strategies for implementing this approach.

REVIEW OF THE LITERATURE ON FAMILY SUPPORT
AND PATIENT COMPLIANCE

There is reasonably strong research evidence linking family support and patient adherence. In their encyclopedic review of studies on patient compliance, Haynes *et al.* (1979) summarize the results of investigations that use variables related to social support (e.g., "influence of family," "interpersonal relations"). The authors report that 33 studies showed a positive relationship between social support and adherence; 18 studies showed no relationship; and one study found a negative relationship between social support and adherence. In the pediatric literature, for example, a number of studies have documented that parents' perceptions of the child's illness and the efficacy of treatment influence the likelihood that they will comply with medication giving and follow-up appointments (Becker, Drachman, & Kirscht, 1972; Charney, Bynum, Eldridge, MacWhinney, McNabb, Scheiner, Sumpter, & Iker, 1967). In the literature on adult medicine, Heinzelmann and Bagley (1970) have documented the influence of spouse support on husbands' compliance with a fitness exercise program related to coronary heart disease. Stuart and Davis (1972) have reported similar findings in the area of weight control. However, as Levy (1980) has noted in her critical review of the literature on social support and compliance, most of these family supports studies have used correlational designs, and most have relied on self-report measures of compliance.

The experimental studies of family support and patient compliance have been centered in the areas of hypertension and obesity. We located three such studies on compliance with antihypertensive regimens. Two of these studies found positive effects of a family support intervention, while the other did not. Levine, Green, Deeds, Chualow, Russell, and Finlay (1979) found that compliance and blood pressure control were enhanced by a home visit to increase family understanding and to elicit their support, although the best gains were found when this intervention was combined with an exit interview for the patient after diagnosis and a small group discussion. Earp and Ory (1979) found similar positive results of blood pressure control after 23 months for a group of patients who received both home monitoring of blood pressure by a significant other and periodic home visits by nurses or pharmacists, as compared to two control groups (a home-visit-only group and a routine clinical management group). Both of these studies were conducted with urban, low-income Black patients in public health facilities. The dropout rate in Levine *et al.*'s study (1979) was quite high.

The third study, by Caplan, von Harrison, Wellons, and French (1979), examined social support from nurses and partners in a racially mixed sample derived from five clinics in urban and suburban settings. (The partners were usually family members.) The investigators examined the impact on compliance and blood pressure control of two interventions: nurse support only and nurse-plus-partner support. These were compared to a routine treatment control group derived from the same settings. Results indicated no improvement in compliance or blood pressure control due to the interventions. Like the Levine study, this experiment suffered from a high attrition of subjects (51%), and the authors admitted that they did not have adequate control over the quality and quantity of the intervention provided by the clinic nurses. The results of the Caplan study are particularly bothersome, because the correlational findings of the study supported the relationship of partner support with patient compliance and blood pressure control. But the experimental intervention appears to have been too weak (the nurses had only two meetings with the partners) and inadequately managed.

If compliance with antihypertensive regimens has been problematic for physicians and patients to achieve, compliance with weight loss advice has been a notorious failure. The record of weight loss treatment even in specialized programs has generally been disappointing (Stunkard & Penick, 1979). When studies have shown statistically significant long-term results, clinical significance has usually been trivial. Primary care treatment results are probably worse still. A chart audit of patients being treated for obesity at The University of Iowa's family practice residency program indicated a median weight loss of approximately zero pounds. The treatment generally consisted of diet and nutritional counseling from the physician and occasionally from a nutritional counselor.

Appalled by such poor results, a number of obesity researchers have turned to family supports as a way to enhance patient compliance with diet regimens. The first such study, conducted by Brownell, Heckerman, Westlake, Hayes, and Monti (1978), compared the weight loss of three groups: a patient-only group whose spouses did not wish to participate; a patient-plus-spouse group; and a third group whose spouses were willing to participate but were randomly assigned to not participate. In the patient-plus-spouse group, the spouses attended the weight loss sessions and were encouraged to modify their own eating behavior along with their partners. Results showed that the patient-plus-spouse group exceeded the other two in meaningful long-term weight loss. Since Brownell et al.'s (1978) ground-breaking study, other reports have generally supported the efficacy of spouse involvement in weight loss treatment (Pearce, LeBow, & Orchard, 1981; Saccone & Israel, 1978). All of the studies, however, have been conducted in specialized weight loss clinics rather than in primary care settings, and the "active ingredients" in spouse support have not yet been clearly identified.

In summary, the family support literature has yielded strong correlational linkages but still fairly skimpy experimental linkages between family support and compliance. It should be noted especially that almost none of this research has been conducted in private practice medical settings where patients and families have an ongoing relationship with the health care team.

In addition, as Levy (1980) has noted in her critical review, most of these studies were marked by three important limitations: first, reliance on self-report measures of compliance; second, failure to specify which supportive family behaviors were associated with compliance; and third, lack of multiple measurements of social support. Despite these shortcomings, the area of family support and compliance holds great promise for an empirical foothold for a family-oriented approach to patient care.

A FAMILY SYSTEMS VIEW OF PATIENT COMPLIANCE

Like virtually all human actions, patient compliance to medical regimens is influenced by its social context. We maintain that the fundamental social context for compliance is the therapeutic triangle consisting of the physician, the patient, and the patient's family. However, there are some compliance situations that may call for expanding the social context of treatment and compliance beyond the therapeutic triangle to include the community as well. In our view, patient compliance emerges in a cooperative therapeutic system from which the patient derives support, resources, and information needed to adhere to the agreed-upon regimen. We propose that certain conditions are necessary for the interaction patterns in the therapeutic triangle to function as an optimal resource for patient compliance. First, there must be congruence in beliefs and expectations related to the disease and the treatment—that is, the patient and the family must agree with the physician on the existence and urgency of the diagnosis and on the potential efficacy of the prescribed treatment; second, the physician and family must know how to support the patient's attempts to adhere; and third, the physician and the family must be motivated to provide this support. Following the work of Caplan et al. (1979) on how social support influences compliance, we suggest that supportive interaction patterns will lead to enhanced patient *motivation* to comply and greater patient *knowledge* of the therapeutic regimen, and therefore to better compliance and clinical outcome. Our theoretical model is outlined in Fig. 9-1.

The therapeutic alliance described in the model can break down at a number of points. The patient may not agree with the physician about the nature of urgency of the diagnosis and treatment. The physician and patient may agree, but the family may disagree and therefore may not provide needed support for the patient to comply. The family "health expert," for example, may believe that the physician is overreacting to a high blood pressure reading ("Harry has just been tense lately, that's all") or is prescribing the wrong medication ("Your sister just got worse on those pills"). Even if the parties in the therapeutic triangle agree cognitively on the treatment plan, other disturbances in this social system may hinder effective social support. The patient or family who does not *like* the physician or is

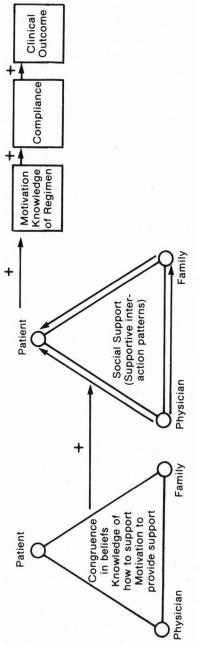

FIG. 9-1. FAMILY SYSTEMS MODEL OF PATIENT COMPLIANCE.

dissatisfied with the bill or with the humaneness of the treatment may not cooperate with a regimen that seems reasonable to everyone else. Patient satisfaction with care is a well-established predictor of patient compliance (Haynes *et al.*, 1979). Less well established is *family* satisfaction with care, but the Korsch and Negrette (1972) study did find that mothers who felt that the physician did not relate well to them as persons were less apt to comply with their child's treatment regimen.

In addition to problems affecting relationships with the *physician* in the therapeutic triangle, disturbances in the family or in the patient's relationship with the family may also undermine the patient's efforts to comply with the treatment. Family dysfunction is likely to lead to poor patient compliance. Steidl, Finkelstein, Wexler, Feigenbaum, Kitsen, Kliger, and Quinlan (1980), for example, found a relationship between compliance with adult dialysis treatment and an observational measure of family functioning. One striking finding was a correlation of .71 between poor compliance and the family's score on the interaction pattern consisting of one parent aligning with a child against the other parent. The psychosomatic families described by Minuchin *et al.* (1978) tend to be too rigidly overinvolved with the patient to provide helpful support.

Even in the absence of general family dysfunction, moreover, a particular patient–family interaction pattern surrounding the medical treatment may undermine compliance. A common example is the nagging spouse and the resentful patient who refuses to comply to spite the partner. Families can be underinvolved or overinvolved in the treatment process. Either way, the patient's compliance is apt to suffer: An underinvolved family does not support the patient enough, and an overinvolved family robs the patient of personal responsibility. Because patients and families vary so much in their abilities and needs, there are no universal formulas for how families should support their members' compliance. Later we suggest a way to individualize family support for each patient and family.

Doherty and his colleagues (particularly Helmut Schrott, MD) at The University of Iowa are conducting research that stems from this family systems approach to patient compliance. In a correlational study completed in 1981, Doherty, Schrott, Metcalf, and Vailas (1982) investigated the relationship among spouse support, spouse health beliefs, and patient compliance to a medication regimen. A group of 150 middle-aged men was drawn from a longitudinal pool participating in a coronary prevention trial that was aimed at reducing serum cholesterol levels. These men and their wives were given structured interviews focusing on health beliefs related to the coronary prevention trial and on the amount of support the wife gives her husband to adhere to the requirements of the program. To fill out the therapeutic triangle in this study, four program staff members who knew the patients well were asked to rank-order the patients on the amount of support each received from his wife. Thus this study measured wife support from three complementary perspectives—the patient's, the wife's, and the staff's. Each wife's health beliefs were assessed by a modified form of the Health Belief Interview (Becker & Maiman, 1975), which yielded scores on her perceptions of her husband's *susceptibility* to problems associated with high cholesterol, the *severity* of the possible health risks, the *benefits* to her husband of participating in the coronary prevention trial's regimen, and the *costs* or disadvantages of his participation.

Compliance was measured by a pill count on the day of the interview. It was hypothesized that men with higher wife support would adhere better to medication taking, and that wives with stronger beliefs in the danger of high cholesterol and the benefits as opposed to the costs of the program would offer greater support to their husbands.

The findings generally supported the hypotheses. Men who had highly supportive wives were significantly more likely to adhere to their medication regimen than were men with less supportive wives. The high-support group (as measured by a consensus of patient, wife, and staff ratings) had a mean compliance score of 96%, while the low-support group averaged 70%—a difference that in hypertension compliance has been shown to be clinically important (Sackett, Haynes, Gibson, & Johnson, 1976). The specific wife behaviors that correlated positively with compliance were "reminders" and "encouragement"; "nagging" correlated negatively with compliance. The other major finding was that a wife's beliefs about the *benefits* to her husband of his participating in the program were associated with higher wife support for his complying with the medication regimen.

With this correlational study as a backdrop, Doherty and his colleagues are designing further experimental research to attempt to demonstrate that family-oriented compliance counseling can improve compliance and clinical outcome in the treatment of hypertension in family physicians' offices. Ultimately, such experimental evidence will be needed to demonstrate the usefulness of the family systems approach advocated in this chapter.

FAMILY-ORIENTED COMPLIANCE COUNSELING

We discuss two issues here: (1) when to involve the family and other support systems directly in the treatment compliance plan, and (2) how to conduct family compliance counseling.

WHEN TO INVOLVE THE FAMILY AND OTHER SUPPORT SYSTEMS

Although virtually all patient compliance occurs within a social context, it is not practical to assemble the family or other support persons to discuss every treatment regimen. Only in the case of pediatric visits is another family member (the parent) usually present when treatment is prescribed, and here the key question is when to involve the other parent or other family members. A further issue concerns engaging support groups beyond the family, particularly community self-help groups. In brief, we propose that the more serious or chronic the illness is, and the more life style change is required for successful treatment, the more important it is to mobilize the patient's social support systems—almost always the family and sometimes community support groups as well. Figure 9-2 presents a continuum of problems with different levels of urgency for engaging social support for the patient. The figure is a modified version of one from Chapter 5 (Fig. 5-1).

On the left end of the continuum in Fig. 9-2 are those illnesses that have temporary, minor effects on the patient and family and that are either time-limited (like the common cold) or have uncomfortable symptoms that lend themselves to high patient compliance (like contact dermatitis). Similarly, routine self-limiting disorders like influenza normally should not require a family conference. These ailments can and should be treated with an appreciation of the family and the therapeutic triangle, however, and the family physician's knowledge of the home environment of the patient can be important for the treatment and prevention of minor illnesses. But the physician ordinarily need not assemble the family in these cases, unless such involvement seems indicated by other information about the patient and family.

Treatment failure or repeated recurrence of routine disorders, on the other hand, should signal the desirability of bringing in a spouse or other family members to find out what is going on and to offer family compliance counseling. Sometimes these family interviews uncover psychosocial problems that are blocking effective treatment, as when poor compliance is associated with depression or chemical dependency. Direct family involvement is even more important when a patient is diagnosed as having a chronic illness such as hypertension or diabetes, which will require some life style changes (in diet, medication taking, exercise) that affect the family and depend in part on the family's support. Similarly, we believe that the family should routinely be assembled to assist in the treatment of (1) stress-related disorders (such as the clinical "red flags" discussed earlier), (2) psychosocial problems, and (3) serious acute illnesses (such as myocardial infarctions, strokes, and bleeding ulcers). Family compliance counseling is a task of the family physician that cannot be referred to a therapist, since most families do not need therapy. They simply need to be involved in the significant health experiences of family members.

When should community groups be actively incorporated into the treatment plan? As Fig. 9-2 indicates, we believe that when the patient is being asked to undertake major life style changes, the patient and family will probably need outside support to comply with the treatment plan. Particularly for obesity and chemical dependency—disorders that are apt to involve

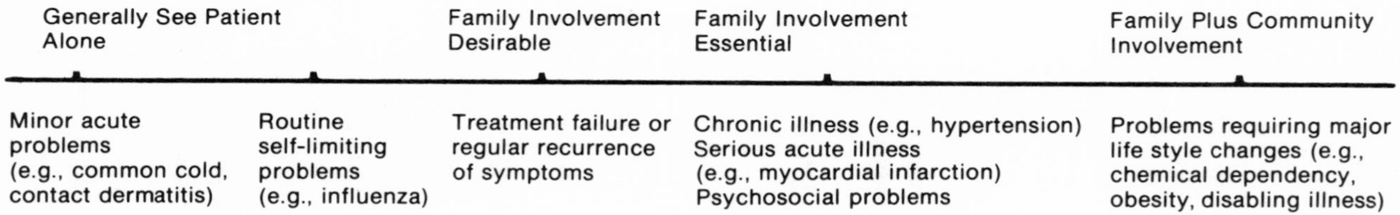

Generally See Patient Alone	Family Involvement Desirable	Family Involvement Essential	Family Plus Community Involvement
Minor acute problems (e.g., common cold, contact dermatitis)	Treatment failure or regular recurrence of symptoms	Chronic illness (e.g., hypertension) Serious acute illness (e.g., myocardial infarction) Psychosocial problems	Problems requiring major life style changes (e.g., chemical dependency, obesity, disabling illness)
Routine self-limiting problems (e.g., influenza)			

Fig. 9-2. When to Involve Social Support Systems Directly to Help Patients Comply.

long-standing family interaction patterns related to eating, chemical use, and stress management—the family might lack the internal resources or adaptability to help the patient modify his or her life style. Often the most effective social support comes from persons with the same problem or who have made the same life style change. For obesity, groups such as Overeaters Anonymous, Take Off Pounds Sensibly (TOPS), and Weight Watchers provide education and encouragement for persons struggling to eat more sensibly. However, we believe that these groups would be more successful if they incorporated families into their program. Like traditional medicine, they are based on an individualistic approach, with inadequate attention to the "weight loss triangle" created by the entry of a family member into a weight loss group. Family members have ways of undermining such "self-help"—for example, by giving gifts of candy, by teasing the weight reducer, and by insisting that no one else in the family will eat all the fish and liver required on some diets.

Since many community programs do not involve families, it is up to the family physician to foster the family's support for the patient who is using these outside groups for support. Support groups for patients with a disabling illness such as cystic fibrosis, on the other hand, usually do a good job of involving and supporting families. To sum up: The best therapeutic system for handling life style change would involve a cooperative "rectangle" of the physician, the patient, the family, and a community support group.

CONDUCTING FAMILY COMPLIANCE COUNSELING

Based on our experience with family compliance counseling, we suggest the following step-by-step approach:

1. *Assemble the family for a family interview by asking the patient to bring his or her family to the next visit after the diagnosis is made and the treatment plan formulated and agreed upon.* Patients will generally accept a rationale that you, as a family physician, like to explain matters to the family and to respond to their questions and concerns. Over time, patients in your practice will come to expect you to invite their families to the office for a conference. You are not suggesting that the family has problems, only that you want to meet with the family to talk about the illness and the treatment. Baird's custom is to ask the patient to bring in the "family" but to let the adult patient decide on whether to bring the children. For pediatric illness, assembling the family should involve at least both parents or a single parent and a primary support person. In the case of the serious life-threatening illness, the patient will usually be hospitalized, and the physician should ask that all available family members attend a family conference.

2. *Begin the family interview with a discussion of the medical problem.* Share with the family the information that you had previously given to the

patient—that is, the course of the illness so far, the etiology if known, the treatment, and the prognosis. Here you are in the familiar expert role that calls for clear, coherent explanations of the facts as you know them and the plan of action that you are suggesting. The advantage of relaying this information to all family members at once is that they can all receive the information unfiltered by the patient's anxious reactions and misunderstandings. Communicating this information to all family members is an essential first step in forging a therapeutic alliance with the family around the treatment plan.

3. *Then shift gears from the role of teacher to that of listener and counselor.* Now is the time to elicit questions and reactions from the patient and family members. It is best to begin on the cognitive level by saying, "I would like to answer your questions now about what I have said so far or anything else about Jim's illness and the treatment plan." Usually family members will have questions about the illness or about the treatment, but if they do not you can encourage them to talk by asking, for example, what they thought you were saying about the hypertensive patient's salt consumption. After fielding questions from the family, you should shift one gear further from the expert role by asking a question such as "I would like to hear your reactions to Jim's being ill." Here you are asking the family members for their feelings, and you should be prepared for them to express emotion, particularly if the illness is life-threatening or terminal. Even though family members may experience emotional pain during this discussion, they will generally be grateful to you for giving them the chance to express their feelings, fears, and hopes. Without a chance to do this, the quality of their family life may become emotionally quite constricted.

4. *After this, shift gears again into a more active problem-solving mode by helping the family and the patient make a contract or agreement about compliance with the prescribed regimen.* The goal is a supportive family interaction pattern. Once you are sure that everyone understands the requirements of the regimen, you can facilitate a family support contract in the following way: First, ask the patient if he or she would like help from other family members to follow through on the treatment plan. If the patient replies affirmatively (most will), then ask the spouse or other family member whether he or she would like to help the patient stay on the therapeutic program. If the spouse, for example, says yes, then tell both partners that you would like to see them work out a way that they would work together on this. It is important that the patient ask for support while at the same time remaining responsible for his or her own compliance behavior. You can help to bring this about by asking the patient, "How would you like your spouse to help you with your medication taking? Some people like their partner to put the pills on the table for them; some people like to be reminded; other people like their spouse to stay out of the medication matter altogether. How about you? How could your wife best help you take your pills regularly?" When the patient proposes a

way for the spouse to help, you should then check out with the spouse whether this is acceptable. You are teaching behavioral contracting here.

Once they get the idea of contracting, the partners themselves may spontaneously generate their own agreements—for example, the wife will stop salting food when she cooks, but the husband will be responsible for remembering not to salt his food at the table. The advantage of a give-and-take contract like this is that the family can provide support without invading the patient's rights or autonomy and without being burdened with too much responsibility. Sometimes the contract may call for the family to keep "hands off" entirely as the best way to support the patient. Each patient and family have their own peculiar needs and wants in this area. Finally, at the physician's suggestion, the family contract may involve participation in supportive community groups.

5. *Then hand out any patient education materials that you think will be helpful for this patient and family.* Ask everyone to read the materials.

6. *Finally, schedule and conduct a follow-up meeting to monitor the progress of treatment and the effectiveness of the family support contracts made during the session.* Help the family to modify and update their contracts as needed. If you involve an office nurse in your compliance counseling, this nurse can provide periodic ongoing family compliance counseling for patients on long-term treatment.

The main purposes of the family compliance conference are to educate the patient and family about the illness and the treatment program; to give the patient and family members a chance to share with one another their emotional reactions and concerns about the illness and the treatment; and to facilitate an explicit agreement among family members as to how the patient will be supported in adhering to the therapeutic regimen. We have found this approach useful in everyday patient care and are proceeding to conduct research on its effectiveness.

CONCLUSION

With their access to the whole family and their participation in the community, family physicians are uniquely situated to try innovative social support approaches to improving cooperation with medical treatment. The evidence is clear that the traditional one-to-one compliance counseling model is not effective with many patients. While the greater effectiveness of the family approach has not yet been sufficiently documented empirically, we believe that it could become family medicine's most distinguished contribution to the delivery of health care.

10 PRIMARY CARE COUNSELING FOR MARITAL AND SEXUAL PROBLEMS

This chapter presents our approach to handling marital and sexual problems in family practice. Like other psychosocial problems, marital and sexual difficulties typically present in covert ways in family practice. When a family physician opens an interview with a question such as "How can I help you today?," rarely does the patient reply, "I need help with my marriage," or even less frequently, "I'm having sexual problems." More often, relationship distress presents as either physical symptoms, general anxiety, or dysphoric mood. Therefore, preliminary assessment of the patient's presenting complaints must accompany the evaluation of relationship problems. Once this assessment is conducted and the general nature of the marital or sexual problems is understood, the family physician can decide whether to attempt a primary care intervention or to refer the couple to a marital or sex therapist. Generally, little is lost and much can be gained by meeting with the couple at least once, since the physician can either begin counseling at this time or make a more persuasive referral recommendation with both partners present. While referral is always an option, this chapter stresses the role of primary care counseling in preventing and treating marital and sexual problems.

MARITAL PROBLEMS

ASSESSMENT

We apply our four basic categories to the primary care assessment of marital problems: stress, cohesion, interaction patterns, and adaptability.

STRESS

Stress is the personal and marital strain stemming from events that tax the coping resources of the couple. Stress may reflect changes over the life cycle, pressure from external events, or challenges from internal family experiences.

Marital Life Cycle Stress

Many of the marital problems physicians see in medical practice are associated with the normal stresses of life transitions. In their early stages of development, these problems respond well to primary care counseling. The two most common life stressors we have confronted in family practice are adjustment to parenthood and adjustment to midlife role changes, particularly the transition to parenting one's aging parents. Marital problems connected with early child rearing often present to the family physician in the form of excessive office visits by the mother with one or more of the children. The mother brings a child to the office every 10 days with cold-like symptoms, or she is hyperalert to signs of allergies, or she complains that her little boy is hyperactive. Observation and physical examination by the physician reveal no medical or behavioral problems in the child. Marital and parental distress is a likely diagnosis in this situation. Many mothers are waiting for the physician to pay attention to their plea for help. It is not hard to get them to tell their story: They are often overwhelmed with young children, stuck at home or carrying two jobs (work and home), feeling unsupported by their husbands, and upset at the increased arguing and poorer sexual relations in their marriages.

With more people living longer into old age, and with more women employed full-time in the work force, the problem of "what to do with Grandma" has become increasingly common for American families. Just as the nest empties for middle-aged couples—when they feel free of parenting responsibilities and can rekindle their marital companionship—they are faced with the prospect of the unanticipated dependency of their parents. Parenting their parents is not in the life scripts of most people. The couple may experience conflict over what to do with the dependent parent, and the wife may feel resentful for having to shoulder most of the burden for the care—especially if it is *his* parent. Such life cycle stresses commonly present to the family physician in two forms: (1) the old person is "dumped" at the office or hospital for the physician to make a decision about future care, or (2) the wife presents with physical complaints, depression, or anxiety. Questioning by the family physician can reveal the underlying life cycle adjustment stress on the patient and the couple. Generally, these couples do not require either marital therapy or tranquilizers; instead, they need primary care counseling.

Externally Caused Stress

One couple we worked with had a satisfying relationship for 25 years until the government took over a portion of their land for a highway. The husband became depressed and withdrew from his wife; she reacted by catering to his need to be alone but then getting angry at him. This couple was responding dysfunctionally to an external stressor that shattered their previous contentment. Most couples probably have a "breaking point" of stress beyond which they are not able to function well as partners. Fortunately, the storm usually passes, and what they need is support through the crisis. Without support, however, the dysfunctional patterns can escalate and the relationship can experience permanent damage.

Internally Caused Stress

Unanticipated events such as illness, death, and major changes in one of the spouses can create marital distress for some couples. If the couple functioned adequately before the onset of the stressful experience, the spouses have a good chance—with proper support—of regaining their balance. Sometimes, however, they need help in forging a new kind of relationship if the internal stressor requires permanent adjustment (e.g., to a handicapped child or spouse). Here the flexibility of the marital system will be taxed strenuously, and the impact of the primary care counseling can be greater. An often overlooked internal stressor for some couples takes the form of a major life style change for one member—for example, drastic weight loss through dieting or an extensive new exercise program. The other spouse may have difficulty adjusting to the "new" partner. We have seen marriages become unstable after an obese wife takes on a new sexy appearance.

COHESION

Some couples with marital problems are struggling against a suffocating closeness that has drained their personal autonomy. Typically, one partner in such an enmeshed relationship tries unilaterally to gain some distance—for example, by getting more involved with work or hobbies or friends. The other partner reacts with alarm, and a series of conflicts begins. On the other extreme are couples whose cohesion has been eroded to the point of disengagement: They live separate lives under the same roof except for occasional flare-ups when someone's disappointment surfaces. One of them is probably contemplating divorce. In between these extremes is a wide range of marital cohesion patterns reflecting various degree of closeness and distance.

It is a common mistake to view highly conflicted partners as necessarily disengaged. They are more likely to be on the enmeshed end of the continuum: emotionally very reactive to each other, constantly "pushing each other's button," reading each other's mind, thinking about each other a lot—and still in love. Their positive energy for each other has turned negative, but they are still very much interconnected. Unless they have worn themselves out in conflict, this couple is a good candidate for marital counseling or therapy, since they still have strong emotional bonds.

A more disengaged couple, on the other hand, may appear calm, reasonable, and not very conflicted—but may have a poor marital prognosis. Classically, one or both of the partners has all but decided to end the marriage or at least to stop working on the relationship. They will have little energy or motivation to salvage a satisfying marriage. In such cases, the counselor's initial task is to help the partners decide whether to stay married and then perhaps to shift gears into divorce counseling to help them separate amicably and justly.

Marital cohesion, then, represents the central issues of emotional bonds and commitment to the relationship. Strong bonds and strong commitment offer the best prognosis for primary marital counseling: The partners are apt to cooperate actively with the counselor. Couples with low commitment need primary care help in sorting out whether they want to work toward a better marriage or toward no marriage.

INTERACTION PATTERNS

Identifying a couple's particular interaction patterns is more difficult than identifying the life stressors that are affecting the couple. Most people— including physicians—have a bias toward viewing marital problems as caused by a fault or flaw in one of the partners. The family systems approach, on the other hand, looks at marital problems as symptoms of the marital "dance." The "dance" metaphor conveys the fluid and cooperative quality of marital interaction patterns. Although individuals do have "flaws" or personality limitations that contribute to marital problems, a physician can only under- stand marital dynamics by taking into account the mutal give-and-take of the couple's interaction. The same individuals with different partners might not have these particular problems.

Although the variety of marital dances is beyond cataloguing, the fundamental assessment issue is the *complementarity* of the partners' behav- ior. One nearly universal complementary marital pattern centers around the roles of the pursuer and the pursued. It is rare in marriage that both partners are equally and simultaneously interested in each other's time, attention, and affection. Rather, one partner is usually wanting more than the other is willing to give, or is wanting to give more than the other is willing to receive. Over time, the spouses can become locked into fixed roles in which one of them is constantly asking for more time and attention from the other, while the other feels intruded upon and guilty for keeping distant from the pursuer. While some form of this chase is probably inevitable in marriage, the dance breaks down when the steps become exaggerated: The pursuer becomes a ceaseless nag, and the pursued becomes aloof and ungiving. If the family physician assesses this problem in its early stages—for example, after the birth of the first child, when the wife wants more from her husband and he is preoccupied with financial burdens—then making the couple aware of the dance may help minimize the damage. Partners who have been locked into this pattern for many years will probably require marital therapy and should be referred after the assessment is made.

Some other common marital dances are these:

1. The jealous–flirtatious pair, in which excitement is maintained by the complementary roles of one partner's pretending to be interested in other sexual relationships while the other partner obsessively watches; the subsequent fighting and making up serve to cement this enmeshed marital relationship in an unhealthy way.
2. The "supercompetent" partner and the "incompetent" partner, in which the strength of one is based on the weaknesses of the other. For example, the husband copes extremely well only when his wife is depressed or ill, or the wife gains the praise of the community for her heroic efforts to maintain the family in the face of her "hopeless alcoholic" husband.
3. The quiet, "nice" husband and the assertive, unsatisfied wife, a pattern in which she gets cast in the role of "bitch" and he in that of the "good guy"; as she complains more about his passivity, he grows more resigned and unsupportive of her. Often he avoids conflict with his own family while she does battle with his parents. This couple's sexual relationship is usually unsatisfying: She is sexually unresponsive with him, and he is not interested in sex very often.

The listing of marital dances or interaction patterns could go on indefinitely, but the fundamental point is that marital dysfunction is a collaborative, complementary process in which there are no "good guys" and "villains," no martyrs and persecutors. Each partner has enormous power to reward and punish and influence the other. The physician should beware the lure of the spouse presenting as an innocent lamb. If the physician sits down with both partners and observes their interaction, he or she will probably see two people struggling to get close without losing their individual identities—no easy task for any pair.

ADAPTABILITY

After stresses, cohesion, and interaction patterns have been assessed, the key diagnostic issue is the partner's ability to change the way they interact and feel in order to overcome their problems. A chief indicator of adaptability is chronicity: The longer the duration of the dysfunctional patterns, the greater the likelihood that the marital system has become rigid. If a life cycle transition merely exacerbates problems that have pervaded the relationship from the beginning, then this couple has low adaptability. On the other hand, if the "supercompetent" wife and the "incompetent" husband have assumed these roles only in the few months since his heart attack, then their relationship may still have adequate adaptability. In addition to chronicity, a second indicator of adaptability is the way in which the partners respond to the counselor's efforts to help them change. When such efforts meet with resistance or increased rigidity—when the dance tempo either does not change or perhaps escalates—then this couple's relationship is probably not flexible enough for a primary care intervention.

A third indicator of the level of marital adaptability is the presence of serious problems such as chemical dependency or clinical depression in one of the partners. Chemically dependent family systems tend to be among the most rigid. Depression tends to diminish the individual's motivation and energy to work on marital problems, and chronic depression is often accompanied by dysfunctional adaptations by the other spouse to a "supercompetent" role. Such couples need a skillful blend of individual and marital treatment beyond the training of most family physicians.

Generally, a family physician should be able to determine what kind of help is needed—primary care or specialized care—after one session with the presenting patient followed by one or two sessions with the couple. Further assessment will continue during the course of the primary care counseling or during the therapy to which the partners are referred.

COUNSELING APPROACHES

The family physician's approach to counseling a couple with marital problems will vary with the goals of the counseling, which can include prevention, education, support, and challenge. Specific counseling techniques have been discussed in Chapter 7. Here, a number of more general approaches or strategies are proposed for preventing and alleviating marital problems through primary care counseling.

PREVENTION

Anticipatory guidance has always been a unique specialty of primary care physicians. Some marital difficulties are predictable, as when a couple faces major life cycle transitions, unemployment, illness, or a housing move. Office visits for routine medical care provide the ideal opportunity for preventive marital counseling. During prenatal visits, for instance, the wife (and preferably the husband as well) can be gently alerted to the changes that the baby will bring. Although these expectant parents may not heed the warning at the time, they may remember the advice later when they begin to experience marital strain. One new father told us that he kept recalling his doctor's words during stressful periods, and that this recollection helped him see the strain as normal. Preventive counseling can help either by assisting couples in avoiding problems, or by normalizing experiences that the couple may be tempted to view as abnormal. Normal marital strain is a well-kept secret in our culture; "other couples" are thought of as blissful after having a baby, happy to retire, fond of their in-laws, and even more in love when facing adversity. Family physicians can perform a valuable service to couples by saying, in effect: "It isn't going to be easy."

In addition to such admonitions, preventive counseling should focus on what partners can do to ward off possible serious strain on their relationship, for example, by retaining time for themselves as a couple after the first child. Family physicians can also help couples to make important decisions that they might be postponing, such as how responsibilities for an elderly parent who moves in are going to be shared. *Preparing for stresses by discussing them in advance and normalizing them after they occur*—these are key strategies for preventive marital counseling.

EDUCATION

Educating couples can take a number of forms. In the sexual area (to be dealt with more extensively below), some couples experience trouble because of ignorance of sexual functioning. When there are no serious underlying personal or relationship disorders, these couples respond quite well to simple teaching and encouragement by the family physician. Similarly, couples who have difficulty solving normal marital disagreements because of poor habits of communication may respond to "coaching" in more effective communication behaviors. No fancy communication techniques should be taught, just a few basics:

1. Each partner should speak for self rather than for the other partner ("I believe" rather than "You seem to believe").
2. Each partner should pay attention when the other partner is speaking (i.e., should maintain eye contact and an attentive body posture).
3. Both partners should make positive, supportive statements as well as critical statements (they should say what they like as well as what they dislike).
4. Both partners should continue communicating about the issue until they resolve it or decide to take it up later.

When counseling partners who lack one or more of these fundamental communication skills, the family physician can demonstrate the skills through modeling or can instruct the couple directly to try the new behavior. For example, after noticing that the partners do not look at each other when talking, the physician can ask them to try facing each other and making eye contact. When one partner is speaking for the other (mind reading), the physician can say, "I think it would be better for you to say what *you* think or feel about this matter, rather than concentrating on how you think your partner feels. When we talk about someone else's feelings, usually we are wrong at least half the time. So try just speaking for yourself." If this educational process does not succeed—if the partners continue to communicate poorly—there is a high likelihood that their marital communication is too rigid for a primary care intervention. Pushing such a rigid couple to communicate more directly and openly may lead to a deterioration in the relationship by "overloading" the marital system. (Such effects have been documented in some couples after a Marriage Encounter weekend, a program that fosters a rapid opening up of feelings between the spouses; see Doherty & Walker, 1982, and Lester & Doherty, 1983.) On the other hand, there probably are many couples who can benefit from low-key instruction in marital communication when their family physician is helping them face problems or decisions.

SUPPORT

In the therapeutic triangle, one of the family physician's most important functions is to support the relationship between the other two members—in this case, the spouses. Marriages need nurturance not only from the partners but also from concerned outsiders. In fact, it could be argued that the stability and satisfaction of any marital relationship depends to an important extent on the quality of support the couple receives from others. This is particularly true in times of trouble or stress, when the coping resources of the couple are severely strained. At such times, the family physician can literally be a "marriage saver" by calling the partners to the office and providing help in a number of ways: listening empathically to them, encouraging them to persevere and to face their difficulties collaboratively, and helping them locate other sources of help and support. Fragmentation is a chief danger for couples under stress: Instead of banding together, each partner becomes more private from the other; pain or fear is not shared with the other for fear of rejection or of overwhelming the other. A concerned third party makes it easier for these couples to face each other and support each other.

> Within the space of 1 year, a husband and wife we know moved a long distance from their families and had a first baby. The wife quit work to care for the baby, who turned out to be quite irritable. The husband took an extra job to support the family, but his income from the first job plummeted because of poor sales; he then increased his hours at the second job, which kept him away from home

from early morning till late night. The wife, without friends or family in the community, became more anxious at home with the fussy baby. Finally, the couple lost their recently purchased house in a mud slide and their car in an automobile accident. (Remember Job?) The wife presented to the family practice office with symptoms of anxiety. The resident asked her to bring her husband back for a joint session. The couple reported a good relationship prior to making the move and having the baby. Supportive counseling focused on allowing the couple to "ventilate" their feelings about the events in their lives, and on helping them plan together what steps to take to get themselves out of the hole they were in. Their morale and confidence improved considerably after two sessions.

Since family physicians generally do not have the time to serve as the primary support persons for many patients, marital counseling should also focus on how the couple can gain access to other support systems. The family physician can then settle back into a secondary support role for the couple by keeping in touch with both partners through routine office visits.

CHALLENGE

These remarks concentrate on the use of challenging statements within ongoing primary care marital counseling, as opposed to challenge that leads to an immediate referral. Several situations lend themselves to such challenges or confrontations within marital counseling:

1. *Challenging unrealistic expectations about family life.* Often one or both partners hold unspoken assumptions about how wonderful and trouble-free married life is "supposed" to be. One common irrational belief is that "My partner should understand my needs without my having to express them." Other common expectations are that the marital relationship should get better without the partners' having to work at it, or that the in-law problems should disappear once the couple moves out of the same geographical area, or that children will necessarily bring the couple closer. The family physician can nonjudgmentally confront the couple about these unrealistic expectations that stand in the way of problem solving: "I get the feeling that both of you thought that once you got married, the rest would take care of itself and you wouldn't have to really work every day at your relationship—you know, happily ever after. Does that sound true for either of you?"

2. *Challenging the partners to act collaboratively.* In the example of the couple whose house was destroyed, the counselor primarily supported the couple at first, but then proceeded to challenge the spouses to work together on their problems. These partners had divided their roles rigidly in the crisis: In order to "protect" his wife, the husband had taken sole responsibility for knowing how badly off they were and deciding what should be done. The wife wanted a greater role but had accepted his monopoly. The counselor challenged the partners to share more information about their situation and

to discuss their options jointly. Their current arrangement was portrayed as too stressful for both of them individually: They needed to act more like a couple. Encouraging couples to behave collaboratively puts the responsibility for problem solving where it belongs—on *them* rather than on the physician. Such a challenge can also free their complementary strengths and resources to deal with their problems.

3. *Challenging the partners to change dysfunctional interaction patterns.* After assessing the couple's transactional patterns, a family physician can supportively but firmly confront the couple about these patterns: "Here is what I see going on. Mrs. T, you try to get close to your husband, but Mr. T, you feel smothered and you move away from her. She doesn't bring up her feelings about this until she blows up, and then you retreat further. You folks have a painful little dance going on here that you can probably change if you want to work at it." A hallmark of a healthy couple will be that the partners can respond constructively to the physician pointing out their dysfunctional patterns. They will tend to "see it" when their dance is described to them, and they will work to change it. For some couples, understanding in a different way what they are doing helps them to change. If the interaction pattern is of relatively recent origin (e.g., if it has begun since a new baby arrived, a new job was taken, or a mother-in-law moved in), then the likelihood of a positive response to this challenge will be even higher. On the other hand, some couples will agree with the physician but be unable to change their habitual styles, while other couples will deny the counselor's assessment of their patterns, preferring their own explanations of their difficulties. The family physician should not continue to counsel these couples alone, but rather should seek a consultation or make a referral.

4. *Challenging the partners to take responsibility for solving their own problems.* As Minuchin once noted, if the physician wants the family members to change more than *they* do, that physician is lost. Failure of couples to keep appointments or to follow through on agreements they have made during the session should be challenged by the physician. Such confrontations should be firm and low-key, with no pleading or scolding: After all, these are *their* marriages to make or break. The physician can let them know that he or she is willing to help but that they must do most of the work. Such firmness from the counselor can serve as a model to spouses of how to confront each other about dissatisfactions.

In summary, to the extent that it can prevent and alleviate marital distress, primary care marital counseling by family physicians offers an important mental health service to patients. Situational and life cycle stresses are particularly suited for marital counseling in family medicine. When these problems do not relent with primary care treatment or when the presenting problems are chronic or severe, then the family physician can guide the couple into the domain of specialized marital therapy and continue to provide backup support and ongoing medical care.

SEXUAL PROBLEMS

Sexual problems are often manifestations of underlying couple problems; hence, they are often handled within the context of couple counseling. Sometimes the sexual difficulty clears up when the partners learn to handle their conflicts in other areas. A rocky marriage does not make for a smooth sex life for most couples (there are exceptions). Except in the case of organic etiology or severe psychopathology, then, a sexual dysfunction in one partner can best be conceptualized and treated as the presentation of a couple's interaction pattern. This systems approach to sexual dysfunction was pioneered by Masters and Johnson (1970), whose work, along with that of Kaplan (1974, 1978), provides the basis for our recommendations. Sexual relationships are by definition mutual, and resolving sexual problems usually requires the cooperation of both partners. We limit our discussion of sexual counseling to a few sexual problems we have encountered often in primary care.

Assessment

As we have highlighted often in this book, psychosocial problems present to family physicians in varied forms—but rarely in straightforward fashion. A sex therapist is accustomed to having patients announce on the telephone that they want help with a sexual difficulty. But a family physician must know how to ask the right questions and then how to listen "between the lines" when the patient replies. In our experience, sexual problems in women most commonly present as discomfort during intercourse, while sexual problems in men present in the form of nonspecific rectal and urinary problems. We recommend that the physician ask during the woman's routine pelvic exam if she has discomfort during sexual intercourse. A positive response to this question or a nonverbal display of tension indicates the need for follow-up conversation after the examination. If there is no objective physical reason for her discomfort (such as a vaginal infection), the most common cause is "relationship distress." She may feel that her husband or partner is not attentive to her emotional and sexual needs, that he is mainly concerned with his own pleasure. Sometimes the woman feels used by her partner: He remains distant from her all day, but then wants to enjoy her sexually at night. She may respond by "shutting down" sexually: She does not lubricate vaginally and is sore during intercourse. She may then conclude that something is wrong with her and feel anxious during subsequent lovemaking, which makes her less responsive. Because she appears less interested in sex and less willing to become sexually aroused, her partner may shorten foreplay to a minimum and proceed to have his orgasm as quickly as possible. This pushes her further away. Their inability to talk about the problem exacerbates the tension. She may be too embarrassed to verbalize the difficulty to her family physician until asked during a routine office visit.

Men are even more reluctant than women to admit openly to a sexual problem. They may carry around from doctor to doctor a questionable diagnosis of chronic prostatitis, until someone finally asks, "Do you have trouble with erections?" If medical evaluation does not reveal a physical cause, an underlying clinical depression, or chemical dependency, then the most likely cause for erections problems is "performance anxiety"—the excessive fear of not achieving or maintaining an erection, and thereby failing to please one's partner. A chief indicator that performance anxiety is the culprit is that the erection problems began after a discrete incident of impotence. The man carries a fear of repeated failure to his next sexual encounter, thereby causing himself to "shut down" sexually. The process then snowballs.

In addition to relationship issues and performance anxiety, a third common cause of sexual problems is ignorance of male and female sexual functioning. In our society where accurate sex information is difficult to come by for young people, many persons never learn about their own and their partner's sexual anatomy and sexual responsiveness. Both partners may be unaware of men's and women's different timing needs for sexual arousal, or that women tend to be more responsive to the emotional context of lovemaking, or that clitoral stimulation is quite important for many women's sexual responsiveness. Finally, they may not realize that a variety of sexual behaviors such as oral–genital contact can be both pleasurable and "normal."

In summary, assessment as a prelude to sexual counseling should rule out a primary diagnosis of organic disease, depression, chemical dependency, or serious individual psychopathology. Primary care sexual counseling is suited for a primary diagnosis of (1) relationship distress (mild to moderate; couples with severe marital distress are not good candidates for sexual counseling or sex therapy), (2) anxiety about sexual performance, and (3) poor sexual practices because of ignorance of misinformation.

COUNSELING APPROACHES

EDUCATION AND PREVENTION

No other helping professional has the physician's regular opportunities for educational counseling to enrich couples' sexual relationships and to forestall possible problems. The best vehicle for sexual education in family medicine is the routine pelvic exam, whether it is associated with an annual Pap smear or with requests for contraceptives. We recommend involving husbands in their wives' pelvic exams for the purposes of teaching both partners about sexual anatomy. If the husband is in the waiting room, the physician can ask the wife if it is all right with her if her husband participates in the exam. Most women are quite willing, and most husbands accept the invitation. In fact, we have begun to find husbands already in the examining room expecting to be part of the proceedings. You can show the husband his wife's genital area, including the clitoris and the cervix. In pointing out the cervix, you can note that he may have felt the cervix with his penis in certain sexual positions or with his fingers during manual stimulation of his wife. Statements like these serve indirectly to communicate to the couple that a wide range of sexual behaviors is normal and that you are willing to talk about sexual behavior with them. We term this whole procedure a "sexology exam" (admittedly only of the woman), and we strongly urge it for all family physicians who want to be involved in primary care sexual counseling.

Additional opportunities for education and prevention occur before and after the birth of a child. Many couples go through a period of sexual abstinence or sexual tentativeness during late pregnancy and after the birth of a baby. They can profit from educational counseling that assures them of the safety of sexual intercourse or points out any dangers, and that communicates the "normality"—if the couple so chooses—of engaging in alternative forms of sexual pleasuring, such as oral–genital and manual stimulation activities. Here it is important not to invade the couple's value system, but merely to indicate that this is how some couples handle their difficulties in having vaginal intercourse. Similarly, new parents can be warned that sometimes one or both of them will be more tired than usual and may not be as sexually responsive. A third common opportunity for education and prevention occurs after a spouse's first myocardial infarction, a situaion discussed in an earlier chapter. Finally, premarital exams present an ideal opportunity to teach about sexuality, provided that the partners are told to expect more than a blood test.

When a patient's sexual complaints are related to the relationship with the partner, we invite both partners to return for further evaluation and counseling. During the couple counseling, we try to determine their level of (dis)satisfaction with the relationship and their level of knowledge about sexual behavior and functioning. Couples without deep-rooted relationship problems often respond well to (1) help in negotiating more time for talking and nonsexual touching prior to lovemaking; (2) recommendations for more companionship time in their relationship; and (3) more specific advice about improving the quality of the lovemaking (e.g., more foreplay or clitoral stimulation). These discussions break the barrier of silence that couples build up over sexual problems. For some couples, open discussion and exploration of alternatives stimulate rapid progress in their sexual relationship. For other couples, such discussions with the family physician will not break the impasse, and a consultation or referral is appropriate.

When a man's erectile difficulties relate to performance anxiety, we have had success with the following primary care counseling intervention: We explain to the man the relationship between fear of failure and subsequent difficulties getting or maintaining an erection. We also explain that it is normal for most men to experience occasional difficulties with their erections and that the biggest problems comes from worrying about it too much. Then we instruct him in a simplified version of Masters and Johnson's (1970) sensate focus exercise. (See the illustrated description of this exercise in Kaplan, 1974.) We ask the man to convey the instructions to his partner. Basically, the couple are asked to refrain from sexual intercourse for 2 weeks and instead to engage every other day in nondemand touching or massage. We keep the instructions simple: "During the first week, I'd like you and your partner to give each other back rubs when you go to bed. Take it slow and easy and don't be concerned about whether you get turned on sexually. During the second week, I'd like you to move to a full body massage, including breasts and genitals. Don't treat this like a professional massage, but just as a way to make each other feel relaxed and cared for. The idea is to get back to touching each other without the pressure of performing sexually. I'll see both of you in 2 weeks and we can decide where to go from there. If you or your wife have any questions about what I want you to do, give me a call."

This procedure is unconventional for sex therapy because of the loose quality of the instructions (sex therapists tend to be more specific about where to touch and not to touch) and because the instructions are given to only one partner. However, we have found this approach quite successful with couples who have a supportive relationship and a problem of short duration. In such cases, the wife is glad to cooperate with the touching exercises; she will do almost anything to help. The husband's morale improves because he can take some leadership to solve the problem and because the sensate focus procedure relieves the pressure on him to perform. Often the erection difficulties clear up and the couple returns to regular sexual relationships prior to the scheduled follow-up session. Other times, a follow-up session or two is needed to reinforce the principles of nondemand lovemaking and mutual cooperation. When a few sessions are not achieving progress, then a consultation or referral is in order. Referral sources were discussed in an earlier chapter. Generally, however, little is lost and much can be gained by a short-term primary care intervention in sexual problems.

SUPPORT

A principal way of supporting couples who have sexual problems is to communicate to them that their sexual difficulties are both understandable and fairly common. People get to believe that they are alone in a world of satisfied lovers, and that having a problem like theirs is strange and shameful. If the family physician deals with them in an empathic but matter-of-fact way, the couple's morale will be helped and their sense of confidence improved. A specific way to express this expectable quality of sexual difficulties is to demonstrate how impotence, for example, is a natural consequence of fear of failure, or that orgasmic difficulty in women is an inevitable by-product of inadequate stimulation during lovemaking, or that premature ejaculation is related to the simple lack of recognition of an approaching orgasm. In addition to "normalizing" sexual problems, the family physician can offer a sense of confidence that the partners can solve their problems by working together and by trying different behaviors such as the sensate focus exercise, or by spending more time showing affection to each other. For many couples, support for dealing with sexual difficulties is terribly difficult to find in any other setting than their family physician's office. And many unfortunately do not find it there.

CHALLENGE

Challenge is especially important at one point in primary care sexual counseling: when the partners do not follow through on their agreed-upon assignment for at-home activities. At this point they need a push either to take responsibility for solving their own problems by committing themselves to the exercises, or to accept a referral to a marital or sex therapist. Failure to follow through after the counseling session is a sign of resistance. The primary care counselor's best move generally is to nudge the partners firmly but gently to see if they will give up their resistance. If this challenging move does not lead to renewed cooperation or to a decision to try a different counseling approach, then a consultation or referral is in order. In such cases, the minimum goal of challenging the couple is to keep the family physician out of the frustrating position of trying to change people who do not want to change or are too afraid to try. It is *their* sexual relationship, and ultimately they may prefer familiar problems to unfamiliar solutions.

CONCLUSION

Counseling couples can be difficult and sometimes unsettling work. We bring into the counseling session our feelings and values related to male–female relationships, marital roles, sexual behavior, emotional closeness, and individual freedom. Everyone who has worked with couples has heard opposite-sex partners sound like the counselor's own spouse or parent. If a *male* family physician gets complaints from his wife about his inattentiveness to her needs and his "affair" with his work, he will be tempted to side with a husband who is receiving similar "nagging" complaints from his wife. If a *female* family physician is dealing with the troublesome complexities of a dual-career relationship, it will not be easy to remain neutral when a wife complains that her husband does not respect her rights to outside interests of her own. If a counselor of either sex has grown up in a family where conflict is avoided and not dealt with, then it will be hard to allow couples to express negative feelings openly in counseling. Unhealthy triangles in one's family of origin are apt to carry over to the therapeutic triangle in marital counseling: The counselor will have trouble letting partners handle their own conflicts without becoming triangulated into their relationship.

The other side of these challenges in marital counseling is the opportunity for stimulation and personal growth. Marital counseling provides a continual source of issues for personal reflection and a continued invitation to learn more effective ways to help people cope with problems. The primary care nature of marital counseling in family practice gives the physician the flexibility to bail out of the counseling when the issues become too stressful for the couple or the physician. This "self-protection" is essential if family physicians are to take the risk of trying to help patients with marital and sexual problems. Given the importance of a satisfying marriage to the well-being of most people, helping couples can be one of the most rewarding aspects of family medicine.

APPENDIX: A SIMULATED FIRST INTERVIEW WITH A RECENTLY MARRIED COUPLE

Following is the transcript of a simulated marital counseling interview that was originally produced for educational television. The couple was asked to demonstrate a common problem that marital counselors run across. In a family practice setting, the wife might have presented with headaches or fatigue. The couple were in their late 20s and recently married. The session contains two abbreviated segments, each followed by comments from Doherty to the TV (and, here, the reading) audience. The opening line is appropriate when the counselor does not know either partner especially well.

INTERVIEW SEGMENT

DOHERTY: Nice to see you, Dee and Rick. I'd like for one of you to begin by telling me what brought you here to see me.

DEE: Well, I'd like to begin. I guess I'm sort of surprised actually that Rick got here on time, because that's sort of a problem that we've been having. It seems that after the first few months that we got married I'm at home a lot and Rick isn't. It's just me. I'm doing a lot of the cooking, a lot of the cleaning, and he's not around and I get phone calls—he's going to be late, there's lots of weekend plans, there's evening classes—I'm really actually surprised that he showed up here. It surprised me a lot to see him come.

DOHERTY: So you don't feel like you have enough time with Rick.

DEE: Absolutely. I feel like I'm just giving a whole lot—I'm throwing a whole lot into marriage—and he's not around to appreciate it. It's really beginning to get me pretty badly.

DOHERTY: Rick, what brings you here?

RICK: Well, I came along because Dee really asked. What she's talking about I just don't see as that much of a problem—it's just one of those things you have to do in your life. You work and sometimes you have to work longer hours than you like but that's about it.

DEE: But, Rick, I just don't see how you can say that you don't know why we're here. I've been talking about it and talking about it for weeks now, and I just can't believe that you would deny there's a problem. I just don't believe it. I really think that what's going to happen from now on is that you just call me if you're planning on coming because otherwise I'm just going to assume that otherwise you're not going to be there till really late. I'm sorry, I just don't believe that you don't think there's not a problem.

DOHERTY: Dee, you're getting pretty disgusted right now—you believe there's a problem. It's very serious to you, and, Rick, you don't see it that way.

RICK: No, I see it as a part of something that you just have to do.

DEE: To work all the time?

RICK: You don't seem to mind it all the time, do you?

DEE: Oh, but geez, Rick, I don't see how you can say that.

RICK: Well, I don't see what you're getting so upset about. I don't hear you complain about having extra money.

DEE: I don't think that's at all fair.

RICK: Well, what's the big difference if I'm home on time or not?

DEE: When we got married, I assumed that I had a certain idea about the way it would be and about what family life is all about and it's just not happening that way. It's just that work has the place in your life that I thought the marriage would be.

RICK: So I'm not being the perfect husband right now because I'm not fitting into all these plans.

DEE: Well, I guess that's true. You're not being the way I assumed you would be. I'm really surprised. I don't appreciate it. I think it's getting time that I should just stop giving so much to it, I think.

RICK: You're really giving a whole lot.

DOHERTY: Let me ask you something. When you discuss these things at home do you stay this low-key, or do you sometimes get into loud arguments about this sort of thing?

RICK: She is the one who usually gets into a loud argument.

DEE: It's true, usually all by myself.

DOHERTY: When he comes home, what do you say to him?

DEE: Well . . .

RICK: Plenty.

DEE: Usually, I look at my watch and remind him of the fact that he mentioned that morning that he would be back at 5 and it's 6:30 and dinner is cold and then it reminds me of all the other things that he hasn't done all that week. Then he'll do one thing—one thing—like rake all the leaves in the yard and that's it. . . . As if that's his contribution for the month. Then nothing else happens.

RICK: You spend an awful lot of time talking about what I don't do. "You didn't do this, you could have come home sooner." Most of our conversations are about what I could have been doing had I come home on time. You don't realize that there are a lot of things that I'm dealing with.

DEE: Why don't you come home on time?

RICK: Because I have work to do.

DEE: Like what?

RICK: And you know that I'm the kind of guy that puts in a lot of time into his work. You knew this.

COMMENTS BY DOHERTY

This couple appears to be going through a difficult adjustment to marriage. The partners have not worked out their developmental task of accommodating each other's needs for companionship and individual freedom. In this sense, they are experiencing life cycle stress. In addition, they have developed the common interaction pattern of a wife pursuing a husband who keeps cool and distant. The rapid-fire intensity of their dialogue suggests a degree of marital enmeshment; Rick may be afraid of being smothered by Dee, who is in return feeling abandoned. Their level of adaptability or flexibility is not yet clear and probably won't be clear for another session or two.

Even though they both work, he's at home less and his wife is feeling neglected. That's a very common problem—even in very early marriages. What's gotten this couple into trouble is the way they're trying to solve this problem. I see problems as universal in marriage. What's happened here is that they are defining the problem as being owned by Dee. She wants more. Rick is saying that there is no problem. "I'm just doing what I have to do." He's being very cool about it. Dee is pursuing him—chasing him and trying to get more out of him—and he's just playing cooler and cooler, and she gets progressively more upset. At home they would be showing a lot more of the upset, and in future counseling sessions when they get to know me will be showing more of the upset. They're in a circle now, with Dee chasing Rick and Rick playing hard to get—very frustrating for them. You may have seen this at times in the discussion where they've both petered out. You know, "Here we go again—we've been this road before." So the reasons why they're here and why they need marital counseling is not because they have a problem with affection and distance, but because of the way they are trying to solve it. They are digging themselves deeper. The more Dee complains and nags—"Why aren't you home?"—the more Rick gets turned off. The more Rick gets turned off, the less he wants to be around her. The less he wants to be around her, the more she pursues him.

One of the things that I would be working on with a couple like this is to get the husband to say what *he* would like to see changed in the relationship. I will, of course, try to get the wife to make her requests in a calm way without nagging, but I also assume (unless I know otherwise) that he's dissatisfied too. So, I try to get him into the counseling by having him say, "This is what I'd like to see improved." The way they're going now, they're going nowhere. I have to get him involved and her making her requests in a straightforward way. The next segment will demonstrate my attempt to work out these short-term goals.

INTERVIEW SEGMENT

DOHERTY: I want you to continue the discussion, but from now on I will interrupt you if I think that I can help you say what you want better or help you express yourself in a way that would be more constructive. What I'm going to ask is for each of you to tell the other something that you would like that person to do differently, some kind of change you'd like to see in the relationship. Dee, since you have a lot of energy coming into this session, I'd like you to start. What would you like Rick to do differently?

DEE: Well, Rick, you're not doing your part in this marriage. You're not giving what I think you should be giving. I think that if that were changed I would feel a lot better. You're not . . .

DOHERTY: (*interrupting*) Dee, what I would like you to do is try to tell him not what he's not doing but tell him something that you would like more of, of what he is already doing.

DEE: That's really going to be hard.

DOHERTY: Some sort of change. What would you like him to do that would make you a happier wife in this relationship?

DEE: I want him to be a good husband. I want you to do what you're supposed to do to be a good husband.

DOHERTY: Give him an example.

DEE: You mean specifics?

DOHERTY: Ask him something that he could specifically do that would make your life happier right now.

DEE: Well, if you could come home when you say that you're going to come home and that if you could be there and not call up and say you're going to be late. There.

DOHERTY: Rick, would you respond to that?

RICK: Well, I try to do some of that. I just think that there are times that I just can't tell when I'm going to be late or not. I think that sometimes in the week I can't tell whether I'm going to be late or not, but I think sometimes during the week I could let you know and then stick to it. You just have to give me a little bit of leeway when something comes up and it's just not my fault if something comes up.

DEE: I think I give you a lot of leeway, and then you take it. Then I'm the one who ends up getting hurt every time.

DOHERTY: Rick, do you want to be home with her in the evening?

RICK: Yes, I do.

DOHERTY: Okay, tell her that.

RICK: I would much rather be home with you; I don't like working late, and I don't do it on purpose or anything. I just find it hard to take care of the things that I need to do with work. I would much rather be home much more than the way things are working out.

DOHERTY: Rick, I know that we haven't finished with that, but let me ask you, what would you like Dee to do different that would make this marriage happier for you? It's not easy to be complained about, and you feel like she's nagging you. What's something that Dee could do that would make life better for you in this marriage?

RICK: Dee, I would like it when I come home whether it's late or otherwise, is that we just start off our conversation with hello, we kiss each other hello—something other than the complaining. That really gets me after long days at work to come home and our first fifteen to twenty minutes of conversation are complaining. I would really like it that if when I just come home, even if you're a little upset, that we would just have a conversation about superficial things. Anything that isn't complaining. That's what I want.

COMMENTS BY DOHERTY

We would be dealing with these issues further, but there are two things that I want to point out that I'm trying to do here. One is that I'm trying to get Dee to make the changes she wants specific—make them positive in terms of her saying what she would like him to do. The way she started out was the way spouses often start out—"Stop neglecting me," "Stop being crude," "Do not do this." The other person does not feel in a mood to respond positively. Rick was threatened, and what I did was ask him to wait and for her to say what positive things she did want from him. Often what you can do is find out whether he does *anything* that she likes—that she would like him to do more of. He does come home on time sometimes and maybe he does give her a kiss. You can ask one spouse to request that the other do more of that behavior, rather than asking for a major personality change. A positive momentum for change might occur if they could settle one issue where both felt like they gained something, like working out a way that he would get home more regularly. If he couldn't get home, how could he let her know in a way that she wouldn't feel put down and then get angry at him later? That's what I was working at with Dee—specific requests, positive requests for a change.

What I did with Rick was to identify with the frustration that he feels. He wasn't putting his own words on that before, but I know that it must be hard to be complained about and that he must feel bad, and so I identified with those feelings. He joined the counseling session more at that point, and then I asked him to make the same sort of request that his wife did. A simple thing like he requested—like "Say, hello to me and let's kiss." It isn't the end of their problems, but it's a start in the right direction. Helping this couple early in their marriage will prevent years of gradually escalating resentment.

11 PRIMARY CARE COUNSELING FOR PARENT-CHILD PROBLEMS

Whether or not they are prepared for the role by training or experience, family physicians are expected by parents to be child-rearing experts. Interesting documentation for this cultural role of the physican has come from a study of the sources of child-care advice among Chicago parents. Clarke-Stewart (1978) found that parents reported they would turn to professionals (mostly physicians) more often than to relatives or friends or to books for help in a large number of problem situations. Table 11-1 reproduces Clarke-Stewart's findings. The problems parents would bring to a physician ranged from thumb sucking to disobedience to refusal to go to school. One other finding was that the more someone reported worrying about being a parent, the more likely he or she would be to consult a professional, most often a physician. For many parents, the family doctor has replaced Grandma.

Many of the problems parents bring to family physicians (and pediatricians) are not serious enough for referral to a therapist, but they are serious enough to merit primary care counseling. In fact, no other professional provides as many natural opportunities as the physician does for parents to raise questions and concerns about their children. Well-child visits and routine childhood illnesses place physician and parents in regular contact for a number of years. Any runny nose can serve as a ticket to talk to the doctor, although the doctor must be able to read between the lines on the ticket; otherwise, parents will be back and back and back. (Or they will find a doctor who can read.) Medical care of the rest of the family also allows for continual observation of the development of the child in his or her environment. But taking full advantage of this role requires explicit assessment and counseling approaches that go beyond the traditional common-sense wisdom of the country doctor. This chapter addresses these assessment and counseling issues.

TABLE 11-1. PERCENTAGES OF PARENTS TURNING TO SOURCES OF CHILD CARE ADVICE IN HYPOTHETICAL PROBLEM SITUATIONS

Specific problem situations when parents could consult an "expert"	Experts		Book
	Relative/friend (other than spouse)	Professional (mostly physicians)	
Infant crying all night, every night	38	94	27
Child slow to begin talking	28	83	23
Child won't do as told	20	29	21
Four-year-old sucking thumb	38	65	38
Toilet training	40	27	40
Child doing poorly in school	10	96	10
Child steals something from store	18	27	19
Child has no friends	29	65	21
Child wetting bed at night	17	85	33
Child wants to watch parent in shower	23	4	19
Child afraid of dark	15	35	33
Child always fighting with parents	17	48	19
Child refuses to go to school	21	64	9

Note. From K. Clarke-Stewart, "Popular Primers for Parents," *American Psychologist,* 1978, *33,* 359–369. Copyright 1978 by the American Psychological Association. Reprinted by permission of the author.

ASSESSMENT

When a parent brings a child-related psychosocial problem to the office, it is important to gather some symptomatic information about the problem. Sometimes it is possible to do this by talking with one parent alone or with one parent and the child together. Other times both parents and the whole family should be assembled for assessment; this will depend on the severity of the problem, the reliability of the reporting parent, and the physician's relationship with the other parent. Since we recommend a counseling approach that works through the parents to help their child, we generally discourage separate assessment sessions with the child alone. While making exceptions for such situations as treatment of venereal disease and adolescent boyfriend or girlfriend problems, we prefer to work with children in the context of their families. In addition, we recommend a problem-focused approach to assessment, rather than trying to understand how everyone in the family relates to everyone else. That is, the focus should be on the presenting problem or complaint—what goes on and what goes wrong. When parents ask for help with a "ping" in their family engine, they generally do not want the physician—the "mechanic"—poking around in their suspension system or kicking their tires. If the physician's efforts to solve the problem eventually lead to the shock absorbers, so be it, but it is best to keep the initial assessment tied directly to the presenting problem. We suggest that the following issues be assessed.

IS THE PROBLEM ONE OF BEHAVIOR OR OF EXPECTATIONS?

Sometimes parents' concerns stem from unrealistic expectations rather than from a problem in the child's development or from a disturbance in the parent–child relationship. Parents with little knowledge of normal child development may become alarmed when their baby sucks her thumb, or their toddler is slow to talk, or their 5-year-old lies when caught in a misdeed, or their adolescent wants to spend more time with his peer group than with the family. We do not wish to speak lightly of the pain that such unrealistic expectations can cause parents, but the family physician's approach to handling this pain will depend on its source. A 10-year-old who is fearful of going to school presents quite a different challenge than a new kindergartener with similar fears does. On the other hand, if unrealistic parental expectations come not from ignorance but from exaggerated needs for their children to be perfect in every way, then the counseling intervention will be far more difficult.

STRESSES ON THE CHILD AND THE FAMILY

When Doherty was a struggling graduate student (is there any other kind?), his 2½-year-old boy suddenly began wetting his bed, crying when left with a babysitter at night, and clutching his parents when left at preschool. The parents, at a loss to explain these new behaviors, consulted with one of the preschool faculty at the university. He inquired routinely, "Have there been any major changes in your family recently?" "Well, yes, come to think about it," the Dohertys replied. "We just had a new baby 3 weeks ago, we moved to a new apartment last week, and our son just started at a new preschool." Enough had been said: The child was responding to stress affecting the whole family. When the stress diminished, so did his symptoms.

External stressors, such as unemployment and a household relocation, affect children as much as adults and affect parent–child relationships in the family as much as the marital relationship. The Atlanta child murders of the early 1980s are a tragic example of the powerful influence of external events beyond the family on the emotional well-being of children. Child abuse experts believe that abuse increases as the national economy declines, leaving more parents out of work and demoralized. External stressors beyond the family's control must be assessed, lest the victim be blamed.

Internal stressors have an immediate, direct influence on children and their relationships with their families. Life cycle changes, such as the birth of a new sibling or the death of a grandparent, can temporarily unsettle children and parents alike. For some families, the very process of coping with the continuous growth and development of children can be quite taxing. As children grow more independent of parents, parents must grow more independent of children—an ongoing developmental task that challenges most families and overwhelms some. Haley (1980) has highlighted the hurdles of the leaving-home stage of the family life cycle. Parents whose marriages have been based on caring for dependent children may have great difficulty letting all the children go. One vulnerable child may "help them out" by not making it in the world and returning to the family nest.

Perhaps the most commonly experienced serious internal stressor in contemporary families is marital disruption. Although scholars disagree about the long-range effects of divorce on children and on parent–child relationships, in the short term it is clear that divorce is painful and emotionally unsettling for most children and adults (Bloom, Asher, & White, 1978). Most family members, however, appear to adjust eventually to their new circumstances and to regain their emotional equilibrium. But the remarriage of the custodial parent calls for difficult new adjustments for the family, which of course create new stresses for everyone. Family physicians would do well to pay careful attention to these family adjustment problems presenting as clinical "red flags" in the adults or the children.

Interaction Patterns

We offer three guidelines for assessing family interaction patterns that can contribute to child behavior problems.

1. *Get the details of the events surrounding the problem behavior.* Particularly important are the *sequences* of behavior that constitute the family's interaction pattern or "dance" on this issue. What is the context of the child's misbehavior—that is, where does it occur, when does it occur, who else is around, and what events does it immediately follow? For example, if Sara will not go to bed when asked to, does this occur every night or just some nights? When both parents are home or just one parent? When the other children are cooperating or not? When a babysitter is in charge or just when the parents are? Does she cause a scene only for Mom, or only for Dad, or both? These questions concern the *context* of the behavior. The second set of questions concerns the actual problem scenario itself: Who says and does what to whom? And in what sequence? How does the scene end? For example, Mom says, "It's time for bed, Sara." Sara goes to bed but keeps returning for another glass of milk or checking to see if she has enough

pencils for school the next day. Mom gets irritated each time, reminding her that it's bedtime. Dad silently reads the paper. Mom finally threatens Sara with a spanking if she comes out one more time. Then Mom goes off to take a shower or do the laundry in the basement. Sara comes out of her room one more time to ask Dad for a glass of milk. He agrees; Mom comes upstairs and threatens Sara, who says, "Daddy said I could have a glass of milk." Dad says, "I told her just one glass." Mom walks away in disgust.

2. *Look for the breakdown in the parents' efforts.* If a child chronically engages in disruptive or other inappropriate behavior, chances are the parents are behaving ineffectively in trying to handle the child. Examples include not informing the child clearly of parents' expectations, not setting up consequences for misbehavior, being inconsistent in enforcing consequences. In the bedtime scenario described above, one of the parents' mistakes is their failure to set up an unpleasant consequence to be imposed when the child comes out of her room. After repeated scoldings, the mother threatens to spank the child, but spanking is a notoriously inefficient method of discipline—not to mention the risk of abuse when the parent loses control. (By the way, we never tell parents to stop spanking their children; we try to help them develop alternative methods.) In summary, when you assess the behavioral sequences described by the parents and children, pay attention to the ways in which the parents behave ineffectively in coping with the child's behavior. Parents can best change children's behavior by changing their own behavior first.

3. *Examine relationships in the adult hierarchy for signs of noncooperation and undermining.* The adult hierarchy in a child's life consists mainly of parents, grandparents and other family members, and outside professionals. Haley (1980) proposes that chronic dysfunctional behavior in a child reflects disturbances in the adult hierarchy in the child's life. When parents do not support each other in dealing with the children, the effect is that of undermining each other's relationship with the children. In the bedtime example, one of the keys is the father's noninvolvement during the exasperating early rounds of the conflict, followed by his undermining his wife's authority by allowing the child to come out "one more time." This couple has probably learned their roles well: She comes on as angry but ineffectual, while he stays above the fray; at the point when she escalates the conflict with threats, he steps in to appease the child. The child carefully observes and takes advantage of this parental division.

Another common example of this parental cooperation problem with older children concerns the use of grounding as a punishment. The father gets angry at the child for misbehavior and sentences the child to an extended period of being grounded at home. But who stays home more to enforce the punishment? It is the mother, who has had no part in the decision to ground the child but who is unwilling to confront her husband about his unilateral decision. After a few days of pleading and manipulating by the child, the mother relents and grants a pardon from the grounding, but does not tell her husband. When the father finds out, he gets angry at his wife for not supporting him and feels more ineffective in controlling his child's behavior. Meanwhile, the mother and the child develop an artificial closeness based on her being the more "reasonable" or "sympathetic" parent. In full form, the family creates a cross-generational coalition of mother and child against father. The parental alliance breaks down, and the child or one of the adults may develop dysfunctional behavior or physical illness.

Sometimes the central problem in the adult hierarchy lies in the undermining influence of grandparents or outside professionals—anyone, indeed, who forms part of a triangular relationship with the child on the one hand and the parents on the other. These persons can be either supportive or undermining of the parents' relationship with the child. (The undermining is usually unintentional.) In one family we know, the husband's parents continually criticized his new wife (by remarriage) for her handling of her stepson—*their* grandchild. They criticized her in front of the child and enforced their own approach when the boy and his parents visited the grandparents' house. By not siding with his wife, the husband was pulled into a passive coalition with his parents. The boy's behavior became more and more bizarre around his stepmother, who, unfortunately, viewed the problem as a mental disturbance in the child. The boy behaved normally in school and other settings, but was caught up in—and playing for all it was worth—a major disturbance in the adult hierarchy in his life.

Outside experts can also unintentionally create problems for parents. Some professionals act like crusaders for children. They tell parents that their children need more love and attention, and they mutter to their colleagues about the child suffering from poor parenting—usually stated as poor *mothering* (fathers get off the hook more easily). Troublesome, too, are child-rearing experts who tell parents that they are hurting their children unless they follow a new, enlightened (and often franchised) approach to raising them. Parent Effectiveness Training (P.E.T.) is a leading example of a program that, in our judgment, can undermine parents' self-confidence by teaching that parents who do not use P.E.T. methods—which are quite difficult to apply consistently—are damaging their child's development and causing mental health problems (Doherty & Ryder, 1980). In the same way, a family's morale can be shattered when it is caught in a crossfire between the department of social services and the school system over school truancy, or between a physician and the school system over a diagnosis of "hyperactivity" versus that of "behavior problem." Outside professionals must cooperate if the family is to be helped and not damaged.

In summary, assessment of the interaction patterns—collaborative or undermining—of the adult relationships in the child's life is a cornerstone for parent–child problems. To give parents advice without knowing something about the adult hierarchy—particularly the parental alliance—is at best to court ineffectiveness and at worst to risk adding one more underminer to the family's list.

COHESION

Highly enmeshed families will overprotect children and overreact to stress affecting children. We have previously noted that this is part of the syndrome of the psychosomatic family. Parents may be obsessively concerned with the child's health and well-being. They will react negatively to other adults such as teachers who reprimand or challenge the child. Such parents labor under great fear of not being perfect parents. They need both support and challenge from their family physician.

Disengaged families at the other extreme, are generally so overwhelmed by stress or so disorganized that they do not take adequate care of their children's health and do not provide adequate discipline. In one family we know, the 14-year-old boy living with his alcoholic father frequently skipped school, rarely changed his underwear, and ate a poor diet. Such extreme cases require that the physician mobilize community resources to help the child and family.

Dysfunctional interaction patterns, such as one parent's undermining the other, are often accompanied by an enmeshed relationship between the child and one parent, and a more disengaged relationship between the child and the other parent. The child may have become a substitute spouse or a loyal friend to use against the spouse. Sometimes a child who is "special" in some way—for example, physicially handicapped, the "baby" of the family, or the first-born child—becomes the object of excessive attention from one parent at the expense of the child's autonomy and relationship with the other parent.

Generally, when one parent is overinvolved with the child and the other parent is underinvolved, the best initial counseling approach is to help the uninvolved parent get back into the parenting role, thereby relieving some pressure on the overintense dyad. In very dysfunctional families, such an intervention will be strongly resisted by the enmeshed parent, and a referral will be needed.

ADAPTABILITY

Assessment of the family's adaptability or flexibility can help the physician decide whether to work with the parent and child who present in the office (if only one parent comes in) or to bring together both parents and the rest of the children—or even members of the extended family. In the case of a single parent, the corresponding decision would be whether to involve the noncustodial parent or other significant adults such as grandparents. The more adaptable the family, the higher the likelihood that working with one parent may be successful; the less adaptable the family or the more severe the problem, the greater the need to call a family meeting. We do not repeat here the discussions of adaptability found in other chapters, except to say that adaptable parents are more willing to accept and follow through with ideas from a number of sources. Like the parents of the boy with headaches discussed in Chapter 8, they will collaborate with each other under stress; they will not label their child as "disturbed" and "hopeless"; and they will be open to alternative interpretations of their problems. Less adaptable parents are apt to have fixed on a single approach that is not working—such as excessive grounding or spanking—and are more likely to resist alternative interpretations and approaches. From them the physician will hear such statements as "I've already thought of that," and "I'll try it, but it won't work," and the perennial "Yes, but. . . ." Such families are generally in great pain and have become behaviorally cramped, as an overextended muscle becomes physically cramped. Their needs are beyond primary care treatment, but their problems must be assessed and referred at the primary care level.

COUNSELING APPROACHES

EDUCATION AND PREVENTION

In modern times, people become parents with less experience with children on the average than people in earlier generations had. As Americans have moved from the eight-child family in colonial times to the four-child family at the turn of the 20th century to the two-child family in the 1980s, many more individuals reach adulthood with little knowledge of the needs and behavior patterns of small children. Nor does a college education necessarily help much: Courses in child development offer little in the way of practical understanding of 2-year-old temper tantrums, 5-year-old stealing, and adolescent moodiness. Family physicians are unfortunately not well trained in these practical areas of parenting, since these issues fall outside the biomedical emphasis of pediatric rotations. However, family physicians usually have children and perhaps grandchildren of their own, and have the advantage of contact with a wide range of children and families. Therefore an experienced family physician can provide helpful educational and preventive counseling to improve the quality of parent-child relationships, to prevent child-rearing problems, and to help families deal with parent-child problems in the early stages. The best opportunities for such teaching occur during

well-child visits or routine illness visits when the parents are not highly
anxious about their child's health and when the physician is not preoccupied
with the biomedical aspects of patient care. Although the content of educational counseling should be specific to each family, we propose two general
categories of teaching: instruction in child development and strategies for
handling misbehavior.

CHILD DEVELOPMENT

Parents' reactions to children are determined to an important extent by the
parents' expectations of how children *should* behave at certain ages. We
have seen parents get quite stirred up at a 10-month-old girl for spilling her
glass of milk in the high chair, a 2½-year-old boy for wetting his pants, a 4-
year-old for refusing to talk to unfamiliar relatives, and an 8-year-old boy
for not being "responsible" enough to do his chores unsupervised. As Doherty
has observed elsewhere (Doherty, 1981a, 1981b), when parents with unrealistic expectations try to explain to themselves the unacceptable behavior of a
child, they tend to believe either that the child has a character flaw (stupidity,
laziness) or that the child is being willfully and purposefully rebellious.
Either interpretation leads to problems between parents and children. Physicians can intervene here by explaining to parents what level of performance
they can reasonably expect of their children. The belief that their child is
"normal" helps parents to relax and avoid overreacting to behavior that they
cannot change much anyway. In teaching child development to parents,
however, it is important to empathize with their frustration and concern
about the child's behavior and not just to say, "Don't worry about it. It's
normal." It is better to say, "I know how frustrating it can be to have to keep
checking up on Joey's work in the yard, but I'm afraid that most 8-year-olds
need pretty close supervision."

STRATEGIES FOR HANDLING CHILDREN'S MISBEHAVIOR

When parents ask their family physician for assistance in handling a problem
with a child, it is helpful to have a framework for how child discipline
problems can be handled. Although there is no universally effective approach, the following steps are ones we have found helpful in educating and
coaching parents to handling child's ordinary misbehavior:

   1. *Help parents define the problem in concrete, behavioral terms if
possible.* "Sara doesn't stay in her room at night" is a concrete and behavioral description of the problem as the parents see it. Avoid intrapsychic
or personality trait definitions of the problem, such as "She is such a
stubborn child that she won't stay in bed," or "She is trying to get back at us
by staying up at night." We recommend avoiding personality terms such as
"low self-esteem" or "overly aggressive" or "terribly shy" in accounting for
the child's behavior. The disadvantage of using these labels is that they leave

parents with little means of coping: They may be able to get Sara to stay in bed, stop fighting so often, or eat her breakfast, but there is little way they can directly change her stubbornness, decrease her aggressiveness, or increase her self-esteem. The other problem with personality trait explanations is that parents are apt to feel very guilty for having caused the personality defect in their child. Speak whenever possible about changing the child's *behavior* rather than the child's personality or attitudes.

2. *Put the child's behavior in a developmental context.* Much parent–child conflict can be understood within the context of the changing needs of the child for establishing autonomy and testing limits. Children will sometimes deliberately refuse to cooperate with their parents because of what the children feel is a more pressing need. Although such behavior is irritating and at times upsetting to parents, they can be helped to understand their children's developmental need to test authority. Parents, of course, have the responsibility of maintaining their authority, and that is why conflict is inevitable. Sometimes an understanding of the child's developmental needs brings forth a solution that helps the children meet their needs in a more appropriate manner. In one family we know, when the 5-year-old boy began stealing money under the influence of an older friend, the parents, realizing that their son needed money of his own, solved the problem by (a) curtailing their son's contact with the older boy, and (b) starting a regular allowance for their son, telling him he was old enough to have his own money. The parents also told him that future stealing would be punished severely. Both parents and child were happy with the outcome. The point is that some problem behaviors clear up when parents discover and respond to the child's underlying need—for example, for attention or for autonomy.

3. *Help the parents look at stress on the child and the family.* This is what the preschool teacher did in the earlier example of Doherty's son. Sometimes a child's behavior problems are a temporary manifestation of family stress. Some of these problems are best left for time to take care of, as when a previously sociable child is reluctant to make new friends after a move. If the problem continues for months, then perhaps help is needed. Other problems, such as Jimmy's beating up on his new baby sister, can be understood in developmental and family stress terms, but still must be dealt with directly.

4. *Help get the parents (and other members of the adult hierarchy) cooperating.* This is the crucial step often overlooked by physicians who advise parents. The triangle involving mother, father, and child must function well for the problem to be solved. In single-parent families, the third member of the triangle might be a grandmother, a friend, or the ex-spouse, but the single parent will need somebody's moral or physical support for trying new ways of handling problems with the children. Unfortunately, most books on child rearing and most child-rearing experts appear to assume that one parent handles one child in a social vacuum. We tell parents that if they work together they can handle practically any behavior problem their children present. And we believe this; it is not just a line. It should be

noted that we do not say that the parents *caused* the problem—only that they can probably handle it effectively if they cooperate with each other.

Helping parents collaborate involves relating to them as partners. This is best accomplished by seeing them together, but the process can be started with one parent alone (usually the mother). Specifically, it is important to stress to parents that it is up to them both to decide what behavior they want changed, and how they are going to handle infractions of their rules. When we see both parents together, we have them talk with each other to reach these agreements, rather than acting like parents ourselves by telling them how to handle their children. In the example of Sara's not staying in bed, we would ask the parents to reach an agreement about rules for bedtime that they could both enforce. Then we would have them agree on how to share the enforcement of these rules. All along we stress the importance of their teamwork, indicating that they can certainly cope with the problem if they work together.

The same principles of parental cooperation can be stressed with one parent seen individually, but then it is especially important to follow up to determine whether both parents have been able to use the counseling funneled through one partner. Flexible parents with generally collaborative relationships will be able to incorporate such input, especially if they both trust the physician. But if the initial interview with one parent reveals strong disagreement between the partners, then we recommend bringing in both parents to try to get the parental alliance working more effectively. Similarly, if a grandmother lives with the family or plays some other important child-rearing role, it may be advisable to invite her to the counseling session. Finally, if the parents are already getting advice or counseling from another professional, then the best guideline is to delay counseling until a division of leadership has been worked out with the other professional. Sometimes the family physician's best contribution can be to call a meeting of the various social agencies and school counselors who are working at cross purposes to help the family. The alternative is to become one more ineffective member of the professional hierarchy in the family's life.

In addition to helping parents (and other professionals) understand the problem and take on a collaborative frame of mind, we also teach several specific guidelines for handling children's misbehavior. The following sequence of actions draws a number of schools of thought on child rearing into a synthesis that seems to strike most parents as valid and commonsensical:

1. *The child should be clearly informed of the parents' expectations.* (Children, of course, should be consulted about their wishes, but the final decision should generally be made by the parents.) Often the rule has not been made clear to the child, in part because it was not clear or agreed upon by both parents. At any rate, the expectation must be clear and concrete: for example, "No leaving your room after 9 P.M."; "Curfew at midnight on Fridays and Saturdays"; "Chores must be done before play on Saturday."

2. *Consequences for noncompliance should be established, and the child should be informed of these consequences in advance.* We prefer the term "consequences" to "punishment" because the former conveys the sense that the child can anticipate an identified reaction to an infraction of the rule. "Punishment" is often what parents decide on impulsively after the misdeed has been done. Although we ask the parents to generate the consequences, we suggest that these actions be clearly spelled out, appropriate to the offense, and consistently enforced. We also suggest that consequences be of relatively short duration, so that the child can get back into the parents' good graces by choosing to cooperate the next time. For example, the child must go to bed early the day after a bedtime rule infraction, or must be grounded the next weekend night after the curfew violation, or must stay home until the chores are done. Some consequences can take the form of parents letting the children face the inevitable result of their nonresponsible behavior, such as letting an oversleeping child be late for school or a sloppy teenager go without clean clothes as a consequence of not putting clothes in the dirty-clothes pile. We discourage long-term consequences, such as a month's grounding, because these tend to be demoralizing to the child, to be difficult to enforce for the parents, and to provide no early opportunity for the child to show a change of heart. A consequence generally does not have to be severe in order to make the point. But it does have to be consistently enforced; in fact, we tell parents to expect the child to test their resolve to impose the consequence. Children will behave like children, and parents must behave like parents.

3. *The behavior should be monitored regularly and parents should stay flexible.* The parents should discuss from time to time how the new system is working. Since no discipline approach is perfect, modifications might have to be made. The parents may have chosen an ineffective consequence, say, if the child does not care about not watching TV or would prefer to be late for school. If a consequence is not working even though it is consistently enforced, then parents should switch to another one or come back in for further counseling to understand what has gone wrong. A common mistake is to keep escalating one consequence—for example, grounding the child for a day, then for a week, then for a month, then till age 18. Particularly if the breakdown has been one in the parents' teamwork, further counseling may be necessary. To repeat our article of faith, parents who work together and stay flexible can handle almost any child-rearing problem.

SUPPORT

Parents need support all the time, but particularly when living through their children's illnesses and difficult developmental phases. A sick child is often a source of guilt and self-doubt for parents: "What did I do wrong? What early sign did I miss? Why is my child getting sick so often?" Parents often feel terrifically responsible for their children's illnesses. They feel especially vulnerable to criticism from other members of the adult hierarchy—physicians and relatives—about their handling of their children's health. Thus opportunities abound for family physicians either to support or to undermine parents of sick children. It is not enough to care for the sick child; the parents need care and attention as well. On this point, the study by Korsch and Negrette (1972) on 800 pediatric patients and their mothers found that 300 of the mothers held themselves responsible in some way for the child's illness. Tape recordings of the resident–child–mother interactions revealed that in most cases the physician gave no attention to the mother's own feelings. Not surprisingly, mothers who felt that their needs were not met tended to be grossly noncompliant with the physician's orders. The physicians had failed to create a cooperative therapeutic triangle.

Supportive counseling for parents of a sick child involves talking directly with the parents about the issue of responsibility. If there is little way the parents could have prevented the problem, tell them so. Listen to their self-doubts, but calmly repeat your assessment of the cause of the child's illness. Parents of seriously ill children may feel guilt that they do not express directly. Ask them if they feel responsible for their child's condition, then counsel them accordingly. In addition to support concerning their responsibility for the sickness, parents also need encouragement for coping with a sick child. For instance, although it is easy for the physician to write a prescription, it can be torture for parents to get the medicine down the child's throat. Medication taking is an issue of control between parents and child; the child needs encouragement and firm insistence from the parents, who need the same from the physician.

A second area of supportive counseling concerns helping parents accept what they cannot change. A sense of compassion tinged with humor helps here: There is nothing to be done to change the willfulness of a 2-year-old, the restlessness of a 10-year-old, a teenager's relentless pursuit of peer acceptance, or sibling rivalry at any age. Parents can change specific disruptive behaviors in their children, but they have precious little control over normal developmental progressions. Parents can be told that these parenting hassles are part of the universal burden of parenthood—the stuff that was not even in the fine print of the warranty that came with the children. At the same time, you can help them understand that most parents—including yourself if appropriate—survive these tribulations, many of which become the funny stories of later family reunions. The multilayered message is this: "I understand you, I know it's hard; however, your child is normal, you are a normal parent, and I think you will make it through together." This message was delivered most often by grandparents in the past; modern parents may turn as readily to their physicians.

An important support that physicians can offer parents is to help them find outside people and agencies to support them during difficult times. Especially useful are self-help groups of parents with common problems such as a developmentally disabled child. Some parents are reluctant to ask family and friends to help them, preferring to cling to their physician. Family physicians can be at best only part-time and expensive grandmothers. It is often better to help the parents get back in touch with the real thing.

To recapitulate, the two generic areas for mainly supportive counseling are childhood illness and normal parent-child concerns. Physicians can both offer personal support and help the parents find outside helpers. Of course, every counseling approach must have a heavy component of support, for without it education becomes pedantic or patronizing and challenge becomes rejecting. Support for people with the world's most complex job—parenthood—is the heart of primary care family counseling.

CHALLENGE

When parents turn to a physician for counseling, the physician takes on a quasi-parental role to the parents and therefore a kind of grandparental role to the children. Put in Haley's hierarchical terms, the expert outranks the parents, who outrank the children. (Unlike grandparents, physicians can be hired and fired by the parents, but as long as the therapeutic triangle is still functioning, the physician holds the elevated status of an expert.) Therefore, the physician has a special prerogative to challenge parents to change their way of handling their children. Such challenges should be made sparingly and cautiously until a physician-family bond has been created. The safest approach is to challenge parents to follow through on what they have already decided to do with their children. In other words, the physician should start with changes the parents already want to make and challenge them to persevere.

MOTHER: Sara just won't stay in bed, no matter what I try.

PHYSICIAN: I am sure that if you and your husband get together on this, Sara can learn to stay in bed.

MOTHER: She's so stubborn.

PHYSICIAN: Not so big and not so stubborn that she can't be handled if you put your minds to it.

When patients are giving up on a problem, one option for the physician is to confront them rather than sympathize with them. In the above example, the physician is behaving firmly with the parents so that they will behave firmly with their daughter. A good rule of thumb for physicians is this: *Treat patients as you would have them treat others.* If the parents need to be more assertive with their children, the physician should be assertive with the parents. In so doing, the physician is effectively using the therapeutic relationship with the parents and modeling a form of caring authority. By challenging the parents and not the child, the physician is acknowledging their primary responsibility for their own children. If the physician personally tries to cajole or frighten Sara into staying in bed, he or she will probably not succeed with Sara and will almost certainly confuse the roles in the therapeutic triangle. The parents will probably report back next week that this effort failed. What does the physician do next—adopt her?

In addition to challenge as part of ongoing primary care counseling, sometimes parents need a challenge that leads to a referral for family therapy. This can be done in a kind of "bad news and good news" format. First, the physician should tell the parents that the problems they are having with their child appear serious enough to warrant specialized help from a family therapist—that the physician may have given all the help he or she can. Second (the good news), the physician should tell them that he or she wants to send them to a well-qualified family therapist who has had considerable success with the kinds of problems they are having. The physician should say this, of course, only if it is true; if it cannot be said, the physician should find a therapist about whom it *can* be said. At this point, the focus of the challenge should be to help the parents see that they need specialized help. Ultimately, the physician can make continued supportive counseling contingent on their accepting the referral. In the case of child abuse, the physician can tell the parents that the law requires doctors to report unexplained children's injuries: "I am not accusing you of being bad parents, but I legally must report my findings." This is certainly bad news for parents. The good news is a promise to stay with them as their physician in order to support them through whatever investigation will follow and whatever help they need. Reporting child abuse while remaining the family physician—this is the sternest challenge in providing primary care for parent–child problems.

Physicians are understandably reluctant to challenge patients' behavior. Even for direct health hazards such as cigarette smoking, physicians sometimes neglect to ask whether their patients smoke and often make only the blandest confrontations of patients who do smoke. In the psychosocial realm, physicians are even more squeamish—partly for good reason, since patients have the right to privacy and personal autonomy. On the other hand, patients are often more willing to accept challenge than physicians give them credit for. If parents ask their physician for advice about handling their children, the physician can presume they are granting permission to challenge them constructively. If they agree to follow through on some new procedure with their child, and then fail to do so, they probably expect to be confronted about their lapse. If the physician tries to be too nice and does not pursue what went wrong, the parents ironically may feel unsupported. There is a primitive sense in all of us that can be expressed as follows: "If you care for me, you will challenge me when I am out of line or when I need a push." This notion captures the place of challenge in primary care counseling.

THE DISRUPTIVE CHILD IN THE OFFICE:
A COUNSELING APPROACH

This chapter concludes with a practical example of primary care counseling for parent-child problems. When the child's behavior in the doctor's office is disruptive, the situation can be irritating and frustrating for parents, physicians, and staff alike. The therapeutic triangle is never more exciting than when a child is tearing up the office, especially when the parent acts helpless and the physician grows angrier by the minute. These situations can be turned into useful counseling opportunities. In the following scenario, the physician demonstrates a variety of counseling approaches, including education, support, challenge, and prevention.

A mother (Mrs. T); a 4-year-old boy, Johnny; and the physician are in the examining room. Johnny has presented with a sore throat. The physician has examined him, has told him what was wrong with his throat, and is now explaining the findings to the mother. Johnny starts to open the desk drawers and rattle them around. His mother ignores him.

PHYSICIAN: Mrs. T, would you tell your son not to play with drawers in the office?

MOTHER: Johnny, stop that.

JOHNNY: I'm not doing anything.

MOTHER: You are so, now cut it out. Don't play with those drawers.

[The physician goes on with the explanation of findings, and then notices that Johnny is still opening and closing the drawers. The mother ignores him again.]

PHYSICIAN: Johnny is still playing with the drawers.

MOTHER: Johnny, stop that this instant.

JOHNNY: I'm not hurting anything.

MOTHER: I don't care, get away from that desk.

[Johnny leaves the desk and then goes over to the door and begins to open and close it.]

PHYSICIAN: Do you have this kind of trouble with Johnny at home?

MOTHER: All the time. He just won't listen.

PHYSICIAN: What would you do with him at home if he were acting like this?

MOTHER: I'd probably wallop him a good one.

PHYSICIAN: Does that work?

MOTHER: Well, it works for a while, but he seems to go right back to it again.

PHYSICIAN: Can I make a suggestion about what you can do with him here?

MOTHER: Sure.

PHYSICIAN: Why don't you tell him that if he won't wait for a couple of minutes until you're finished without bothering anything in the room, you're going to make him sit in your lap?

MOTHER: Okay, Johnny, If you don't get away from that door, I'm going to make you come over here and sit in my lap. You won't be able to do anything in the room.

[Johnny walks away from the door and sits down in a chair. The adults go back to the conversation. A minute later Johnny is back over at the door turning the knob. The mother looks over and sees him but says nothing.]

PHYSICIAN: Mrs. T, one of the things that may go wrong when you discipline Johnny is that you tell him you're going to do something and then you wait until he pushes you really far before you act. Does that happen at home?

MOTHER: Yeah, I guess it does.

PHYSICIAN: Now that you see him over there, turning the doorknob, why don't you follow through on what you said you were going to do?

[The mother walks over to the door, picks Johnny up, and brings him back over to her chair. Johnny struggles for a moment but then settles down. The physician and the mother finish the conversation. The physician and Johnny chat for a while. Before they leave, the physician adds another bit of advice.]

PHYSICIAN: The next time you bring Johnny in, why don't the two of you talk about some kind of treat that he could get if he cooperates when he comes here, so he feels like he has some reason to cooperate? You could also bring a coloring book for him. If he doesn't cooperate, you can tell him what's going to happen—what sort of consequence there will be if he doesn't settle down. The one you used today of having him on your lap seemed to work. He would rather sit in his own chair, or maybe color, then have to be confined. It would be up to him whether he would be confined to your lap. He can bring that about by tearing up the office. You've got a challenging little boy here.

MOTHER: You're telling me.

PHYSICIAN: Does your husband have trouble controlling him too?

MOTHER: No, he does what his daddy says. He's afraid of his daddy. But I couldn't handle him the way his father handles him.

PHYSICIAN: How's that?

MOTHER: His father is so big and strong that he just has to look cross-eyed at Johnny and Johnny shapes up.

PHYSICIAN: Well, I bet you're also home a lot more with Johnny. You know, the effect wears off when somebody is around a child all the time.

MOTHER: That's right.

PHYSICIAN: So you have to find your own style of dealing with Johnny, and it may not be one that is based on physical size. I hope your husband comes in some time with you so I can see how he handles Johnny. Anyway, we can talk about those things some other time if you like. Meanwhile, I think it would be a good idea if you continue to let Johnny know what you want of him the next time he comes into the office—what you expect from him. And follow through with him if he doesn't cooperate. If you can help this boy channel some of this energy, he's going to be a great one.

MOTHER: Energy, he's got plenty of. I just hope we can handle him.

PHYSICIAN: I think you can.

This vignette demonstrates a way to do primary care family counseling during interactions that occur when a parent, a child, and the physician are together in the same room. The physician's office is different from home, and parents may not be sure of their authority there. But if the child is out of control and the parents are ineffective in gaining control in the doctor's office, chances are that this occurs at home as well. We recommend putting the parents in charge of the child's behavior when they are in the physician's office. This keeps the hierarchical relationships clear. The physician is in charge of the office, and the parents are in charge of the child. The physician controls the child through making expectations clear to the parents. In the above vignette, the physician's counseling finally is successful in helping the mother gain control of her child. If this counseling does not work, however, the physician must intervene directly to handle the child's behavior. Otherwise, the child is in control of both the parents and the physician. The physician's discipline of the child should be done in such a way as to model the kind of discipline that the physician is suggesting to the parents. Subsequently, every effort should be made to get the parents back in control.

The physician's office is the best laboratory available for primary care parent-child counseling. In the case of the disruptive child, such counseling stands to benefit everyone in the therapeutic triangle, including the physician and all who work in the office.

12 TREATING CHEMICAL DEPENDENCY IN A FAMILY CONTEXT

Most family physicians see patients daily who abuse, misuse, or are dependent upon alcohol or other drugs. The national incidence of alcoholism is estimated at 5 to 7% of the general adult population (Clark & Midonik, 1980; Zarafonetis, 1972). This does not include dependency upon other drugs. A recent survey in hospitalized patients in a large metropolitan area recorded that 20% of the general hospital patients were chemically dependent as measured by standard alcoholism questionnaires and specific laboratory tests (Briggs, Malerich, Hafner, Magee, & Michaelson, 1980). A 1975 study of diagnoses on hospital discharge summaries listed 424,000 cases of alcoholism for short-term hospital stays (National Center for Health Statistics, 1975). This does not include admission for alcoholism treatment centers. Baird's practice surveys have shown a 7 to 8% incidence of chemical dependency problems in office patients. Each day the impact of chemical abuse and dependency touches a family physician, but the problem may not always be apparent.

ASSESSMENT

DIAGNOSIS OF CHEMICAL DEPENDENCY

We begin with a functional definition of "chemical dependency," a term synonymous with "substance abuse." A person is chemically dependent when he or she demonstrates preoccupation with using alcohol or other chemicals to the point of producing substantial continuing or recurring interference with a major life area—especially family, work, or health. If problems in these areas are associated with chemical use, then chemical dependency is an appropriate diagnosis (Criteria Committee, 1972). Physical dependency suggests serious withdrawal effects and is estimated to be present in less than 5% of alcoholics (Criteria Committee, 1972; Seixas, 1976). This functional definition of "chemical dependency" is more sensitive than a definition based upon physical dependency and subsequent withdrawal effects. Frequently the first sign of dependency is recurring serious conflict with other family members (Weinberg, 1976). Eventually a rigid interaction pattern of nonresolution of conflicts is created. Family coping skills become diminished. Hope, self-esteem, and optimism gradually become rare commodities in these families (Wegescheider, 1981). *If the family physician fails to review family relationships in the assessment of patients, then the ability to diagnose early stages of chemical dependency is essentially lost.* Only when late complications occur—such as obvious health deterioration—can the routine physical or history reveal chemical dependency. For adolescents, some experts believe that chemical "abuse" is a more appropriate term than "dependency" because of shorter duration of chemical use among younger persons (Donovan & Jessor, 1976). However, we use the term "chemical dependency" when referring to both adult and adolescent problems related to drug use.

Physicians are often reluctant to risk early intervention for chemical dependency problems because of the uncertainty of a diagnosis based on a routine day-to-day history and a routine exam. Reluctance based upon this type of information is justified, since clear evidence will be lacking until very late in the course of the illness. It is parallel to diagnosing breast cancer only by looking for metastatic axillary nodes while avoiding the examination of the breast itself. To repeat, the traditional history and physical exam will only uncover chemical dependency late in its course, after it has seriously damaged family structure and begun to influence the patient's occupational, economic, and physical health systems negatively. At these later stages, the prognosis in chemical dependency is less optimistic. There are often irretrievable physical and emotional losses even with the best of treatments. The physician and patient may then rationalize a passive, nonintervening approach based on mutual fatalism. A common patient plea is "I can't change now, Doc, I've been drinking for 20 years." A physician who views chemical dependency problems as untreatable will not challenge such a statement. Many physicians have never seen the excellent results of early intervention and have seldom asked relationship questions that reveal the true pain of the illness in its early stages. Since early intervention is an unfamiliar activity to most physicians, and since physicians also rarely see excellent outcomes from later diagnosis and treatment, it is no mystery that chemical dependency is underrecognized in its early stages and usually treated with pessimism late in its course. The upshot is that physicians avoid dealing with the problem at all.

Even late in the course of chemical dependency, physicians may still not recognize the problem unless the family is included in the interview. A case in point is the occurrence of blackouts. Blackouts provide conclusive support for the diagnosis of alcoholism (Weinberg, 1976). Even though the dependent person looks awake, speaks fairly clearly, drives a car, and generally appears to be functioning well, that person will have no memory for events that transpire during the blackout. Great skill in disguising these memory lapses will be developed by these patients and their families. Many are not fully aware of why this frustrating amnesia occurs or even that it is caused by long-term alcohol or drug abuse. Although such blackouts are a common problem late in the course of alcoholism, family physicians often fail to recognize this symptom. A careful history taken from the entire family may be needed to uncover such a puzzling problem. These symptoms will almost never be discovered from talking only with the dependent person alone. Denial of the illness, fear of discovery, and a real lack of understanding block such disclosures. However, a family interview focusing on the patient's failure to recall conversations, assigned tasks, and everyday events can reveal this symptom unmistakably. In the absence of other neurological diseases, the history of blackouts should erase all doubts as to the diagnosis of alcoholism and/or other chemical dependency (Criteria Committee, 1972). (Even then the diagnosis will be missed unless the physician carefully considers chemical dependency in the differential diagnosis; see Weinberg, 1974). Since blackouts indicate advanced chemical dependency, treatment should be aggressive and should be initiated as soon as possible.

"Alcoholism" and "chemical dependency" are sometimes avoided as diagnostic terms because of their negative connotations. The diagnosis of "hypertension" faced similar obstacles as recently as 10 years ago. The patient with mild to moderate elevations of blood pressure was treated gingerly with advice to "slow down" or "relax," or was asked to return endlessly until one normal blood pressure was recorded. The perceived economic and social impact of the label "hypertension" encouraged physicians to avoid the diagnosis. Identified hypertensive patients were usually hospitalized, given extensive laboratory workups, and put on harsh treatment regimens. Such aggressive treatment was reserved for patients suffering late complications such as congestive heart failure, stroke, or myocardial infarction. Fortunately, a massive public and professional educational program over the past decade has taught physicians to make an early diagnosis of hypertension, to perform reasonable outpatient evaluations (which rarely prove an etiology for the hypertension), and to begin a rational therapy plan that is convenient enough to ensure compliance. Now physicians readily diagnose hypertension at earlier and earlier stages, with less disruptive impact upon the patient and with documented improvements in longitudinal outcome.

A parallel approach could be effective for chemical dependency, but the massive education campaign has not yet begun (Council on Mental Health, 1972). For chemical dependency, as for hypertension, we have a clinical condition for which an exact etiology is still unknown (Eckardt, Harford, Kaelber, Parker, Rosenthal, Ryback, Salmoiraghi, Vanderveen, & Warren, 1981). The negative implication of the diagnosis still causes many physicians to hesitate to use it. Treatment is often initiated only after late complications have occurred. Few physicians are trained to investigate the early signs of chemical dependency, particularly the health of the patient's close relationships. Even fewer physicians have had the opportunity to observe the impact of successful early intervention in a chemically dependent family. It is a rare physician indeed who has a working knowledge of the therapeutic process involved in chemical dependency treatment and recovery programs. Therefore, the idea of early intervention and treatment for chemical dependency is unfamiliar or unpopular with many physicians. Because of the high incidence of this illness and its devastating impact on patients and families, chemical dependency education deserves a high priority in the training of family physicians. The key to this training will not be to develop more sensitive liver function tests to establish the diagnosis of alcoholism. The key will be to help primary physicians to view individual patients as part of a social context. Then train the physician to evaluate that patient and his or her social and family systems for significant disturbances that commonly occur in chemical dependency. By evaluating the presenting patient in a family context, the primary physician has the means to discover chemical dependency in early stages when treatment options are less disruptive; when outcome is improved; and when emotional and economic losses to the patient, family, and community are reduced. Early family-centered intervention is an effective and achievable task that can result in many rewards for patients, families, and physicians (Wegescheider, 1981).

FAMILY ASSESSMENT

How can the family physician interact with the patient in a manner that would lead to early diagnosis and treatment of chemical dependency? Viewing the patient as part of the family system is an essential first step. The myth of the physician–patient dyad and the functional reality of the triangular patient–physician–family relationship should be recalled. With the "shadow" of the family always present, the physician can move from reviewing individual health and psychological systems to reviewing family relationships (Ireton & Cassata, 1976). The family physician will be in contact with the nonusing members of the dependent family. Some ways to learn about disturbed family relationships, mentioned in earlier chapters, are appropriate here. During a routine examination of a married male for insurance purposes or a general health maintenance physical examination, a physician can inquire about his wife's or children's health. During periodic gynecological and Pap smear exams, a physician can ask about the woman's relationship with her husband. In this setting, a question about sexual discomfort or dyspareunia can provide helpful information for evaluating the marital relationship. At other times, "How is your husband's health?" or "How is your husband feeling these days?" is a benign opener. If there is hesitation or other communication of tension in the patient's response, it may indicate something stressful about the marital relationship. Responses such as "I don't know, I rarely see him," "Okay most of the time when he behaves himself," or "Fine, except for Monday morning, when he's hung over," may indicate significant conflict and the possibility of chemical dependency. Gentle follow-up questions such as "What does he enjoy doing for fun or relaxation?" can sometimes allow the spouse to describe the partner in a nondefensive manner. A direct question such as "How do you two get along?" is rarely productive unless the patient already has a trusting relationship with the physician; a common response is "Oh, just fine," even when serious problems exist.

If major family conflict is revealed by the index patient, the physician must be careful not to accept a unilaterally described villain role for any family member. The family systems perspective described in this book implies that all family members play a role in the maintenance of and recovery from relationship problems. An empathic physician can listen carefully to harsh complaints about another family member without absolving the primary patient of responsibility for part of the problem and for seeking change. If the patient acknowledges recurring conflict, then the physician must ask if alcohol or other drug use is associated with the conflicts. In Baird's own practice survey, major family conflict was accompanied by alcohol or drug use in nearly 80% of the cases. Interestingly, the incidence of chemically associated conflicts seems to be much lower in Baird's practice for patients referred from churches, schools, and social agencies where the referral originates outside the primary physician–patient relationship. These different rates of chemical problems may be related to the high use of medical services and avoidance of underlying conflict by chemically dependent families. Families with less rigid, short-term conflicts may utilize other nonmedical resources to resolve conflicts more directly and may not see physicians as often. Or more advanced chemically dependent patients may get physically ill and then seek medical care.

The following sections discuss how our formal family assessment categories can be used for viewing chemical dependency in a family context. Major variables to be discussed are stress, cohesion, adaptability, and observable interaction patterns.

WHAT ARE THE STRESSORS THAT HAVE AFFECTED THIS FAMILY?

External stressors such as job dissatisfaction, recurrent auto accidents, school problems, and chronic financial difficulties may be more prominent in chemically dependent families where organization and ability to perform daily tasks are impaired. Life cycle transitions such as adjustment to new children in the family, children leaving the home, or retirement are common times for latent chemical dependency problems to surface. Adaptation to these internal stressors is difficult for many families but may be totally impossible for a family impaired by chemical dependency. If the family seems overwhelmed by internal and external stressors and unable to cope with life cycle challenges, the physician should look carefully for chemical dependency somewhere in the family.

HOW ADAPTABLE OR HOW RIGID IS THIS FAMILY?

By taking a history of the growth of the family unit and its experience over time, the physician may see a picture of the family's inability to change as its environment changes. In severely impaired families where conflicts have been unresolved for many years and the drinking problem has been entrenched for two or three generations, there may be very low adaptability. Such inflexibility may show itself in the family's inability or unwillingness to comply with simple physician requests such as arriving at a requested family meeting. Extreme resistance to any physician intervention may indicate inability to adapt not only to the physician's request but to any new demand on the family. If this is the case, the physician and family must be careful not to expect quick results. A long-term but optimistic stance is the only helpful approach. If the physician has expectations of rapid changes in this family, the intervention is doomed. A long-term intervention is more helpful, especially one involving generous support to the family during its struggle for recovery. Even minor changes are important and demonstrate improvement. This patience is especially difficult for physicians accustomed to treating acute illness; in addition, the physician will need support from chemical dependency counselors and other mental health professionals. On the other hand, if the chemical dependency pattern is of recent origin, the family may be fairly adaptable and may respond quickly to requests for change. There is generally a close relationship between the level of family adaptability and the degree of chronicity of the chemical dependency.

HOW COHESIVE IS THIS FAMILY?

Is the family enmeshed to the point where treatment of one person is threatening to all family members, and all collaborate to avoid therapeutic intervention? Is one spouse reluctant to confront the other because both spouses are drinking? These are common problems in resistance to early intervention. An extreme level of conflict between an adolescent and a parent may signal an enmeshed relationship that would make treatment of one party difficult without working with both of them simultaneously. A classic example of such a family would be one with a chemically dependent father who has a very hostile, explosive relationship with a 15- or 16-year-old daughter. The mother in this family may present with fatigue and/or depression while struggling with her caretaker role, which denies her own needs and prevents other family members from facing their conflicts in a realistic fashion. In such a family the caretaker/mother may be the most difficult to engage in a new behavior pattern. It may be extremely useful to begin with Al-Anon training and support for her even before the other relationships are addressed or the drinking behavior is challenged. If sexual abuse is discovered, it should be managed with an additional focus on the chemical dependency. Such compounded problems are best treated by a therapeutic team rather than by the family physician alone.

At the other end of the spectrum, extreme levels of disengagement are sometimes demonstrated when the nondrinking spouse presents with concrete plans of divorce prior to any intervention by the physician. Engaging a couple with disengaged boundaries—when neither feels involved with the other—is quite difficult. It is useful to encourage education and supportive involvement in Al-Anon prior to making final decisions about ending the marriage. The chemically dependent spouse may be interested in "changing for the sake of my spouse." However, unless the chemical use behavior is changed for internal purposes as well as for the purpose of "saving the marriage," the treatment plan may become a manipulation whose purpose is simply to save the marriage and not to really change the nature of the relationship. This type of problem—like serious family enmeshment—requires intervention beyond the primary care level. The physician can seek help through experienced chemical dependency counselors and/or family therapists with experience in chemical dependency.

WHAT ARE THE FAMILY'S PROBLEMATIC INTERACTION PATTERNS?

The interaction patterns of chemically dependent families are the primary basis for the diagnosis. How has the family's interaction become stabilized around chemical dependency? Are conflicts chronically unresolved or buried? Do conflicts frequently occur at the time of chemical use by one member? Do spouses express their feelings for each other only when one of them is drinking, as Steinglass, Davis, and Berenson (1977) found in their study of alcoholic spouses? If so, the alcoholism may be functional for maintaining marital cohesion. If one spouse is chemically dependent, a teenage child in the family may have assumed the role of a spouse or parent. There may be physical or sexual abuse within the family system. Previously described blackout interactions may be occurring but left disguised or hidden by those involved. A common pattern is for the father to be drinking in an irresponsible pattern, acting out through violence or verbal abusiveness, and ending up feeling more and more isolated from his family. His wife may be both angry at him and protective of him, alternatively pleading with him to stop drinking and buying him liquor (Wiseman, 1980). He may present to the physician's office with fatigue or nonspecific sexual dysfunction. The context of his symptoms cannot be easily evaluated without interviewing the other spouse. In another example, a mother who is chemically dependent may be withdrawn and unable to do normal household activities or may be failing at work outside the home. She may initially be diagnosed as depressed. A careful family interview is needed to uncover covert prescribed medication or alcohol ingestion. In these and many other cases, a family interview is necessary for an accurate assessment not only of chemical ingestion but also of the family interaction patterns that dominate the lives of chemically dependent families.

To repeat our perspective: If the family's conflicts occur primarily at times of alcohol or drug use, or are precipitated by use, then the most likely diagnosis is chemical dependency. If other types of conflict such as parent–child violence or child behavior problems cannot be discussed without drug or alcohol use being mentioned, then the chemical use may be the underlying problem. Any serious conflict that recurs again and again, despite lay or professional intervention, warrants a careful family interview to evaluate chemical use in the family.

ASSEMBLING THE FAMILY

After establishing a preliminary diagnosis of chemical dependency, the physician should ask that the entire family come in for an interview. The more people who can come, the more information that can be obtained. In reality it is often difficult for an entire family to attend. The problem of noncompliance with the request is minimized if the physician is interacting with the family from a hospital setting. Here the social power of the physician is maximized. A hospital family conference is most helpful if the chemically dependent person is the identified patient. Under these circumstances, attempts to assemble the family are almost always successful. If hospitalized, the dependent person has less opportunity to avoid the interview. Other family members usually perceive hospitalization as a major family event and are geared for action. The inconvenience of the interview can often be overlooked under these circumstances.

In a clinic (office) setting, the dependent person may not come immediately upon request but will arrive eventually, if repeatedly invited in a nonaccusing manner. The physician must remember that there are no family villains, even those who stay away from family counseling. A series of family visits can be scheduled without the dependent member. Each visit can offer support for changing family interaction patterns, despite the dependent member's lack of participation. These visits may be kept brief until the absent member finally arrives. It may take weeks or months, but most people will participate eventually out of curiosity or a need to defend themselves. A calm family systems approach is of the utmost importance in this setting, with the emphasis placed upon the role that every family member plays in the maintenance of this illness.

Let us assume that the family is assembled. The group as a whole is tense and uncomfortable. In a hospital environment there may be a feeling of urgency in the air; however, in the clinic there may be skepticism about the need for the meeting. The physician may recognize these and other "moods" as the interview begins. The session should begin as all family counseling sessions should: Introduce yourself and other staff members, have a brief time of social conversation, and then recognize all family members present. We suggest beginning with the question "What is it like to live with this family?" Ask the question and then let them talk. The goal is to help the family face the conflict. The physician can become a too active member of this group and can stifle any meaningful conversation the family members may have among themselves.

After the initial silence or cautious statements that everything is fine, usually someone in the family will be honest enough to discuss the problem. If the physician can allow the discussion to proceed with minimal interference, most families will interact honestly. Ask each family member for his or her perspective; do not permit family members to speak for someone else or interrupt one another. It is often helpful to paraphrase what each member has expressed.

If the conflict seems to be recurrent, upsetting to more than one person, and associated with the use of alcohol or other drugs, then you will probably confirm the diagnosis of a chemically dependent family. One member of the family may be identified as "the drinker" or "the user," but all members play a role in the drama. If the person identified as dependent is not offered some support during this initial interview, the villain role will be perpetuated and the next stage of treatment may be handicapped. The identified user is as much a victim in this process as other "abused" family members are. There may also be more than one chemically dependent person in the family. Resistance and anger toward the diagnosis may be forthcoming from these uncomfortable persons during this interview. Other members may have reasons for vehemently objecting to the diagnosis of chemical dependency and will need an equal amount of assistance in overcoming their contribution to the problem. Remember, it is easy to underestimate the impact of inappropriate chemical use in family conflicts. If conflicts over money, child discipline, sex, or other issues not related to chemical use are brought up, it is important to assess carefully whether these problems occur primarily during drug or alcohol use or are associated with them in any way. Since a key symptom in dependency is denial of the primary problem, probing for the extent of the chemical involvement is most useful after the family members have spontaneously opened the door in presenting their own versions of what is happening.

PRIMARY CARE FAMILY COUNSELING
FOR CHEMICAL DEPENDENCY

If the family interview confirms the presence of chemical dependency, then the family physician must suggest a treatment plan that is realistically capable of helping the entire family. We think it critically important to recommend some form of action immediately. The available chemical dependency resources must be well known to the physician before the family interview and assessment occur. A chemical dependency counselor is usually available through a local mental health center, hospital, or private clinic. Immediate consultation with this professional may be a reasonable option as the first step in the treatment plan for most family physicians. This professional can assess the situation; can determine whether diagnosis is appropriate and whether outpatient or inpatient treatment is needed; and can perhaps arrange for initiation of appropriate treatment. However, the family physician must be familiar with all of the treatment resources available and be capable of assessing the severity and rigidity of the family's chemical dependency problem in order to recommend *any* treatment options beyond consultation with a chemical dependency counselor. As physicians come to work more closely with chemical dependency counselors and treatment centers, they can achieve a confident, optimistic style for handling consultations, referrals, and recommendations for treatment.

We urge physicians not to recommend abstinence alone as a first, isolated treatment step. If the request for abstinence is not accompanied by skilled therapy intended to adjust rigid roles and interaction patterns, it is often futile. How many times have students and residents seen a senior physician ask an alcoholic to stop drinking? The alcoholic patient often says, "No problem, Doc." The same person is readmitted a few months later for recurrent medical complications of alcoholism, with no change in drinking behavior. This scenario is also painfully familiar to most chemically dependent families. They despair at their family physician's recommendation for abstinence without accompanying therapy. If the physician alone cannot competently work with the family—treating it as a complex system that has been organized around drugs and/or alcohol—then the physician needs a consultant to help with planning this intervention and a referral source to carry out the principal treatment. If abstinence is the only element of the treatment plan, then the index patient and family are doomed to uncomfortable and incomplete recovery at best. It is more likely that the family system will not be altered in the least. The physician and the family then begin to view the entire matter as hopeless. It is better to seek consultation before recommending any steps of treatment—even abstinence—unless the physician has knowledge and skill in the specialized family therapy required to treat chemically dependent families.

This is not to say that abstinence is not important—it is critically important. It is central to recovery. There is a controversial body of literature that suggests that social drinking is not harmful to some alcoholics that have undergone alcoholic treatment (Ewing, 1974; Pattison, Headley, Gleser, & Gohschalk, 1968). However, the question is far from settled. For the practicing family physician to help the largest group of chemically dependent persons and families, it is probably best to view total abstinence as the most reasonable approach for most recovering dependent persons. Maintenance of long-term contact with AA and Al-Anon groups is still the most successful long-range treatment plan. This means total abstinence from alcohol and mood-altering drugs, except in unusual hospital situations such as those following major surgery. Abstinence by itself, however, is only part of recovery, and sobriety is only a limited goal of treatment. Improved personal and family functioning is the highest goal, but is more difficult to measure, study, and achieve (Steinglass, 1977).

If the family assessment suggests chemical dependency and the family physician wishes to begin an intervention process, we have found several guidelines helpful during the first interview. Many family physicians may wish to stop here and ask for consultation from a chemical dependency counselor.

1. *The physician should avoid protracted discussion of how much alcohol or how many other drugs are being used.* The significant issue is the impact of this drug on the family relationships. A discussion of the amount and frequency of use is mildly helpful, but frequently leads to a distracting and unsolvable debate about what is enough and too much chemical use.

2. *The family and the physician/counselor should come to some agreement on the seriousness of the family conflict and on whether chemical use is really a principal factor.* If it is a significant problem, it needs appropriate intervention; if it is a minor or secondary problem, perhaps a period of observation would be helpful. If the physician is convinced that chemical dependency is a signficant problem, then he or she should state this clearly so that all members of the family understand the position, especially the person who is being challenged to change a use behavior pattern. The importance and urgency of the chemical dependency issue needs to be agreed upon before the intervention is established.

3. *There should be several indicators for the need for formal intervention and probable inpatient or extensive outpatient treatment.* First, repeated discussion and conflict revolving around drug or alcohol use during

attempts to manage other problems in the family suggest that chemical dependency may be the primary problem. Even with skillful family therapy, relationship problems and multiple other issues will be difficult if not impossible to treat if they are constantly clouded by conflict over alcohol or drug use. If that occurs, *the drug issue must be addressed before continuing to treat other problems.*

4. *If the physician requests abstinence, he or she should specify that it be for an extended period of time, such as a year.* Many alcoholics have quit drinking for short periods of time many times in the past. However, the goal should be for an extended period of sobriety; on the other hand, proposing lifelong sobriety during the first interview would be asking for too much too soon. If the allegedly dependent person agrees to an extended period of sobriety and achieves it, then perhaps dependency really was not a serious problem in the first place. Then the other family problems may be addressed appropriately. An alternative explanation is that the intervention has been extremely helpful or that the person is one of those few who can simply decide to stop using or abusing a drug or alcohol without further intervention strategies. Baird leaves the door open for this "will power" occurrence in recovery from chemical dependency by stating that perhaps 1 to 2% of drinking people quit drinking with no other type of help other than a request for abstinence; however, most people will require an ongoing, supportive treatment plan in order to recover self-esteem and healthy family relationships in addition to simple abstinence.

This "will power" option is raised only when it seems useful to delay a more complete intervention plan. For example, if a husband denies that his drinking is a problem, and his wife has not yet become involved in Al-Anon, and the problem seems to be tolerable to the point that divorce is not an immediate issue, then the confronted dependent person may agree at least to prolonged abstinence. This allows the nonusing spouse time to understand his or her role in the problem through Al-Anon. Future family interviews should be planned in order to monitor progress. It is quite likely that a later interview will establish the need for further help because of failure to maintain the period of abstinence. The stage will then be set for more meaningful intervention because the nonusing spouse will have increased awareness of a role in the problem. On the other hand, if prolonged abstinence is achieved but the abstaining person feels punished, and if chronically angry family relationships have not improved, then further treatment is warranted. This "dry drunk" syndrome may be as painful as the primary chemical dependency for some families.

5. *If abstinence is agreed upon by the allegedly dependent person, then a minimum effort expected of the nonusing spouse should be participation in Al-Anon.* Resistance from the nonusing spouse about Al-Anon is a poor prognostic indicator for that person's willingness to change and for rigidity

in the family system. The chemically dependent individual should be urged to attend AA meetings; however, this participaton initially may not be as important as Al-Anon attendance for the nonusing spouse or other family members. If family members do not agree to either Al-Anon or AA, they may be locked in the rigid pattern of chronic substance abuse. In this situation, any changes will be slow to occur. The physician's expectations must be adjusted accordingly to a long-term intervention plan that will include ongoing support for this dysfunctional family. This strategy will also offer a continued challenge for compliance in initial treatment steps such as involvement in AA and Al-Anon. It is probably not helpful to try to deal with more specific conflicts such as child behavior problems or marital or sexual conflicts if the family is not willing to comply with requests for initial chemical dependency treatment.

6. *If a family interview reveals a chemical dependency problem that has been in existence for two to three generations and is associated with low outside family support systems, low family adaptability, and severely enmeshed or disengaged cohesion patterns, the physician must be careful to structure a long-term strategy.* Changes will be slow to come and small in nature, but an ongoing supportive yet firm stance by the physician can be helpful. The physician must remember that chemical dependency is a progressive and occasionally fatal disease. The intervention is so important that a "never give up" attitude is appropriate. Although initial attempts at intervention may seem frustrating and ineffective, every attempt is potentially useful and may pave the way for a later successful family-centered intervention.

7. *Community issues may be appropriate to raise during the first interview.* Sometimes an employer can be an ally in initiating a treatment plan. Some companies have a formal policy whereby an employee cannot be dismissed for alcoholism unless he or she refuses treatment. Schools may have a similar program. A family may request a court hearing to force treatment via the legal establishment of inebriety. The usefulness of this latter procedure depends upon many variables such as local attitudes about chemical dependency, the specific language of state laws regarding the definition of "inebriety," and the willingness of county attorneys to become involved. It can be very helpful as a last resort in obviously severe cases, but it should rarely if ever be used for early intervention where no one outside the family can easily verify the problem.

When a family wants to resort to court intervention, the physician may be looking at a disengaged family in which there is no "family glue." Unless the family system can be moved to a more supportive and intimate level, treatment of the individual involved may occur without the involvement of the nondrinking spouse or other family members. In this case, the achievement of sobriety may be accomplished without really improving family functioning; the disengaged family will probably go on to separation, divorce, or continued dysfunction in the face of sobriety. Evaluation of treatment outcome should be based on the whole psychosocial picture, not just on the elimination of chemical use from the patient's life.

FORMAL TREATMENT OPTIONS

If formal chemical dependency treatment is offered, it should be presented as a helpful and nonpunitive option that involves the entire family in the process of change. This is the first step toward recovery for the whole family. It involves difficult, emotional work but is an opportunity to recover hope, self-esteem, and honesty in a family now lacking these qualities. We find it difficult to recommend initial outpatient treatment as the best option for most families with long-standing chemical dependency problems. The family and the dependent individual are asked to make major changes in life style and social habits, to decide to make new friends who do not abuse or use drugs or alcohol, and to alter styles of personal relationships that have been long established, sometimes over two or three generations. We consider this initial change a full-time task for at least 3 to 4 weeks in an inpatient family-oriented treatment center. If a working person is asked to confront these issues initially in addition to handling normal job responsibilities, either the job or the recovery process will suffer. In some instances, however, outpatient treatment is the only option—and not necessarily a poor option if supported by strong AA and Al-Anon programs. If the patient and family are in the early stages of the course of chemical dependency and are optimistic, and if excellent outpatient resources are available, then outpatient family-oriented treatment is a realistic option.

If the physician chooses to suggest inpatient chemical dependency treatment, several points can be emphasized to help persuade the patient and family to disrupt their lives by such hospitalization. Untreated chemical dependency is a progressive disease; as time passes, the disease does not get better. This illness is fatal; people and relationships die early from it (Eckardt et al., 1981). In our culture, automobile and other vehicular trauma is a major risk to those that abuse chemicals and alcohol. In the very late stages, the physical and medical complications of alcoholism and other drug dependency take their toll. In the meantime, close relationships are distorted so as to become intolerable; many relationships eventually die. In the face of other progressive and potentially fatal illnesses, physicians readily request hospitalization, expensive treatment, surgery, and appropriate recuperation time. For example, if someone presents with appendicitis, the physician explains the serious nature of the illness, the possibility of finding something other than appendicitis, and the need for immediate surgery and hospitalization. The patient undergoes anesthesia and surgery, awakes with a painful incision, and eventually goes home to recuperate.

The family and the physician readily accept this scenario for treating serious biomedical disease. No physician would knowingly send the patient home and accept the risks of an occasional spontaneous recovery. In fact, if the physician did recommend such home treatment, most families would reject that advice and seek help elsewhere. However, the setting for chemical dependency is far different. Few families troubled with this illness have an accurate concept of how to initiate recovery. If the physician recommends an inappropriate treatment plan for this progressive (and in a sense fatal) illness, the family will often readily comply with this poor advice. Recovery chances are reduced to whatever rate of spontaneous recovery exists in the community. It is parallel to sending the appendicitis patient home to take aspirin. In underrecognizing and undertreating chemical dependency, physicians are ignoring or are suggesting home treatment for a progressive and potentially fatal disease.

If formal chemical dependency treatment is recommended, it should involve all family members in a significant way (Steinglass, 1976). If a patient is being referred to an inpatient treatment center, the physician should ask for a copy of a typical treatment plan to see if other family members are included. Many centers offer a "family week" that consists of at least 3 to 5 days of intensive family involvement. A few centers have fully parallel treatment efforts for all family members and focus on the family's "codependency." The program's family perspective should be evident in the treatment outline. This is far from the simple "drying-out" centers common in the early days of chemical dependency treatment. Modern treatment focuses on honesty in relationships, self-responsibility, recovery of self-esteem, and changes in the rigid family roles that have maintained this illness over a period of time. The principles of AA and Al-Anon are usually apparent. A central concept is that in the disease state all family members participate in a pattern of interaction that contributes to and maintains the problem.

The referring physician who emphasizes the importance of family-centered treatment reinforces the treatment process by setting up appropriate expectations. It is counterproductive to encourage individually focused treatment by "sending off" one family member to treatment as if being sent to prison, while other family members become bystanders. Insisting upon total family commitment to the treatment process is so critical that it may be wise to delay treatment if no other family members except the index patient will participate. The risks of delaying initial treatment should be explained to families. The risks of a poor outcome without meaningful family involvement should also be discussed; such risks include the "dry drunk" syndrome (self-pity, irritability, resentment, but no chemical use), increased marital and family conflict, and the nonusing spouse's jealousy of the "AA family" that occupies so much of the recovering alcoholic's time.

AA, Al-Anon, and, whenever available, Alateen groups for young family members will almost always be a part of the follow-up treatment plan. Families who do not cooperate with such group support, however, should not automatically be considered treatment failures. On this issue, Steinglass (1980) has discussed two types of successful outcomes of chemical dependency treatment. Most families recover by continuing to think of alcohol and drug nonuse as *the central focus* of the family; this is the "abstinence model." This usually involves continual contact with AA, Al-Anon, and Alateen. Abstinence accompanies a major change in life style, new friends, social activities that do not emphasize alcohol and drug use, and help offered to other families in a similar path of recovery. A smaller group of patients and families, however, have been observed to recover by simply avoiding the excessive use of alcohol. Some alcohol use may occur, and the family makes other major changes in life style. Conflict persists in those families, but they appear to be more stable than before chemical dependency treatment. Perhaps future research will demonstrate that the latter recovery model is realistic for some families and is not doomed to eventual failure. The Al-Anon, AA, and Alateen model, however, is the most generally recommended and most successful aftercare program in common use (Wegescheider, 1981).

PREVENTION OF CHEMICAL DEPENDENCY

What can the family physician do to prevent chemical dependency? First, treating the primary disease by including the entire family is a very efficient preventative measure. Chemical dependency occurs most commonly in families with previous generations of the same problem (*Journal of the American Medical Association*, Editorial, 1975; Goodwin, 1976). Primary treatment in this case may result in primary prevention within the family by influencing more than one generation. Second, physicians can stop encouraging chemical dependency with prescription medication. In the United States in 1978, there were 68 million prescriptions filled for benzodiazepines (Valium, Librium, Ativan, Serax, etc.). Approximately 10 million Americans took these medications. Twice as many women as men used these anti-anxiety drugs. Family physicians and osteopaths wrote nearly half of the prescriptions (*FDA Drug Bulletin*, 1980). Consumer concern about this issue has been emphasized in numerous lay publications describing the hazards of prolonged use of sedatives (Hubbell, 1980; Klemme, 1977).

In this climate, it is common to have patients refuse all psychotropic medications even when legitimately indicated. The public has been aroused. Meanwhile, physicians have been slow to see the hazards of this new generation of sedatives. Lethal overdose of these agents has proven rare, but there are other problems. The medical literature on this topic commonly offers only reassurances as to the benign nature of benzodiazepines (Abuzzahab, 1979; Hollister, Conley, Britt, & Shuen, 1981). However, there is a powerful though initially subtle hazard to benzodiazepines—psychological dependency. The dynamics of the dependency for the family are no different for prescribed medications than for alcohol. If the medication is used over prolonged periods of time as a means of coping with stress, then the family mechanisms of stress and conflict resolution may become dysfunctional.

Third, physicians can avoid exacerbating chemical dependency problems by taking a careful history of alcohol and medication use before prescribing sedatives. It is known that 5 to 7% of the population is alcoholic and that alcoholic families have disproportionately high rates of contact with the medical system. But do physicians carefully screen patients before prescribing these medications? Based on simple prevalance rates, at least 1 out of 20 prescriptions for benzodiazepines would be given to a person who is already an alcoholic. If physicians agree that prescribing a benzodiazepine for a person who is already an alcoholic is not appropriate, then the medication should be withheld, except for initial detoxification in a treatment center or hospital. Actively drinking alcoholics should be offered help, not substitute drugs. Fortunately, there are many nonpharmacological methods of reducing anxiety, such as regular exercise, relaxation techniques, biofeedback, and family therapy to improve the ability to resolve family conflicts. If the decision is made to stop benzodiazepines after long-term use, one must do it very slowly in order to avoid significant withdrawal effects (Pevanik, Jasinski, & Haretzin, 1978). Even "normal" doses of 30 to 40 milligrams of diazepam can be associated with significant withdrawal such as tremors, sleeplessness, and anxiety. It should be noted that the withdrawal symptoms are similar to the symptoms for which the medication is usually prescribed (*FDA Drug Bulletin*, 1980).

CONCLUSION

This chapter has stressed that the family physician can discover chemical dependency in its early stages by including a review of close family relationships at appropriate times when seeing an individual patient. When major conflicts are discovered, it is appropriate to take a careful history of drug and alcohol use to evaluate any association that may exist between chemical use and family distress. The second step is to interview the entire family in the hospital or the office. If major conflicts are associated with drug or alcohol use, if the conflicts significantly affect more than one family member, and if the family's interaction patterns lead to no resolution of the conflicts, then there is a high probability of a chemical dependency in the family. The third step is treatment. Physicians trained in specialized chemical dependency intervention and treatment may proceed with recommendations for management for this complex family illness. Most other physicians operating in a primary care mode can be most effective by seeking immediate consultation with a chemical dependency counselor or a family therapist trained in chemical dependency issues. It is probably not helpful to recommend abstinence without a supportive, skilled therapeutic plan that emphasizes the entire family. For serious cases, the treatment plan will probably call for initial inpatient or outpatient therapy for the index patient and the family. Finally, we have emphasized that family physicians can offer preventive care for chemical dependency problems.

APPENDIX: CASE EXAMPLES

The following case studies have been selected from over 80 cases of chemical dependency encountered in 3 years in Baird's practice. Since there is no formal cross-referencing system in the current charting system, more examples are undoubtedly available, but these cases were selected from charts that could actually be retrieved with a primary diagnosis of chemical dependency in which Baird interacted with the family. Names, ages, and some specific descriptive details of the families and occupational details have been changed in order to insure confidentiality. Each case is presented briefly in terms of the presenting situation; the family assessment; the type of intervention planned; and the lengths of time between first contact, assembling the family, and the treatment intervention. Follow-up information is also given for each case.

CHEMICAL DEPENDENCY: CASE 1

The first is an example of an early diagnosis of chemical dependency where there was excellent compliance, good family cohesion and adaptability, and minimal emotional and economic loss to the family. Mr. A was a 35-year-old male who presented with complaints of chest pain and diffuse anxiety. He was treated for several months with several different kinds of antianxiety agents without change in his symptoms. Then he was referred from another family physician to Baird for family evaluation. Mr. A was married. He had three children aged 10 through 17, all in good health and with no significant behavioral problems. Mr. A and his wife were both in excellent health and rarely saw physicians until this episode. New family business ventures were beginning to go poorly over the past 5 to 6 months, and Mr. A began to have more and more sleeping difficulty and trouble concentrating while at work. His wife noticed that he was gone from home more and more frequently and was becoming agitated and irritable. All family members agreed that current attempts at treatment of the anxiety were unsuccessful. They had not had any difficulty with any previous life events, such as birth of children, moving to a new home location, changing occupations, or caring for their aging parents. They wanted very much to work on this problem as a family unit and were eager to attend family therapy. After five visits marked by continued symptoms—despite diligent attempts to change troublesome interaction patterns in the family, along with other nonchemical treatments—a more careful chemical history was taken. Then it was discovered that Mr. A. had begun drinking more heavily about 3 months prior to seeing a physician. Once he saw the physician and combined the prescribed medication with alcohol, he described a feeling of great security and comfort only when taking the prescribed medications and alcohol simultaneously. At those times he was "numb" and felt no anxiety or emotional pain. His family noted that since seeing the physician initially, he had become more withdrawn and less involved in family topics. None of this had been discovered in the previous attempts at family therapy. Baird suggested that chemical dependency might be the underlying problem and asked that the family return in 2 weeks to discuss formal chemical dependency treatment if all still agreed upon this as the diagnosis.

About 5 days later Baird got a call from both Mr. and Mrs. A, who requested immediate placement in a chemical dependency treatment center for Mr. A. All family members agreed to participate, and the treatment center was contacted immediately. Mr. A. attended an inpatient treatment center for 1 month. His family participated fully in the treatment program and the "family week." When Mr. A was discharged, he agreed to follow up with AA and his family with Al-Anon. After about 6 months' involvement in AA and Al-Anon, Mr. and Mrs. A came to the office and stated that they would feel more comfortable in a different type of support group that was not oriented around chemicals. They have been doing quite well and on succeeding follow-up visits have continued to succeed at resolving the other interactional problems that had seemed unsolvable in the past.

None of the As' problems needed the attention of a therapist once the chemical issue had been resolved. Since Mr. A had experienced unusual and harmful drinking patterns for only several months prior to treatment and had functioned quite well until the drinking problem was compounded by prescription medications, the As and Baird made a cautious decision to allow limited use of alcohol in the future. The As were cautioned that this is a relatively experimental treatment plan, but they were comfortable with that option. Both Mr. and Mrs. A agreed to return if problems reappeared and also agreed that if future problems did occur in relation to alcohol use, total abstinence and continual AA participation would be required and definitely needed. This has been the only family in Baird's 3 years of practice for whom it seemed reasonable to allow continued moderate use of alcohol, and for whom continued AA and Al-Anon participation was not deemed essential. This family has found a supportive group of persons outside AA whose life styles do not rotate around alcohol and with whom they can discuss meaningful topics in confidence. The length of follow-up for this family has now been 2 years, and there has been good compliance with the long-term treatment plan.

CHEMICAL DEPENDENCY: CASE 2

This is an example of an early chemical dependency problem associated with poor family cohesion, more than one family member's showing inappropriate use of chemicals, and a treatment outcome that has ended in divorce.

Mrs. B was a 38-year-old female who presented with complaints of depression, multiple crying spells, and difficulty in sleeping. She stated that she had a great deal of difficulty with a 16-year-old daughter, Cindy; the girl seemed to be failing in school, was uncooperative at home, and had recently been in a car accident in which the driver was drinking, although no one was seriously hurt. Further family history revealed that Mrs. B had three daughters, aged 14, 16, and 18; she was remarried to a 39-year-old man who had two daughters by another marriage who were not living with this couple. The couple had one child of their own, an 8-year-old son who was difficult to control. Mrs. B had been divorced about 11 years ago from a husband who had a chronic drinking problem, although no formal assessment or intervention had ever been attempted. Mrs. B and her new blended family had been together for about 9 years. During that time there had been intermittent serious family arguments with occasional family violence in which Mrs. B would be struck by her husband when none of the children were thought to be awake, although the children had commented to her that they were upset about these fights. Mrs. B had contemplated a second divorce many times but felt that she should stay together to "provide a father" for her daughters and son. She stated that her husband did not appear to have difficulty with drinking alcohol, although they did have more family arguments during times when he had been drinking. Physical violence had occurred only at the times of Mr. B's drinking.

Mrs. B's primary concerns at this time were her own symptoms and the fear of more problems with her 16-year-old daugher, Cindy. She agreed to return with the entire family, primarily for assessment of the daughter's chemical behavior, which had already been a topic of discussion with a school counselor.

One week later Mrs. B returned with her three daughters, her son, and Mr. B. The family interview suggested that the 16-year-old daughter's condition indeed had deteriorated over the past half of the school year. She was no longer working up to her potential in school. She was unwilling to comply with family requests to return home by midnight and had been involved in the accident noted above. She saw no problem at this time with her chemical use pattern, but her parents were nervous about it. She said that all of her friends used alcohol frequently and that many were using pot; she said she was not upset about any of that. She had no intentions of continuing on in school and was generally quite defiant.

Baird's assessment, which he stated at that time to the family, was that there was a chemical abuse problem with the 16-year-old daughter but that treatment would require the entire family to participate. There was general agreement on this approach from everyone except Mr. B, who seemed somewhat hostile, although he would not express himself openly. Within 5 days, Mrs. B's daughter was enrolled in a family-centered chemical dependency treatment plan. All family members attended during the next month-long therapy program. Mr. B remained hostile. Upon return from the treatment center, Cindy was cooperative. She seemed to be positive about maintaining a nonuse pattern in the future and was no longer a discipline problem at home. Cindy and her mother seemed to be getting along together quite well, as were she and her two biological sisters. However, there seemed to be increasing antagonism between Mrs. B's children by her first marriage and her husband and son. When this became apparent, further family interviews were called. At that time Mr. B's chemical use was discussed and identified by all family members as a potential problem.

Mr. B refused involvement in AA as well as evaluation by an outside chemical dependency counselor. He did agree to quit drinking for 1 year but remained quite angry. About 1 month later, Mrs. B returned with her daughters and son, stating that she and her daughters were getting along better and that her son was somewhat more controllable. However, Mr. B seemed to be getting more and more distant and uninvolved in the family. At this time she finally described her desire to "have a father" for her daughters. Once this was aired, her daughters stated that this was not important to them; they felt upset that their mother had had that motive for remarriage. After an emotional discussion, it was apparent that Mrs. B had felt little personal involvement with her husband for many years. She would now consider what she had tried to avoid thinking about for many years—divorce.

At the time of this writing, approximately 6 months later, there has been no legal divorce, but Mr. and Mrs. B are living separately. Mrs. B has custody of the children; there are no behavior problems with the children at this time; and Mrs. B no longer feels depressed or seeks medical attention, except for rare acute illnesses or routine examinations.

In this case, the remarried mother presented with a complaint of depression. The family assessment occurred about 1 week later. Chemical dependency treatment for the 16-year-old daughter was instituted within 1 week of the family assessment. Within 6 months of that time it was discovered that the father also had a problem definable as chemical dependency (i.e., serious problems created within the family, primarily at times of drinking or chemical abuse). This family had a characteristically low level of cohesion; therefore it was impossible to keep the family together while they were adjusting to the multiple problems cited. The progression toward separation and/or divorce was probably set in motion long before the intervention process was begun. The outcome of the intervention was to stabilize the interaction for five members of this blended family. However, the father of the family has not yet understood his difficulty with alcohol and with relating to his family. It may be hoped that he will confront his problems and be open to a more successful intervention sometime in the future.

CHEMICAL DEPENDENCY: CASE 3

In this example, a 35-year-old female married to a very successful businessman presented with a complaint of anxiety and sleeplessness. Further history revealed that her husband had been drinking heavily for many years and that they had been in frequent arguments recently. No family violence had occurred, but there were many threats of violence. Mrs. C had three children, aged 5 to 11, who had stopped having friends come home to visit because of repeated family fights. Mrs. C agreed that it would be a good idea to invite the entire family in for furher assessment.

At the time of the family interview, Mr. C was very cooperative initially and seemed to be very persuasive in denying any problem in the family. However, when the children described the family arguments and their occurrence only when Mr. C was drinking, it was difficult for him to deny the existence of the problem. After about a 30-minute discussion, Mr. C agreed to 1 year of sobriety, although he did not think he had a drinking problem. Mrs. C agreed to attend Al-Anon.

Three weeks later, the family arrived for the follow-up interview. At that time, Mr. C had maintained his sobriety and felt that there was no problem that required any further intervention. Mrs. C had begun attending Al-Anon. However, Mr. C had refused AA attendance. Only at this time was it revealed that Mr. C had been confronted some 10 years previously about his drinking and had been asked to attend AA meetings by a counselor who saw him in reference to a citation for driving while intoxicated. Mrs. C now expressed more dismay that the problem would go unsolved. No progress was made at this meeting. Another meeting was planned in another 3 weeks.

Three weeks later, the family again arrived intact. However, it was now revealed that after the last meeting, Mr. C had become drunk and disrupted the entire family late at night. The children were now quite upset and frightened at their father's behavior. Mr. C still insisted that drinking was not the problem, but Mrs. C had begun legal proceeding toward divorce, a move she had not discussed previously. In a very emotional session, the three children and Mrs. C asked Mr. C to give up his drinking behavior and to seek inpatient chemical dependency treatment in order for the family to stay together. Mr. C asked, "I'm not really an alcoholic, am I, Doc?" Baird replied, "Yes, you are." With tears in his eyes, Mr. C still refused treatment for his chemical dependency and literally left his family. Within 3 months, Mrs. C and her three children had moved out of town. About 2 years later she remarried, and she is currently doing quite well.

About 6 months after that interview, Mr. C called to say that he had talked to several acquaintances who were in the local AA group and that he now wanted inpatient chemical dependency treatment. This was quickly arranged, and Mr. C entered treatment. One year later he also had a 5-day stay in a treatment center to deal with his anger and frustration over losing his family. However, after 3 years, he has not resumed drinking, is currently engaged to be married, and is a leading force in an AA group in another community. He has adjusted quite well to the loss of his family and accepts responsibility for his life in the future. He and his ex-wife have maintained positive attitudes toward each other. The three children see him on a regular basis and have reestablished a trusting relationship with him.

In this example, the index patient was the nondependent spouse. There seemed to be no unusual precipitating stresses. The family system demonstrated some rigidity: the problem had continued for at least 10 years without discussion from within or help from the outside. There appeared to be a moderate amount of family cohesion. However, the rigidity of the problem and the denial seemed to overcome that level of cohesion and resulted in divorce. The time from initial contact to family assessment was only a few weeks. The time from family assessment to intervention was approximately 7 to 8 months. However, in the interim the family was divided. Follow-up for 3 years has shown good adaptability and good family functioning for the divided family, whose members are now establishing new family interaction patterns on a healthier basis.

CHEMICAL DEPENDENCY: CASE 4

This is an example of a much later diagnosis in which the index patient was chemically dependent and was hospitalized on first contact. Mr. D, a 54-year-old male, was first seen in the emergency room for vomiting, jaundice, and abdominal pain. He had had multiple previous admissions for alcoholic hepatitis and pancreatitis and had been asked to quit drinking many times over the past 10 years. His drinking history went back at least 20 years, and he had had intermittent problems ever since adolescence. He was admitted with alcoholic hepatitis, cirrhosis, and pancreatitis. He was jaundiced on admission, and his prognosis was guarded initially.

After about 1 week in the hospital he began to improve, and a family conference was called. Family members had never previously been invited for any kind of discussion and were eager to participate. No previous effort at instituting a formal chemical dependency recovery program had been offered until this time, and all members of the family, including the primary patient, were eager to participate. However, when the reality of a prolonged inpatient treatment program became apparent to Mr. D, he became very reluctant and stated that he would not go to inpatient treatment. He felt that he could quit drinking by himself. The family discussion continued, and Mrs. D stated that she would not accept Mr. D back home unless he agreed to participate in a formal inpatient treatment program. Mr. D's two daughters also stated that they loved him very much but were greatly distressed that he would not agree to a plan that might help him recover from his difficult problem. Subsequently Mr. D agreed to treatment; he was discharged from the hospital about 1 week later and entered an inpatient family-centered chemical dependency program. All family members participated eagerly, and Mr. D was discharged approximately 5 weeks after admission to the chemical dependency treatment program. He returned to an active AA group. Mrs. D participated faithfully in Al-Anon, and all generally went well for about 6 months. Then Mr. D began to miss work, and Mrs. D suspected resumption of alcohol use.

A third family interview was called. Mr. D agreed to participate and at that time reluctantly admitted that he was again using alcohol. This he admitted only after there was concrete evidence of his use presented by his family. Rather than reenter treatment, Mrs. D asked that Mr. D leave the house until he was capable of living without alcohol. He was absent from their household for about 2 weeks and lived with an AA friend, and then returned and has not had another episode of alcohol use for 1½ years. He is now working and has not missed work in approximately 1 year. He continues to participate in AA, and Mrs. D continues to participate in Al-Anon to a full extent. Their daughters are participating in school programs for children whose parents are chemically dependent.

In this example, the length of time from initial contact to formal chemical dependency treatment was approximately 3 weeks, during which time Mr. D was in an acute care hospital. The family meeting was called after his medical situation somewhat stabilized, 1 week after admission to the acute care hospital. The second family meeting approximately 1 week later was needed to reinforce the need for inpatient chemical dependency treatment. His inpatient treatment lasted for approximately 5 weeks and was instituted immediately upon discharge from the acute care hospital. Mr. D did not return home even to pick up clothing. He was taken to the treatment center by family and AA friends.

For this family, the major stressor at the time of the intervention was recurrent hospitalization for Mr. D. They were also having family financial problems because he was unable to maintain a steady work role. Numerous family arguments had been occurring for years with no progression toward solution, and the entire family affect at the time of this first interview was depressed.

This family demonstrated reasonable adaptability, as evidenced by the fact that the daughters had developed no apparent problems and Mrs. D had carried the health care responsibility for her aging parents, who are now deceased, without faltering in her work role outside the home. The family responded quickly to requests for a family interview and requested that Mr. D seek inpatient treatment at the same time they were expressing love for him. All this was done without prior training or even warning that this problem would be the topic of discussion when they met with their family physician in the hospital.

As noted, Mr. D did resume use of alcohol about 6 months after his treatment was begun. However, this was quickly changed when Mrs. D stated again that he could not live at home if he could not follow a reasonable AA program. This includes total abstinence for this family.

Finally, this family showed good family cohesion, as witnessed by the fact that although Mrs. D requested that her husband live away from home temporarily, she did not discuss divorce and was not contemplating divorce at any time. This cohesion was also demonstrated when all family members presented for the initial family interview.

13 TWO INTERVIEWS FOR CHEMICAL DEPENDENCY PROBLEMS

INTERVIEW 1: FIRST INTERVIEW WITH WIFE OF AN ALCOHOLIC

INTRODUCTION BY BAIRD

This was my first professional contact with this person, although I see her and her husband regularly as a customer in their family business. I interviewed her at the request of one of my partners, who had repeatedly seen the husband falling down drunk while trying to work in the evening in their family business. His behavior had become worse over the past 2 years, and, according to his spouse, had become particularly bad over the past 6 months. I obtained the woman's permission to tape-record the interview. Identifying information has been altered in the transcript.

THE INTERVIEW

DOCTOR: Let's get an idea of what is happening. Fill me in.

PATIENT: Well, it's his drinking problem.

DOCTOR: Let me back way up and start from things with you two as a couple. I don't know anything about that. How long have you been married?

PATIENT: It will be sixteen years in October. We went together for four years—two years in high school and two years out.

DOCTOR: You've known each other a long time. You have children?

PATIENT: We have four children. A girl who's a freshman in college and three boys.

DOCTOR: How old is the youngest?

PATIENT: Eight.

DOCTOR: When did you become aware of a problem?

PATIENT: Well, probably the last couple years he's been drinking more. But it was only on weekends when we'd go out or something. Well, he'd come home from work and have a few beers or something.

DOCTOR: Is it obvious to you now? Is it obvious to other people?

PATIENT: I don't know. I know Dr. X noticed it. He thought it was in his family too.

DOCTOR: That makes him more sensitive.

PATIENT: I don't think other people see him every night, so when they see that he's been drinking they think that he's just had a few beers. That's about it. It's getting worse now (crying). He drinks much more now than before.

DOCTOR: What happens to him then?

PATIENT: He gets very ornery. Everything is my fault, and he's just a completely different person.

DOCTOR: What has this done to you? Better hold that box of Kleenex.

PATIENT: It's been very hard on me.

DOCTOR: Does anyone know what it's done to you?

PATIENT: No.

DOCTOR: Have you shared it with anyone?

PATIENT: Nancy and I are best friends and I haven't even said anything to her about it.

DOCTOR: What about your children—how is it affecting them?

PATIENT: They are beginning to notice it. Bill got mad one night and he said something about it. I said that I was going to have his dad punish him and he made the remark that he's nothing but an old drunk.

DOCTOR: Bill is how old?

PATIENT: He's in the seventh grade.

DOCTOR: That's a bitter comment.

PATIENT: Yeah, it was. Especially if I've been working at night and when I come home and put the kids to bed or something and different times Joe will stay out drinking. The two youngest ones really don't say too much. Jason, just the fact that our life style has changed too much this year—it's been hard on him.

DOCTOR: What did you do before the new job?

PATIENT: My husband was a furniture maker. He worked at it for ten years and then he managed the factory.

DOCTOR: That's a pretty big operation.

PATIENT: Yeah.

DOCTOR: What were you doing? I know you were managing a household, but were you working outside of the home?

PATIENT: No, except a little bit last year I worked part time for Kay at the clothing store, but it was only two days a week.

DOCTOR: So this is a big change for you too.

PATIENT: Oh yeah, definitely. Day and night most of the time.

DOCTOR: What does that mean for your schedule?

PATIENT: Mostly, when we first opened up we would go down at 7 or 8 in the morning and get home at 2 A.M. And then it got to the point where we had to hire someone for the cleaning and now we go down between 10 and 11 A.M. I usually try to get out of there between 4 and 6 in the evening and go home and I usually try to stay home with the kids and get them in bed. Then I'll go back down and get home between 1 and 2.

DOCTOR: Pretty busy day.

PATIENT: Yeah. I can stay home at least two nights a week, like last night, and go back down next Thursday. Those are the nights I try to clean house and do the washing and then it's 2 A.M. or so before I get to bed.

DOCTOR: This is seven days a week?

PATIENT: Seven days a week. So, in October or November we took a weekend off, and two weekends ago we were gone from Friday to Sunday night. Well, we went to the state tournaments. Friday night he was real good. Saturday afternoon he started drinking and by 5 P.M. he had gone to bed and he was out. At 7 P.M. I tried to wake him up because we were all going to meet and go to eat at 7:30 and he's like this (*gestures*). I tried to wake him up and he doesn't know where he is. He thinks he's somewhere. Like when I tried to wake him up he thought he was at the restaurant.

DOCTOR: No idea.

PATIENT: No idea, like he blacked out. I did wake him up. Everybody was going to go eat.

DOCTOR: Did he remember that night the next day?

PATIENT: I don't think he remembered.

DOCTOR: Have you ever had times when you talked with him when he seemed to have lots to drink and he doesn't remember what you told him? You might mention something to him and the next day you expect him to know what you said that night.

PATIENT: I don't know if it's because he hasn't been paying that much attention.

DOCTOR: Is that a source of discomfort or arguments that you think he knows something?

PATIENT: Not too much.

DOCTOR: This is a blackout symptom. A blackout is where someone has had something to drink but is apparently not drunk, and yet a blackout would mean that they are functioning okay as far as you and I could tell, but they say they have no recollection of that period of time.

PATIENT: No, when he starts drinking, especially any more, he can have just a few beers and I can tell he's drunk right away.

DOCTOR: So he's not subtle?

PATIENT: No. It's obvious then. If I say the next day, "Don't drink any more, please. Why don't you have a cup of coffee instead?" It's then when he gets mad. Just like on Monday night. He worked late at the store and so I came down to help out with the second shift and to help close up and he had started drinking. I had talked to him. We had talked over the weekend. I thought that he was drinking too much and I thought he should get some help and he said no. He didn't drink hardly at all that weekend. I thought, "Maybe he realized that he is an alcoholic. Maybe he is going to quit." But he started drinking again on Monday night. Last night he had too much. He also has a problem and he wets the bed.

DOCTOR: On those nights?

PATIENT: He had his kidney removed about eleven years ago. So he only has one kidney left, but that isn't why. He never did before unless he has been drinking a lot.

DOCTOR: Why did he have his kidney removed?

PATIENT: He had started out with an infection and he went to the clinic and they decided that it had never functioned—it was deformed.

DOCTOR: What kinds of things happen to you when he's drinking? I know it's very upsetting, but I want to know specifically, is there any abuse?

PATIENT: No, he's never hit me. And it has only been within the last few months that he's gotten ornery and mean.

DOCTOR: Verbally mean? He says what will hurt the most?

PATIENT: Right, everything is my fault. Like I was going to say, Monday at the store, he wasn't doing very well. I didn't say anything to him until toward the end of the evening. I said, "You shouldn't drink any more." When he got through he came back and said, "It's all your fault. You come in and start nagging at me and yelling at me because I'm drinking too much. I can't concentrate with the customers." And so he got mad and went home.

DOCTOR: This situation where things are your fault—did this happen over the past two years or did it happen before?

PATIENT: No, it's only been the last few months.

DOCTOR: Anybody in his family have a drinking problem?

PATIENT: Not that I know of. We don't get to see them that much. He has a brother that his parents say has a problem. We're not that close to him so I don't know.

DOCTOR: At least their parents are concerned about it.

PATIENT: Yeah. I don't know if it's a one-night-a-week thing. I just don't know.

DOCTOR: What about your family?

PATIENT: No.

DOCTOR: Have you ever known anyone who had a drinking problem?

PATIENT: Yeah, when I was in high school, my parents moved away at the middle of my junior year, so I lived with my grandparents; and so that they wouldn't have to drive me back and forth all the time, I stayed with a girlfriend whose father was an alcoholic. It's really pretty weird, because her mother was almost like my second mother and I was going with Joe at the time. Oh, he'd go out with the boys and drink and I can remember her saying to me—well, he ran around with older boys and they drank an awful lot and she said that she wished he wouldn't. She said that that's the way Roger started out. She said, "I'd hate to see him end up like Roger." And I think of that so often.

DOCTOR: That's usually how we learn to drink pathologically in this country. With the boys—being antisocial, loud, obnoxious, and we learn that pattern of behavior and it never changes whether you're a boy in the alley or in a fancy dining place, anywhere. The behavior is always the same. When you go out to eat, is it a problem? Do you get tense when the waiter or waitress comes around asking for drinks?

PATIENT: No, usually it doesn't bother me when we're out or something. We don't get to go out that much anymore. But before, no. Once in a while he'd have too much, and he'd come home and be drunk and have too much to drink. As a rule, no, it never bothered me. Really, since we opened up the store, it's there all the time. He can find alcohol any time. (*Patient cries briefly.*)

DOCTOR: What would you like to do to change it?

PATIENT: I don't know. He has a chance to go back to our home town and the factory. I don't know if it would help or not. Just get him away from this.

DOCTOR: What do you think?

PATIENT: Well, he's not happy here. I know that. I'm not happy any more. It can be fun meeting the people at the store, but the hours are too long.

DOCTOR: Thirteen hours a day?

PATIENT: No. Well, I don't have any time with him. I miss that. And Joe was always such a good father. He always did things with them and now he doesn't any more. Now is the time they need it the most.

DOCTOR: Is there a big economic penalty for going back to your home town?

PATIENT: Actually, it would be to our advantage if he would go back. The wages are good there. We don't know what the summer is going to bring—it's going to be a very slow one, I'm afraid. I worry about whether we'll make it through the summer or not. So, financially it would be better to go back.

DOCTOR: Did you talk to him about that?

PATIENT: Yeah, we have. He misses the old business and I know that he has said that he doesn't care for it here. The people complaining all the time get to you. The last fall he had a chance to go back because they couldn't find anybody to replace him, and he decided and told them he would. Then he said, "Oh I can't leave you alone here, and we couldn't find anyone to come in and take care of the machines and stuff." So he didn't. The guy they hired has not worked out and they called him again and I don't know. He doesn't talk about it. He talked a little bit and I thought that after a while he would decide to go back, but the last week or two he just doesn't talk about it.

DOCTOR: It's hard for you to spend enough conversation time to know what he is thinking about.

PATIENT: That's just it.

DOCTOR: Previously, until two years ago when you started this new occupation, did he share feelings?

PATIENT: Yeah, most of the time. He's always been one to keep everything to himself. It's kind of hard to find out what he's thinking. Once he did start to talk, then it was fine. He's always one where he was going to do what he wanted to do.

DOCTOR: He was always a little headstrong?

PATIENT: Yeah. Very stubborn. Even when we were going together, when he wanted to go out with the boys he'd go out, even if he had asked me out on a date it was always what he wanted to do first. It hasn't been that big of a problem until recently.

DOCTOR: Have you ever known anyone who has gotten better from a drinking problem? Who seemed to survive it and do well?

PATIENT: Well, the Joneses did fairly well, and Donna seems to be doing very well, and Susie seems much better.

DOCTOR: Do you have any concept of what they might have gone through?

PATIENT: Not really.

DOCTOR: Let me explain my concept of a drinking problem. I have an idea that your husband's headstrong nature was there early, and maybe it was appropriate at that time to be carefree and footloose, but somehow things have changed after sixteen years of marriage. Now he has more responsibility. My understanding of a drinking problem is that once it becomes fully developed it is progressive. You've observed that over the past two years. The pattern of behavior becomes more abnormal or more intolerable. If you or I had a drinking problem, we would probably project blame onto other people—never looking in or presenting it in any way to anyone else's inspection. It can be fatal. Usually it's not initially, but ultimately people die early with this kind of problem. The thing it is really fatal to is relationships. It is really hard to have a meaningful time, as you are describing now, with someone who is not able to share. Even if he were not drinking on a given occasion, it is hard to get close to a person who is that defensive, who projects that much blame.

Therefore, my understanding of how to recover from this sort of problem is more than abstinence from drinking. It is not just to remove the alcohol. You have to put something in its place. Something to help him understand himself and accept his own feelings and share them with some people. Being free to admit mistakes. That's the only way I know how to do it, and that usually involves a lot of hard work and confrontation initially.

Confrontation usually means that we have to ask someone to change in some way, such as you have probably experienced when you have said maybe it would be better if he would not drink so much. It would involve some support and changes on your part as well. You have to understand how not to aggravate the problem—which you are trying very hard not to do—and how to recover from this pretty devastating situation. Those are areas where Alcoholics Anonymous and Al-Anon come in very handy. It isn't universally required, but I haven't seen very many people do very well without them. Now people do it, and some people indeed are good at recovering. AA and Al-Anon are uncomfortable for some people. However, for most people I know, those are the groups that are most helpful. What is your reaction to this? An honest reaction?

PATIENT: My first reaction is that he would never do it.

DOCTOR: I guess I would worry about him later. What about you? Time is a problem, I know.

PATIENT: I guess I hate the thought of everybody finding out, but if it will help him, that is all I care about.

DOCTOR: What about helping you, would that be important too?

PATIENT: Yeah. I don't want to go through this again, it's too painful.

DOCTOR: One of the concepts that AA and Al-Anon work at is that you and I are responsible for ourselves. We probably can't be responsible for anyone else. So it isn't that you or I can force him to stop drinking. Somehow we have to take care of ourselves and allow him the opportunity to take care of himself—which makes sense but it is hard to do. Those are some of the principles which Al-Anon especially works on. You have to take care of yourself, protect yourself from this hurt—possibly withdraw emotionally a little bit to protect yourself until he becomes more invested in his own recovery. What would happen if you asked him to come in here and the three of us chat? He knows me a little bit.

PATIENT: He'd probably refuse.

DOCTOR: Do you think you could try?

PATIENT: I'd try.

DOCTOR: Do you think it would be all right with you if you let him know that we talked today?

PATIENT: I'll tell him.

DOCTOR: I don't like secrets. He'll be angry initially. I think—I don't know how your schedule is—this is a miserable schedule. I think it would be helpful if you could begin understanding the concepts of Al-Anon. I don't really know whether this is going to be something that is going to require inpatient treatment or not, but it may, in order to achieve all these other areas of recovery, aside from just abstinence. One has to recover one's self-esteem, one's ability to share feelings, to be human and to actually say—at the end of full recovery and with a high head (without the head hanging low), "I have a drinking problem and I'm an okay person." It doesn't help a lot if someone quits drinking and drags it out forever and always apologizes for himself or herself. That's not my goal anyway. Joe has a right to feel good about himself. He is a fine person. He has a very difficult problem.

We should look at this as a problem that is treatable—and it is—at least you have one example of someone you know who has successfully quit. We approach it confidently and with the understanding that with certain kinds of techniques that are available now—they may change in ten years—but right now we know what will work, though we may not always understand why. If we use those techniques people get better—generally. At least that is my experience. But it is as if someone comes with appendicitis; they expect to go to the hospital, have surgery and anesthesia, and have a painful scar. Most of it heals up, but there is a little scar, and that is all accepted. But with chemical dependency, which is what we are dealing with here, it is a complex problem, and if we approach it appropriately I think people do pretty well. If we resist by saying, "Maybe we can just ask him to quit drinking and maybe it'll get better," we would get into trouble because it is too difficult a problem. It is more than just a little problem; it is a complex problem, but it is treatable. My understanding of it is that we must incorporate the whole family into the recovery process, because it affects everybody. Then it's not a mystery to your children or to you about how things are now and how they are going to get better. What I would like to do is give you a few booklets just to start with. Have you ever seen any booklets from Al-Anon?

PATIENT: No.

DOCTOR: That will be a relief to you because in all the things you are going through—you are not alone. And then my recommendation would be as soon as possible for you to take the time to go to Al-Anon, whether he goes to AA right away or not. I expect you may have difficulty in doing that. It is part of the denial. I would like to set up another meeting for a few weeks from now, with him invited. But even if you and I meet just briefly alone, it's still helpful. This brings pressure to bear—for him to accept his own responsibility. It doesn't mean that you or I think less of him; it just means that we know he has a problem that is treatable and we're just asking for the initiation of treatment.

PATIENT: Is there an Al-Anon here in town?

DOCTOR: Yes. You bet there is. Tuesday nights at 8 P.M. it meets in the church—the church right down the street. There are open meetings, I believe the last weekend of the month, and there is an Al-Anon number in the local newspaper. I know the number for—the call number/help number for AA. I think the Al-Anon people are at the same number. You can call and they will give you the details and maybe you can call someone to help you get to the first meeting, so you could go with someone. Let me get some reading material. My view of this is optimistic. Out of all the things I see that create family conflict, this is the one for which we have the most resources to call into play. I find there is a very successful outcome most of the time.

PATIENT: What do we do while I come but he won't come into the office?

DOCTOR: I expect this at first. But I give him the chance, I never know. Maybe after the first request someone will come in and talk. Maybe six months later. But I am always optimistic. You are the one that is in charge. You accept not having to be responsible for his drinking and you just do what you're doing and take care of yourself and the best you can. You don't make apologies for him when he is not behaving well; you just let him go.

PATIENT: That's my—when he gets drinking—that's when I worry about him making a fool of himself or I want to be there to take care of him.

DOCTOR: That's the first thing we resign from—taking care of him at those times. That way it hits him in the face a little bit. He realizes that he is responsible for himself. It is kind of like if you or I keep pulling children's hands away from the hot water and they never quite learn that the water is hot—stick their finger in there and they learn. You have to let him learn the consequence of his own behavior and that is part of the role of Al-Anon to give you the courage to do that. That is a very difficult thing. I'll go get some booklets.

POSTSCRIPT BY BAIRD

After I took the initial history of the severity of the problem, I essentially gave her my usual approach to chemical dependency, which requires her participation in Al-Anon before her husband really catches on to the fact that he needs help. My expectation at this writing is that she will indeed carry through with Al-Anon activity, and I predict that within 4 to 6 months I will be interviewing him as well, unless there is a crisis in the meantime, which will hasten the changes that are required.

In my view, her changes will probably have to come first through Al-Anon in order for her to bring enough sincerity in her request for change to convince him that he needs help. I find that our local Al-Anon group is very helpful; however, I continue seeing the spouse alone on an infrequent basis, either until a crisis arises or until I have a better leverage position for some other reason over the drinking individual. At that point I would probably request inpatient treatment for him at a center that has family participation. I would probably achieve that after some type of family confrontation involving the children as well as both spouses.

I have learned over the past 3 years that it is probably just as well that I wait for a crisis to arise or wait for her to become more convinced through Al-Anon that treatment is necessary, rather than immediately calling a family gathering (unless there is imminent physical danger). It should be noted that this interview was done at the end of a very busy morning schedule, and I purposely cut a few corners because of the time demands that were upon me that day. I will be seeing this couple frequently between now and her next office visit, again because of the proximity of their establishment. Obviously, I plan not to bring the topic up during social conversations, but I will not discontinue seeing the husband during the week in order to avoid this contact. I face the dilemma frequently in a small-town practice of either choosing to avoid contact with someone I am confronting or recognizing that I must go about my daily activities with some contact with people in transition or in the early stages of treatment, during which time they might be quite uncomfortable in seeing me. However, I have become accustomed to this, and I am not personally uncomfortable in seeing them. But it does prevent me from completely relaxing in their presence, because I am never quite sure when they will begin asking for help. They may do it on the spur of the moment or suggest that they would like to see me the next day in the office.

INTERVIEW 2: FIRST INTERVIEW WITH ALCOHOLIC HUSBAND AND HIS WIFE

INTRODUCTION BY BAIRD

The transcript to follow is an interview with Emily and her alcoholic husband. I had initially seen Emily when she presented with complaints of feeling tired and depressed about 6 months prior to this interview. I requested a family interview, at which time all of her six children arrived but her husband remained absent. It very quickly became apparent that the husband, Fred, had had an escalating drinking problem for several years. The older children then became involved in support groups that had previously been established at school for families of chemically dependent parents. I had three other interviews over the intervening 6-month period with the family. Each time Fred was invited but failed to attend the meetings, citing last-minute excuses. Emily and her children described a story of increasing family discord and failing farm activity, which had developed over the 2 years coinciding with Fred's increasing drinking history. He had frequently not accomplished routine farming tasks because of waking very late in the morning or around noon. He had several crop-planting failures, which had been noticed by neighbors and by his own family. He frequently had hangovers and was growing more irritable. Fred had become more verbally abusive over the past several months prior to the first interview. He was frequently either drinking or remorseful about things that were said or done during a drinking episode. Since the beginning of our family interviews, he had reduced his drinking frequency, but was still severely inebriated and belligerent when he did drink.

At the time of this interview, Fred elected to come in with his wife and without the children. The first 10 minutes of the interview were spent in reviewing the farm history and generally getting acquainted. Fred concentrated on his difficulty in dealing with his father, who had always been rather dictatorial toward all family members. Recently, Fred and Emily had decided to move away from the family farm and buy a nearby different farm in order to escape his influence. The only reason that Fred agreed to come to the office was that Emily refused to cosign the loan guarantee notes for the new farm unless Fred agreed to talk to someone about his drinking problem. Emily had been attending Al-Anon meetings since our first visits and was feeling fairly comfortable with herself. After the farm and family material was reviewed, Fred finally agreed to focus on the drinking issue.

THE INTERVIEW

DOCTOR: Now, Emily and I have talked a few times, as you know, and I am just interested in helping in any way I can. But I would like to understand how things are right now and in what way things might change.

HUSBAND: We're trying to buy a farm right now, and her feeling right now is that if I don't stop drinking, she won't help me buy the farm. She won't cosign the papers. We have decided not to buy my father's farm. He has always been such a dictator. I need to get away from him.

DOCTOR: Okay, so the new decision is that you're going to go on your own. That's been kind of brewing this winter?

HUSBAND: Longer than that.

DOCTOR: I understand something about what you say about a dictator, I know that. But some of those things are beyond our control. I guess what I would like to understand is, how are you two doing and are there any things in your relationship that we could work on? That's where I come from to help you with, anyway. What's been the nature of the conflict?

HUSBAND: The nature of it?

DOCTOR: Let's speak just within your own family.

HUSBAND: I guess it all boils down to she thinks I'm drinking too much. I'm not home too much.

DOCTOR: I don't know either, that's why I'm listening. What happens under those circumstances? I'm not there, so I don't know. What's your perspective on what happens?

HUSBAND: This isn't a common everyday occurrence; it's a thing that does not happen often.

DOCTOR: What happens when you come home and you've been drinking? How do people react?

HUSBAND: How do people react? You mean my own family?

DOCTOR: Your own family.

HUSBAND: They probably despise me.

DOCTOR: That's what you'd feel? What do you see in them—I mean what actions do they do? Do they go away or do they not talk to you? From your perspective.

HUSBAND: They try to keep their distance.

DOCTOR: What else happens?

HUSBAND: I don't know. That's about it, I guess.

DOCTOR: In what way aren't you at your best when you've been drinking?

HUSBAND: If you had a little too much when you came in here and tried to sit down and talk to somebody, you wouldn't be at your best.

DOCTOR: So it's hard to concentrate.

HUSBAND: Well, it's probably hard to concentrate on the problems.

DOCTOR: What about your mood at those times? What's inside of you? Everybody stayed away and you're out doing chores. How are you feeling at that time of a typical day?

HUSBAND: I don't feel any special way.

DOCTOR: Are you feeling happy or sad? Or angry or anything like that?

HUSBAND: I don't think I'm feeling happy or sad either. I don't know.

DOCTOR: Kind of numb.

HUSBAND: Not really numb either.

DOCTOR: Now, have you talked a little bit before you got here?

HUSBAND: I don't even talk to her.

DOCTOR: (*to Emily*) What do you see on those days? I know it's not every day, it's every once in a while. What do you see in him?

WIFE: In him? He's feeling a lot of anger.

DOCTOR: How do you know that?

WIFE: Just the way he speaks. I know just for myself, if I know that he's been drinking I set the whole stage—I know that I do that.

DOCTOR: How do you do that?

WIFE: "You kids do what you're supposed to do, get going, do your chores—do this and do that," so as not to agitate him more. Because I know that at certain times something might set him off and make him more angry.

DOCTOR: What happens when he gets set off? What do you see then?

HUSBAND: Do I get physically abusive?

WIFE: No, he's never done that. Sometimes words can hurt just as much.

HUSBAND: I probably say things I shouldn't say.

DOCTOR: (*to Fred*) How do you feel after those kinds of days? Say it's three days later or a week. Let's say it's some time later and you've been thinking about it, how do you feel?

HUSBAND: Oh, I don't know. I suppose maybe I said something—I suppose maybe if you only had a few drinks maybe you could figure out a better way to say it.

DOCTOR: We're not usually as clever as we think we are when we're drinking.

HUSBAND: No, I guess not.

DOCTOR: How serious do you think the problem is?

HUSBAND: Myself, I don't think it's something I don't have control over.

DOCTOR: That's a tough question. That's why I asked that. Maybe we can have a look at the kinds of problems that seem to be associated with it. What kinds of problems do you think are maybe not caused by it but associated with it? What kinds of problems do you think are associated with your drinking?

HUSBAND: I suppose it goes back to my father. You're rebelling against authority or whatever. Probably goes back a long time. My father would drink a few years back.

DOCTOR: Do those things stick in you yet?

HUSBAND: I guess it kind of gets to you once in a while. See, three years ago we rented a farm, that was after his stroke thing. This was going on before his stroke and he came back from New York—well, he's always figured that between the banker and real estate agent and us, me and Emily—that we gave him a raw deal. Well, the banker just told me that the other day that it's still in the back of his mind—he thinks that after his stroke we gave him a raw deal. This keeps surfacing all the time. It gets to you. He'll criticize—this has always been the case. He'll never give credit, unless he can take it himself.

DOCTOR: I know that's a tough person to relate to.

HUSBAND: We went with a little different tillage process than he was used to, and this was no good. It was too modern. He would criticize us for doing that. Well, then the crops turn out good—of course he was always a seed farmer. He wouldn't tell us that but he'd tell everyone else about the good corn I had. If my practices are so bad, then how come my corn turned out so well? I never hear from him that I have such good crops.

DOCTOR: So you're probably not ever going to get any positive feedback? I think we recognize that. Let me ask again—all of this is very complicated and I'm not at all saying that your problems in your life are from only one issue. I'm not saying that at all. But what kinds of problems do you think seem to happen more often when you're drinking?

HUSBAND: What kinds of things?

DOCTOR: I'm picking up that this family conflict gets uncomfortable at those times. Does that sound reasonable? Any other kinds of problems? What about financial? Has it caused any financial problems?

HUSBAND: Well, the old man will say, "What the hell did you do with all your money?" We added it up just the other day and in the last three years we gave him $125,000 and more.

DOCTOR: Okay, so it hasn't caused financial problems. You two agree on that?

WIFE: I think he manages quite well.

DOCTOR: You look pretty healthy.

HUSBAND: Right now I am, besides a cold.

DOCTOR: But besides that, has the drinking caused to your knowledge any health problems?

HUSBAND: Health problems, no.

DOCTOR: (to Emily) Are you aware of problems you observe in Fred?

WIFE: Flushed face more. (pause)

DOCTOR: So the major conflict is within your own immediate family. Now your father and your conflicts will be there, whether you were having any conflict or drinking or not. That was existing long before. Whether that contributes to the thing or not is beyond my power to know. But what happens between you two when you have conflict? Just between you and Emily? How do you resolve things? Do you talk about them? Can you let her know when you're feeling something?

HUSBAND: I suppose not all the time.

DOCTOR: Does it make you uncomfortable not to have her understand how you feel?

HUSBAND: No, I don't think so. I think she pretty much knows how I feel.

DOCTOR: Do you think, Emily, that Fred understands how you feel?

WIFE: No, I'm stubborn.

DOCTOR: You're stubborn, too. So, what happens, Fred, when you've been drinking? You say some things that you don't like, and you're coming back feeling like you wished you hadn't said some of those things. What does that do to you? Or how do you get over that? Or don't you? Do you ever express those kinds of regrets?

HUSBAND: Yes, sometimes. I'm not the kind of person that apologizes for a lot of things. Take things in stride and bury things and hold in things. It goes back—neither one of us are from loving, kissy-type families. If we are with a family and they see each other and have to kiss and hug and all that— well, that's never been my way. Say, for instance, two weeks ago I was up to my sister-in-law's and they're more of an outgoing kissing-type family. We know this woman quite well, and when we walked in there we didn't know what to say—maybe that's a better way of expressing yourself. They come over and they hug and they kiss and everything else, like an old Russian— kiss on one cheek and then the other.

DOCTOR: It doesn't mean anything to you?

HUSBAND: Well, that time it did. It eased me up, I didn't have to say anything. They do their talking that way. I wasn't that lost for words that I would have to say. That's never been our way, the way we were brought up, and I don't think that her family was kissing and hugging.

DOCTOR: What about—there are more than you two in your family—you have several children.

HUSBAND: Six.

DOCTOR: I met almost all of them. I'm not sure what the impact on them is for this particular problem; again, we're still assessing what the nature of the problem is. I'm not sure if it's the drinking or anything else, but something is having an impact on them. Do you have any feeling for how big of an impact this has had on them?

HUSBAND: I think maybe—I think that it boils down to more than just alcohol—see, we have two farms. The kids go to one farm to do chores. If I want to keep them under my control for my purposes, they don't want to do chores at the home farm. Unless I give them a specific job, they're all somewhere else. That irks me. I say when we do something, we're going to do it. It isn't right to have these kids away all the time. The oldest one is all stretched out. His grandfather talks to him at length.

DOCTOR: How did you get along when you were growing up?

HUSBAND: Oh, I don't know.

DOCTOR: That's what your brother had done a little bit, just turned away, walked away from him.

HUSBAND: I suppose that's what I'm doing. I'm trying to do my own thing. Trying to break away. I suppose that's one of the hardest things I'm doing after forty years.

DOCTOR: You have some strong feelings about that. What's that feeling inside right now?

HUSBAND: It bothers me real bad. (*Fred cries briefly; there is a pause.*)

DOCTOR: What's the feeling inside right now? It's kind of overwhelming.

HUSBAND: I don't know, to tell the truth. I despise him so bad. I don't want my kids to get that kind of feeling.

DOCTOR: Anger is okay, though? Is it anger?

HUSBAND: I don't know if it's anger, just after forty years he's a rich man. I have a lot of things stuck in that farm. But I ain't going to let it ruin me. We aren't that bad off financially. We have around $300,000. I just have to learn to pick up without him. That's probably what I'm feeling inside. Just have to have the courage to get up and do it. Nobody has really had the courage—my sisters and brother—they haven't had to stand up to the man. He's a hard man to stand up to. He does things his way. And that was it, I guess.

DOCTOR: And when you confronted him?

HUSBAND: He's just a hard man to deal with.

DOCTOR: He might mean well; I'm not sure that he is aware of his impact on you.

HUSBAND: I suppose the last couple of years, we got to the point where we would have Thanksgiving or Christmas and I flat out told her we would not invite that man to our house. He would in his way—he calls it teasing—he can intimidate people just so much and I don't feel comfortable around him. Maybe he has some smart comment to her mother or something. They all know he's teasing. But that kind of got to me. That he would sit there and you know what I mean by that.

DOCTOR: Let me change the focus again, because you were just starting to express some opinions about moving off the farm. It's anger, but in a way it's the first time you've ever changed anything this big.

HUSBAND: It's the first time since 1959 that I missed field work and was in the service. This is the first spring, so far, that I haven't turned any soil. I thought pretty hard that that was imbedded in me that I'm not a golden-type person. I just saw that it was impossible to be any place else. Now I get the feeling that maybe you're not so bad—you have something you can call your own. We've got all this cattle, this machinery, and all these kids and a wife, and here I sit. They can sit here and be led by him some more. He's got them; he says, "You can stay there and the boys can help me."

DOCTOR: So you're planning to change that for the first time in your life? That's a pretty big moment.

HUSBAND: I'm looking forward to it now. I thought for a long time that I couldn't be any place else. I'm sure some thought—oh, you'll be there ten years from now. As a matter of fact, when I get off there I have a five-dollar bet to collect.

DOCTOR: I'd like to hear about you collecting that bet. Now, we can talk about that for a while, and I can see the determined set in your jaw when you start talking that way and that's good, because I have a feeling that that's part of what needs to be done is to gain your independence and move into a new situation where you are in control and relatively untouchable by someone who can run your life. That's one issue. That might be the big one. The second one is the drinking. I don't pretend to know the cause of any drinking problem, but I do know that it really gets in the way of family relationships, and of your ability to function as a responsible businessman. And heaven knows, it takes a lot of business sense to have a farm.

HUSBAND: I don't think that it's ever gotten to the point where drinking has gotten in the way of my business. Every now and then—usually in the evening—maybe a lot of times on Sunday—that was the free day.

DOCTOR: What comes to your mind, Emily, when you think of a Sunday, which is his free day and a time when he would drink? Does it churn you up in your guts?

WIFE: Everybody enjoyed coming to our place, it seemed like it was a gathering place. It was Grand Central Station at our place all the time. I remember that within the last couple years it got so that I assumed when it came to Sunday afternoons—well, he wasn't doing anything wrong—and by supper time he was maybe not an alcoholic, but he was drunk enough to affect me and the kids.

HUSBAND: I usually drank when I did my chores and the rest of the guys did, you know.

DOCTOR: Maybe it changes you more as a person. Even if you're not flat out drunk, it might make you say things and do things that are offensive to your family just because they love you.

HUSBAND: Maybe what I should have done a while back was set aside a certain time for vacation. I think that within the last three years we've went to Hastings once. We should have a day off, every other week or so a day off. We have somebody hired to help but I couldn't do that.

DOCTOR: Well, you're going to break free of that; I can sense you're going to do that. It's going to be a terrible risk, but I don't see any other way out.

HUSBAND: Why is it a terrible risk?

DOCTOR: It's changing things. Most of us get a little nervous when we change our whole life after forty years. That's what I mean by "terrible risk." Personally, not economically. You know more about the economics than I do.

HUSBAND: I think it's more a terrible risk to stay there [on the family farm].

DOCTOR: Probably so. I trust in your judgment on that. But what I'm saying is that the risking part as a person is to change your life for the first time after you've been under someone's thumb. In a way, we have to look at that as being responsible. If we look at that honestly, we all do the same things. I'm not immune from this either. But what has happened is in a way you've agreed to be under someone's thumb at least the past few years, though maybe not when you were fifteen.

HUSBAND: Well, I suppose.

DOCTOR: That's water over the dam. Anyway, we accept responsibility for our own happiness; you're changing now. You're taking the ball and running with it. That's great. I know that that's contingent on this relationship stabilizing. That's why I come back to really what we've seen is typical, whether it's me or you or anyone else with a drinking problem. I think it is. I don't care if we call it "alcoholism" or not; to me, I don't care about labels. What I see and hear is that your family—just you and your children and wife—have tension and conflict relating around drinking behavior. Now whether that drinking behavior is the same as a hundred other people you associate with, it doesn't matter. The fact is that it is causing conflict here, and if it's going to get better, it's going to take just as big a change as it did for you to break free from your father. That change being that you can talk about it, which you are doing now with me. But, it is so sensitive; it's a life style change. None of us like to change our life style. I think there has to be a major change so that the knot goes out of her stomach on Sunday afternoons, and the kids don't cuss you again when you promise to do something and don't, and you chew them out not because you are hung over or irritable but because they deserve it. They've got to trust you that way. It's going to take a while to gain their trust back. That's a magical thing, almost. It takes time to get that back.

HUSBAND: I don't think it's bad that I've lost their trust that much.

DOCTOR: Don't underestimate that.

WIFE: To a certain extent these past few years have been bad.

DOCTOR: No, I'm not saying that they're going to walk away, but what I'm saying is that you've got to have a big enough change so that they can see it. Otherwise, they won't trust you; they will say they've heard this before.

HUSBAND: I think it gets to the point that, once you've had a bad day, like, and say you have a couple beers, well, they can smell it on you. Even if they get to the point that they see me with a can of beer in my hand, it sets the light on them. I can stop in the liquor store and walk out. I have the sense not to have the next one.

DOCTOR: But what I'm saying is that it is so frightening for the people and the families. It's so upsetting. All you have to do is to have a beer can in your hand and they will go through the same feeling as if you were four-plus drunk. They're not going to be able to distinguish one from the other. They're going to have the same reactions. It's like a reflex. That's why if the change isn't big enough for them to see, it's not going to work. In reality, people can't separate the two. They're going to have the same knot in their guts whether you have one can of beer in your hand or have had a dozen. It's not all that easy to change, but if you change, it's got to be big enough for someone to see it.

Now, to make a long story very short, I'm picking up from each of you that there is a lot of conflict in your family that you grew up in. You're making positive steps now, in this point of your life, to change that. You've actually shown that. My caution is that unless something inside your *own* family changes so that everybody is working on the same team, more or less, it will fall apart. Young people are always rebellious. I was; you were. So when you tell a fifteen-year-old to do chores, there is going to be some flack and that's never going to change. But if you can feel like you're trusting each other, it's going to work a lot better. The only way I know to do that, even though you have perhaps an early drinking problem, is to really be serious about how to change that. I think that means abstinence. At least for the foreseeable future—I don't know about forever.

HUSBAND: I don't know—I don't see myself cheating or nothing like that.

DOCTOR: No.

HUSBAND: I don't find myself being more nervous without a beer.

DOCTOR: No, because it's not a physical addiction with you.

HUSBAND: On occasion I have had too much. If it takes abstaining to gain the trust, then that's what I'll have to do, but there shouldn't be a problem with that.

DOCTOR: So we agree on that. I know it seems like it might be tough from your perspective and an overreaction, but I don't think it's going to work without that. Does that seem like something we can agree on? Abstinence?

HUSBAND: I don't know if it's going to take necessarily abstinence. It's in my mind to quit or something, so I won't worry about the drinking problem.

DOCTOR: I worry about that, because it's easy to underestimate how difficult that is. If you're downtown and your friends are having a beer, your family's reaction is going to be the same, whether you come home with one beer on your breath or thirty.

HUSBAND: That's true.

DOCTOR: So that's what I'm saying, it's not that easy. Because it's going to create conflict even with a little bit of drinking, at least for the foreseeable future. They've gone through things, and you have too, that we have not fully explored today. I think it is easy for you and I, especially, to underestimate the impact of this on your family. I think it's been a big impact. We are taking a few short cuts; we haven't sat down with the rest of the family members today. I think if we did they would tell us in no uncertain terms, it's been miserable! Not a little, but a lot. That's not to say that anyone is an awful person in your family, but the problem that has been created is miserable. It's almost intolerable. It is so frightening to people that they're going to react dangerously any time they're threatened. Now, again, I have to cut a few corners. We seem to agree on abstinence. Is that correct?

HUSBAND: I think like you say that without abstinence they get the same fear as if I drank a lot.

DOCTOR: Now, I've got another thing that I think is going to go along with that, and that is recognizing part of the problem has been a drinking problem with you as a family unit. I know the big conflict with your father, I'm not ignoring that. I'm saying that this drinking is one problem internally that you have. To me I don't know how to treat that successfully other than AA and abstinence. That's where the lumpy throat comes in.

HUSBAND: AA? I don't think—I don't feel a need for AA.

DOCTOR: I know that.

HUSBAND: I have no—they're probably doing a great thing for a whole lot of guys. I suppose after I watched my brother go to AA—he's had more goddamn drinks than I've had in my whole lifetime. I don't want to get myself with something that I'm going to break the rules that often. Hell, I might as well forget it! (*very angry response*)

DOCTOR: I would agree, but I'm not using him as a model.

WIFE: Don't use him as a model.

DOCTOR: I wouldn't use Ralph as a model.

HUSBAND: I see nothing that they could offer me that I couldn't do myself.

DOCTOR: I agree. Let me make it more clear. I'm offering that, I'm not insisting on it right now. I would, if you can't maintain abstinence.

HUSBAND: I would agree to that. If I cannot gain the trust of my family, then I would say that I need it.

DOCTOR: I understand you, Fred. But what I'm saying is that right now I would let you know if I was insisting on AA, and Emily knows you pretty well. Right now she is probably thinking that I'm a soft touch. But I would like to move in fairness. We've agreed that there are two parts to this plan. One of them is abstinence, let's say arbitrarily for a year. Is that agreeable? (*nods from Emily and Fred*) And if that isn't maintained? We can agree on that. Either it is or isn't. I trust you're honest with me on that. If that isn't, then AA is absolutely the only way to go. Now what I am saying is in addition to that. The only way I know successfully to bet on the situation is to make it a sure thing. That's because I'm not a farmer and can't gamble very well. If I asked a family to try to recover from the kinds of conflict you've had, I'd like to make it as sure a bet as possible. If someone is changing their life style enough to gain the trust back from the family, it is not easy. And what I would think AA would offer is not magic but at least a chance to discuss your own feelings on this whole change with other people who aren't going to say you're crazy. If you go to your best friend right now—I don't even know who that is—but I'll bet you it'll be someone who's going to think you're crazy if you *stop* drinking.

HUSBAND: I don't know who I could call my best friend.

DOCTOR: Well, let's say in a social group—a lot of them are not going to understand how important it is for you to turn down a drink. They are more likely to give you grief about it.

HUSBAND: Oh, I don't know. The other day I was offered a beer and turned it down—I suppose we've been drinking for a few years and I don't think he cared. I guess my dad got to the point where a couple of people would stop by his place regularly and it was natural. Even if we were drinking coffee they would think we must have been boozing. That isn't the case all the time.

DOCTOR: I understand. I'm going to say a couple things and call it quits for the day. One of them is that you've been very straightforward and I appreciate it. I know it must have been tougher than hell to get you in here. I've been telling you everything I'm thinking so I'm not holding back any punches. Now Emily has been trained through Al-Anon and she knows what I'm thinking, and I'm thinking that sobriety of which we're speaking means several things, including feeling good about oneself, feeling like you or I can express feelings.

HUSBAND: Well, I feel good about myself now. If I can make the bread from that farm . . .

DOCTOR: I agree, and I'm anticipating that. I'm saying there's several things involved. The trust in your family is involved, expressing your feelings honestly—maybe not to everybody on the street, but I mean at important times. Those kinds of things are hard to accomplish. I think that AA is one place to accomplish them. It's not the only place, and for some people, indeed, AA is not helpful. But I'm saying that if we want to make a safe bet, that's the best place to make it. The second thing is that, yes, indeed, it has been a significant drinking problem, but it isn't the only problem. It is a major problem. My training and beliefs are that if you don't make a serious effort at the drinking problem, the rest of those problems are going to stay there, and your efforts to emancipate yourself are not going to work. That's why I like to bet on a sure thing. I like not to set this thing up on a shaky foundation. You're going to face some big changes now if you change all this, and it's going to be enough to handle all by itself. If we don't have a real solid program to maintain sobriety, I'm worried that the whole thing will fall apart. That's why I'm recommending AA. Now I want you to think about this for a while, and I know you don't like it right now. That's what I'm saying.

POSTSCRIPT BY BAIRD

The purpose of this interview was to initiate positive change in a family with a difficult problem. There seemed not to be enough of a crisis to request inpatient or immediate outpatient chemical dependency treatment at this time. My recommendation for attendance at AA was received with great anger, but this person did agree to a prolonged period of abstinence. I used the abstinence only as an entry into the family system; I expected that he would not be able to maintain abstinence for the agreed-upon length of time. This would allow at a future date a confrontation that could be more forceful and probably more effective for precipitating a reasonable recovery attempt.

Fred clearly wanted to focus on his conflict with his father and farm-related topics. It was somewhat difficult to keep the focus on the drinking issue; however, his attention was well captured by the time I mentioned AA and prolonged sobriety. I did not review much of the painful history of this problem, partially because the children were not at this meeting. I had agreed to the marital dyad interview without the children in order to set the stage for a more powerful intervention at a later date.

Approximately 6 months after this taped interview, Emily called me and asked for further intervention. Fred had not resumed drinking but was belligerent and morose, expressing feelings that everyone was against him. This fit the pattern of the "dry drunk" syndrome and signaled the need for further intervention. With the help of school counselors, a family interview was arranged. Following that intervention, Fred reluctantly agreed to attend

AA meetings. At this writing, he is still struggling with issues of anger and low self-esteem, but is beginning to admit that he has a drinking problem. I think that his future progress will depend a great deal on his ability to establish meaningful relationships with other people in AA, or it may require formal inpatient treatment. This is a classic example of incomplete recovery, in which abstinence from chemical use is achieved with little or no improvement in family interaction patterns or individual self-esteem for the dependent person. In retrospect, it might have been more fruitful to demand an entire family attendance at the initial interview with Fred in order to make a more forceful request for formal chemical dependency treatment as a first step. This may have avoided the pain of his abstinence without other aspects of recovery. However, he might not have agreed to such a powerful intervention at that time.

14 TREATING DEPRESSION IN A FAMILY CONTEXT

According to a survey of mental health activities of family physicians in two states, depression is the mental health problem most often encountered in family practice offices (Cassata & Kirkman-Liff, 1981). The diagnosis of depression is also one of the most common reasons for psychiatric consultation among primary care physicians (Katon, Williamson, & Ries, 1981). Epidemiological evidence suggests that clinical depression is quite common in the general population. In their review of studies that used recent diagnostic techniques, Boyd and Weissman (1981) reported that the prevalence of depressive disorder in industrial countries is 3% for men and 4 to 9% for women, and the lifetime risk is 12% for men and 20 to 26% for women. Along with chemical dependency, depression is the most serious mental health problem encountered daily in family practice. This chapter first reviews the diagnostic criteria for depression and then concentrates on the assessment and treatment of depression in a family context.

DIAGNOSING DEPRESSION

Several challenges confront the family physician in making a diagnosis of depression. First, feelings of sadness and disappointment—a so-called "depressed mood"—are nearly universal human experiences, particularly after a significant loss. But these depressive *symptoms* may not indicate a depressive *disorder*. Second, as Widmer and Cadoret have demonstrated, depression is apt to present in family practice in the form of multiple, ill-defined somatic complaints (Cadoret, Widmer, & Troughton, 1980; Widmer & Cadoret, 1978). Third, anxious-appearing patients may be primarily depressed and may be harmed by inappropriate treatment with antianxiety medications (Taylor, 1981). Finally, the physician must rule out underlying primary causes of depression such as endocrinopathy, dementia, and neoplasia, as well as adverse effects of drugs such as reserpine, methyldopa, propranolol, alcohol, sedatives, and anticholinergic medications.

Although there is no clear demarcation between normal depressive symptoms and a major depressive disorder requiring treatment, the latter is generally distinguished by the intensity, pervasiveness, and persistance of the symptoms (Boyd & Weissman, 1981). A depressed patient will show evidence over at least a 2-week period of several of the following symptoms: sleep disturbances, appetite disorder, decreased sexual interest, loss of interest in ordinarily pleasurable activities, self-reproach, psychomotor retardation, thoughts of death and suicide, and vague somatic complaints. If encouraged to express their feelings, many depressed patients will also admit to a hopeless, helpless despair. Table 14-1 presents the formal criteria for "major depressive episode," found in the most recent *Diagnostic and Statistical Manual of Mental Disorders* (DSM-III) (American Psychiatric Association, 1980).

There are no universally agreed-upon subtypes of depression. Over the years, different terms have been popular—for example, "endogenous" versus "reactive" depression, or "psychotic" versus "neurotic" depression. The distinctions seem to be based on the criteria of severity, chronicity, and the presence of identifiable stressors. DSM-III attempts to bring order to these conflicting categorizations by distinguishing between a "major depressive episode" (Table 14-1), a "dysthymic disorder" or "depressive neurosis," and "adjustment disorder with depressed mood." "Dysthymic disorder" is essentially a chronic but mild or moderate depression. "Adjustment disorder with depressed mood" refers to mild or moderate depression in response to an identifiable psychosocial stressor. The latter two disorders involve less severe somatic and psychological disturbances than does a major depressive episode. Table 14-2 contains the formal DSM-III criteria for dysthymic disorder. Table 14-3 gives the criteria for an adjustment disorder when the predominant manifestation involves depressive symptoms such as low mood, tearfulness, and hopelessness.

The etiology of depressive disorder is not clearly established, nor is there complete agreement on how to treat it. Current thinking on causes and treatment seems to be moving toward a pluralistic approach that acknowledges genetic, biochemical, psychological and social/environmental factors (Usdin, 1977). Calling on Engel's (1977) biopsychosocial model, Grolnick (1981) has articulated well the interconnectedness of different sources of depression:

> Dysfunction occurs on one or more hierarchical levels, from brain cell receptor site to community. If not contained on one level, dysfunction spreads intersystemically, up or down. For example, genetic predisposition to affective

TABLE 14-1. DIAGNOSTIC CRITERIA FOR MAJOR DEPRESSIVE EPISODE

A. Dysphoric mood or loss of interest or pleasure in all or almost all usual activities and pastimes. The dysphoric mood is characterized by symptoms such as the following: depressed, sad, blue, hopeless, down in the dumps, irritable. The mood disturbance must be prominent and relatively persistent, but not necessarily the most dominant symptom, and does not include momentary shifts from one dysphoric mood to another dysphoric mood (e.g., anxiety to depression to anger), such as are seen in states of acute psychotic turmoil. (For children under 6, dysphoric mood may have to be inferred from a persistently sad facial expression.)

B. At least four of the following symptoms have each been present nearly every day for a period of at least 2 weeks (in children under 6, at least three of the first four).
  1. Poor appetite or significant weight loss (when not dieting) or increased appetite or significant weight gain. (In children under 6, consider failure to make expected weight gains.)
  2. Insomnia or hypersomnia.
  3. Psychomotor agitation or retardation (but not merely subjective feelings of restlessness or being slowed down) (in children under six, hypoactivity).
  4. Loss of interest or pleasure in usual activities, or decrease in sexual drive not limited to a period when delusional or hallucinating (in children under 6, signs of apathy).
  5. Loss of energy; fatigue.
  6. Feelings of worthlessness, self-reproach, or excessive or inappropriate guilt (either may be delusional).
  7. Complaints or evidence of diminished ability to think or concentrate, such as slowed thinking, or indecisiveness not associated with marked loosening of associations or incoherence.
  8. Recurrent thoughts of death, suicidal ideation, wishes to be dead, or suicide attempt.

C. Neither of the following dominate the clinical picture when an affective syndrome (i.e., criteria A and B above) is not present, that is, before it developed or after it has remitted:
  1. Preoccupation with a mood-incongruent delusion or hallucination.
  2. Bizarre behavior.

D. Not superimposed on either schizophrenia, schizophreniform disorder, or a paranoid disorder.

E. Not due to any organic mental disorder or uncomplicated bereavement.

Note. From American Psychiatric Association, *Diagnostic and Statistical Manual of Mental Disorders* (3rd ed.) (Washington, D.C.: Author, 1980). Copyright 1980 by the American Psychiatric Association. Reprinted by permission.

disorder directs a psychobiologic disruption of the person, with impact upon his/her interpersonal networks. A major corporation moves out of state, creating a ripple effect upon those in it employs. In either case, it is important to examine the function which altered mood of one member serves in the family emotional system. (p. 244)

While acknowledging the many causes of depression, our discussion in this chapter focuses on assessment of the family context of depression and on the combination of pharmacological and primary care family counseling treatment.

TABLE 14-2. DIAGNOSTIC CRITERIA FOR DYSTHYMIC DISORDER

A. During the past 2 years (or 1 year for children and adolescents), the individual has been bothered most or all of the time by symptoms that are characteristic of the depressive syndrome but that are not of sufficient severity and duration to meet the criteria for a major depressive episode.

B. The manifestations of the depressive syndrome may be relatively persistent or separated by periods of normal mood lasting a few days to a few weeks, but no more than a few months at a time.

C. During the depressive periods there is either prominent depressed mood (e.g., sad, blue, down in the dumps, low) or marked loss of interest or pleasure in all, or almost all, usual activities and pastimes.

D. During the depressive periods at least three of the following symptoms are present:
   1. Insomnia or hypersomnia.
   2. Low energy level or chronic tiredness.
   3. Feelings of inadequacy, loss of self-esteem, or self-deprecation.
   4. Decreased effectiveness or productivity at school, work, or home.
   5. Decreased attention, concentration, or ability to think clearly.
   6. Social withdrawal.
   7. Loss of interest in or enjoyment of pleasurable activities.
   8. Irritability or excessive anger (in children, expressed toward parents or caretakers).
   9. Inability to respond with apparent pleasure to praise or rewards.
   10. Less active or talkative than usual, or feels slowed down or restless.
   11. Pessimistic attitude toward the future, brooding about past events, or feeling sorry for self.
   12. Tearfulness or crying.
   13. Recurrent thoughts of death or suicide.

E. Absence of psychotic features, such as delusions, hallucinations, or incoherence, or loosening of associations.

F. If the disturbance is superimposed on a preexisting mental disorder, such as obsessive–compulsive disorder or alcohol dependence, the depressed mood, by virtue of its intensity or effect on functioning, can be clearly distinguished from the individual's usual mood.

Note. From American Psychiatric Association, *Diagnostic and Statistical Manual of Mental Disorders* (3rd ed.) (Washington, D.C.: Author, 1980). Copyright 1980 by the American Psychiatric Association. Reprinted by permission.

ASSESSMENT OF THE FAMILY CONTEXT
OF DEPRESSION

In a review of research on the role of life events in precipitating depressive disorder, Lloyd (1980) found evidence from a number of controlled and uncontrolled studies that depressed patients have a higher incidence of family death, marital separation, family conflict, and family illness in the months preceding the depressive episode. Weissman and Paykel (1974) found that the marital relationship was the most impaired area of functioning in depressed women as compared to their neighbors. A series of follow-up studies on these women showed that marital problems persisted even when the patients were asymptomatic (Bothwell & Weissman, 1977). In a population study on the social origins of depression, Brown and Harris

(1978) found that the presence of a "confidant" relationship with a husband was a strong buffer against depression for women who had experienced major stressful life events. Finally, Widmer, Cadoret, and North (1980) showed that the spouses and children of depressed patients presented to their rural family physician with complaints of pain, functional disorders, and anxiety that were very similar qualitatively to those of the depressed patients and higher in frequency than those of the control families. While the causal links between family problems and depression are not clearly established in any of these studies, there seems little doubt about the importance of the family context of depression. We discuss this family context using our assessment categories of stressors, adaptability, cohesion, and interaction patterns.

STRESSORS

It is first important to see if the depressive symptoms are a reaction to specific stressors that have affected the patient or family. Major changes in the patient's occupation, income level, health status, or family situation may contribute to a recent onset of depressive symptoms and may suggest a good prognosis. Sometimes, the presenting patient may be grieving for the loss of something precious, such as a loved one, a job, a friend, or previous good health. Here the intervention task for the physician may be different than for long-standing depression with no associated precipitating event. In the case of grief- or loss-related depression, the physician can use a supportive mode of counseling while calling the family together to allow a grieving reaction to get unstuck and to proceed. A long-standing depression with no apparent precipitating life event, on the other hand, may signal the need for a consultation and a therapeutic team approach.

TABLE 14-3. DIAGNOSTIC CRITERIA FOR ADJUSTMENT DISORDER

A. A maladaptive reaction to an identifiable psychosocial stressor that occurs within 3 months of the onset of the stressor.
B. The maladaptive nature of the reaction is indicated by either of the following:
  1. Impairment in social or occupational functioning.
  2. Symptoms that are in excess of a normal and expectable reaction to the stressor.
C. The disturbance is not merely one instance of a pattern of overreaction to stress or an exacerbation of one of the mental disorders previously described.
D. It is assumed that the disturbance will eventually remit after the stressor ceases or, if the stressor persists, when a new level of adaptation is achieved.
E. The disturbance does not meet the criteria for any of the specific disorders listed previously or for uncomplicated bereavement.

Note. From American Psychiatric Association, *Diagnostic and Statistical Manual of Mental Disorders* (3rd ed.) (Washington, D.C.: Author, 1980). Copyright 1980 by the American Psychiatric Association. Reprinted by permission.

It is especially important to review the emotional and physical health of other family members to identify possible sources of stress. The presenting patient may be reacting to a dysfunctional family situation and may arrive in the office as the "squeaky wheel" for the family. We have observed that chemical dependency frequently presents first in the depression of the nondependent spouse. Without a family-centered approach and/or a family interview, it may be impossible to discover this important source of the patient's depression. A common example follows:

> A 35-year-old woman, who has two children and has been married for 15 years, has had multiple previous clinic visits for depression and ill-defined somatic complaints; she now presents to the office with a complaint of fatigue and not being "well" for many years. Approaching this index patient from a family systems orientation can be extremely helpful. Her symptoms, history, and physical exam may suggest depression as a primary diagnosis. A routine family interview should then be requested. Important information can be gathered just from who arrives at the meeting and who does not. With an appropriate interview structure, which has been previously discussed, the subject of her husband's alcohol abuse or dependency may surface. This may have been a previously well-kept family secret. The mother may have been the family symptom bearer and self-sacrificial martyr. The family equilibrium has been stabilized by her helpless "patient" role. The powerful and rigid husband has always been difficult to engage in the medical care system. The children may have become involved as supercompetent caretakers, or they may have become entangled in the legal system through behavior problems.

In this example, the patient's major stressor is the family's entrenched interaction pattern, which requires specialized treatment. However, the problem at least becomes understandable when viewed in a family context. This may be contrasted with the difficulty of resolving the index patient's depression through individual treatment alone. The very process of involving the entire family in the evaluation of depression can offer encouragement for the identified patient, may reduce frustration for the other involved family members, and will introduce the concept that the entire family is involved in the evaluation and treatment process to follow.

ADAPTABILITY

During the initial assessment of the primary patient's depressive symptoms, the physician can direct the history taking in a manner that reveals how flexible and adaptive the patient and family are in responding to life events and life cycle changes. This may give a clue as to the resources available within the family to cope with the current depression. It is quite likely that patients with long histories of depression will reveal family histories that suggest low adaptability. Conversely, depression of recent onset may be associated with a more adaptable family system; however, this is not always the case. The presenting patient may have never previously experienced a major depression, but a review of life cycle events may reveal the patient's and family's difficulties in adapting to job changes, birth of children, children leaving home, or other classic life cycle stages or events.

If low adaptability is evident in either recent-onset or long-term depression, the family physician must be patient in the approach to the family system. Appropriate treatment may involve not only office intervention but also community support activities, such as home visits from mental health workers, in order to deal more specifically with the low adaptability of the family. The recovery process may be slow, and responsibility should probably be shared with other mental health professionals in order to maintain one's enthusiasm over the long-term treatment that might be necessary in this situation. On the other hand, if the family has demonstrated good adaptability through life cycle events or other major stressors that can be identified through taking a family-centered history, the primary care physician may be more optimistic and may focus the treatment plan on office-based procedures with less need for community-based support. These considerations are important whether or not the treatment plan involves antidepressant medications. By identifying a base level of family adaptability, the physician is in a better position to establish an adequate treatment plan for the depressed patient.

COHESION

If the identified patient is clearly depressed, how do other family members react to the physician's diagnosis and treatment plan? In a family with a middle range of cohesion, other family members will probably react with concern, yet remain functional in their daily activities. If the family is enmeshed, the primary physician may have difficulty in identifying the most depressed member of the family. All members may feel the symptoms of the index patient and react with extreme concern and discomfort to any intervention program. The physician may hear statements such as "I can't eat or sleep when my mother is so depressed." In this case, clearer boundaries and more autonomy must be established between the index patient and other family members in order to allow adequate treatment. In fact, establishing these boundaries may be the fundamental part of the recovery plan.

If the index patient presents to the office with no visible support from other family members, and the index patient's symptoms seem to have no impact on other family members, then the physician might be seeing a family with a disengaged family system. In this case, it is common for the physician to have difficulty in finding other family members with whom to interact. There may be few or no visits to the primary patient in the hospital. The generalized sense of isolation within a family will generally become apparent to the family physician. The depressed patient in a family that has been disengaged for many years presents a complex treatment challenge to the physician. These patients and disengaged families may best be served by a team approach in which other mental health professionals and community support programs are incorporated into the treatment plan. The recovery process may be slow and may end in family breakup or divorce, an unfortunate but not always unwelcome outcome. The physician's intervention may not have *caused* the divorce, since divorce may have been inevitable prior to any intervention, but the process may have been accelerated by attempts to solicit the spouse's support for the depressed individual.

INTERACTION PATTERNS

By observing the family, the family physician can gain insight into the typical interaction patterns characterizing the family of the depressed patient. These patterns are most visible through direct observation of the family and can be only estimated, sometimes inaccurately, by interviewing the index patient alone. Family interaction patterns can both lead to depression and be distorted by depression. The physician should look especially for patterns of overresponsibility and underresponsibility for self and other family members. If the index depressed patient is usually the problem solver for the family, other family members may be extremely upset and anxious during the time when the family leader is dysfunctional; the family leader's depression may signal the need for more sharing of responsibility by other family members. Do family members generally speak for themselves, or are there family "mouthpieces" whose usual custom is to speak for everyone in the family, including the depressed member? If a usually inexpressive and functionally "speechless" family member is the index patient with depression, the family physician may find that taking a direct history from the index patient is complicated by constant answers from the family spokesperson.

Unspoken family rules that relate to the therapeutic triangle are important considerations in assessing the family context of depression. For example, in some families it is unacceptable to seek outside help for any problem. This must be addressed if the physician is to become significantly involved in the treatment process. Otherwise, the physician's interaction with the index patient may be constantly undermined by family leaders' trying to reinforce the unspoken family rule of not accepting outside help.

A common interaction pattern in depression is for family members to avoid any direct confrontation that can cause pain; therefore, they communicate through intermediaries. When someone becomes depressed, this pattern is enhanced even further. Once involved in the treatment process, the physician becomes part of the family system and must be careful not to become incorporated into this dysfunctional interaction pattern. For example, people will contact the physician to tell him or her their concerns about other family members—concerns that they say are too "sensitive" to bring up to the individuals involved. If this pattern is not successfully challenged, the depressed member will continue to live in a family cocoon where no one speaks straightforwardly for fear of causing pain. By observing the physician's modeling of appropriate communication in family counseling sessions, the family may understand new and more functional ways of relating to one another. Obviously, this cannot be done in an interview with the single family member. It requires time spent with families and may indicate a need for family therapy if patterns are rigid and not easily challenged.

Whether or not family interaction patterns have helped precipitate a depressive disorder, they can get in the way of a natural or treatment-induced recovery—and may sometimes enhance the severity and persistance of the depression. A common such pattern has been articulated by Watzlawick, Weakland, and Fisch (1974): Family members first try to cheer up a depressed person who responds by feeling worse. Family members then increase their efforts to help the patient "see the silver lining in every cloud." This amounts to pressure on the depressed person to feel different, leading him or her to feel misunderstood, ungrateful, or like a failure. We have seen families veer back and forth between false bubbly optimism and angry outbursts at the patient to "snap out of it." The patient usually snaps deeper into it, thereby eliciting feelings of frustration, despair, and anger from the rest of the family. As Watzlawick et al. (1974) state, this interaction pattern may stem from well-intentioned "common-sense" attempts to solve a problem that does not lend itself to such direct solutions.

PRIMARY CARE TREATMENT OF DEPRESSION IN A FAMILY CONTEXT

Involving the family in the treatment process has already begun if the physician has interviewed the family during the evaluation steps. If the depressive symptoms are of recent origin and the assessment suggests an adequately functioning family system, then the family-centered treatment process can begin with optimism. If the assessment reveals chronic depression or a rigidly dysfunctional family system, the family physician may want to remain involved in the treatment process but seek a consultation or referral. While each case presents a unique clinical picture, we suggest that the primary care treatment of major depressive episodes can frequently involve a judicious blending of antidepressant medication and family counseling. When somatic or vegetative symptoms are not pronounced, as in dysthymic disorder and adjustment disorder with depressed mood, counseling without medication may be sufficient. These suggestions are based partly on the demonstrated efficacy of antidepressant medications for symptomatic relief, the documented importance and persistance of marital problems for depressed persons, and the positive results of the one clinical trial that combined drugs and marital therapy (Friedman, 1975).

ANTIDEPRESSANT MEDICATIONS

Antidepressant medications, especially tricyclic antidepressants, have been demonstrated to be effective in alleviating the depressive symptoms of many patients (Jackson & Bressler, 1981; Morris & Beck, 1974). Morris and Beck's (1974) extensive review of double-blind studies found that tricyclic anti-depressants were more effective than a placebo in 61 of 93 comparisons. In another review of predictors of tricyclic antidepressant response, Bielski and Friedel (1976) concluded that the following patient factors are predictors of positive response to imipramine and amitriptyline: relatively high socioeco-nomic status, insidious onset of depression, anorexia, weight loss, middle and late insomnia, and psychomotor disturbance. Patients who showed poor response were those with predisposing personality traits, multiple prior episodes, and delusions. Bielski and Friedel concluded that tricyclic anti-depressants are more effective with depressions that used to be termed "endogenous" (those with no clear precipitating events and a strong somatic component to the symptoms) and less effective with so-called "reactive" or "neurotic" depressions (those with sudden onset, environmental precipitant, or long-standing negative personality predispositions), which are now termed "dysthymic" and "adjustment reaction" disorders.

   Thus the evidence suggests that antidepressant medications, while effec-tive for many symptoms of depression, are not a panacea for all depressed patients. *We urge the physician not to rely exclusively on pharmacological treatment when the context of the depression suggests that the family may have stabilized around a depressed member.* In addition, there is increasing evidence that pharmacotherapy helps with temporary symptomatic relief but does not prevent relapse or recurrence. Two recent studies found that the majority of treated patients became symptomatic during the year following generally successful treatment with tricyclic antidepressants (Kovacs, Rush, Beck, & Hollon, 1981; Weissman, Klerman, Prusoff, Sholomskas, & Padian, 1981). Murphy, Woodruff, Herjanic, and Super (1974) reported that all patients in a 5-year perspective study who were continuously taking anti-depressant medications had relapses. Weissman, Kasl, and Klerman (1976) found that about 60% of patients on maintenance treatment with amitripty-line experienced recurrence of symptoms within 1 year after acute treatment ended. Research is needed to determine whether depressed patients recycle less often through primary care and psychiatric treatment if their initial treatment more directly addresses the social context of their depression.

We have found in clinical experience that many patients with short-term depression improve with no medication if they are given adequate support from the family and the physician. Furthermore, some patients refuse medication treatment or have medical conditions that rule out such treatment. On the other hand, we have found antidepressant medication quite helpful for patients who are not sleeping or eating regularly and who cannot concentrate on daily tasks. The medication restores their bodily functioning to the point where they can work on the problems that confront them. But as the documented relapse rates suggest, pharmacological treatment provides a beginning but not an end to the treatment of depression.

When medications are used, other family members should be included in each office visit for the ongoing management of this problem, and the patient must be given the primary responsibility for recovery, with the support of the family. The medication is a support to help patients get physically stabilized—especially eating and sleeping regularly—in order to work on their problems. The combination of medication and primary care family counseling will help counter the entrenched hopelessness of the seriously depressed patient. After the primary patient and the family have become stable and new interaction patterns have been achieved, the medication can be tapered off slowly, a process that can be done more confidently because the medication has been described to the patient as only one part of the treatment program. This approach can help alleviate the patient's and family's fears of recurrent depression. If the family system does not seem to change in a helpful direction, it may be wise to continue the medication while patiently challenging the family system. An alternative is to suggest that the patient and family enter therapy.

THE PSYCHOSOCIAL TREATMENT OF DEPRESSION: RECENT DEVELOPMENTS

In recent years, two university centers (Yale and Pennsylvania) have developed individual psychotherapeutic interventions that rival tricyclic antidepressants in the treatment of nonpsychotic depression and surpass such drugs in enhancing some areas of psychological and social functioning (Kovacs et al., 1981; Weissman et al., 1981). In addition, most of the studies that combine drugs and these psychotherapies have shown the combination treatment to be more effective than either treatment alone or no treatment (Rounsaville, Klerman, & Weissman, 1981; Weissman, 1979). The drugs appear to affect vegetative symptoms, and the psychotherapy appears to affect psychosocial functioning; no negative interactions between the two treatments have been found (Rounsaville et al., 1981).

Despite this newly found status of psychotherapy (alone and in combination with medication) for treating depression, two nagging problems appear in the literature: relapse rates and limited impact on marital problems. The 1-year symptom recurrence rates for psychotherapy (specifically, cognitive therapy and interpersonal therapy) are comparable to those of medication alone, with 10 to 15% of patients becoming chronically depressed after either drug or psychotherapy treatment, and over half having some recurrence of symptoms even on maintenance treatment (Weissman et al., 1981). In the words of the cognitive therapy research team at Pennsylvania, "Our one-year follow-up suggests that for a distinct portion of patients, cognitive therapy or pharmacotherapy on a short-term basis may offer temporary symptomatic relief but not prevent relapse or recurrence. This somewhat discouraging finding echoes the results of other short-term and longitudinal studies and has several implications" (Kovacs et al., 1981, p. 38). One of the two implications the authors mention is the importance of the patients' social context; the other refers to distinguishing between a relapse and a new episode.

The second problem with individual psychotherapy for depression concerns the issue of marital/family problems. The Yale research team has shown (1) the predominance of marital problems among depressed women; (2) the relatively poor prognosis of depressed women who do not resolve their marital problems; and (3) the lack of effect of either pharmacotherapy or interpersonal therapy on marital problems (Rounsaville, Weissman, Prusoff, & Herceg-Baron, 1979; Rounsaville et al., 1981). It should be kept in mind that "interpersonal therapy" as practiced at Yale is an individual intervention, even though it focuses on the patient's social problems. These researchers have begun to suggest that conjoint marital therapy (with both partners present) might be the psychotherapy treatment of choice for depressed women with marital problems. As mentioned before, one study (Friedman, 1975) did find that marital therapy improved the marital functioning of a group of depressed patients and enhanced the effectiveness of drug treatment.

Given these research developments in the treatment of depression, we believe that it is wise for the primary care treatment of depression to include medication where indicated and marital or family counseling where possible. Although research is needed to show the efficacy of this family-centered primary care approach, we believe that such an integrated treatment strategy is the most rational one at this time.

SPECIAL ISSUES IN PRIMARY CARE FAMILY COUNSELING
FOR DEPRESSION

Following the individual and family assessment for depression, and in conjunction with the medical treatment of depression with antidepressant agents if indicated, the family physician can begin primary care family counseling for depression. The information gained in the individual and family assessment will be utilized heavily in planning a strategy for the counseling sessions. If the primary patient is depressed in reaction to a relatively recent stressor and the family shows good levels of cohesion and adaptability, the physician's main task may be to address family interaction patterns that hinder the resolution of depression. The depressed family member, for example, may express increased hopelessness and lack of interest in normal activities, which initially is countered by unusual cheerfulness or "stiff upper lip" recommendations from other family members. In such a case, the counseling strategy might be to recognize the primary patient's mood and affect as very uncomfortable, but also to inquire as to the feelings of other family members. They may express a range of feelings from frustration to anger to extreme pessimism. Such expression of feelings can lead to a suggestion from the physician that family members stop focusing all their energies on "curing" the depressed member and instead start taking better care of themselves as well. The depressed member can be encouraged to ask for support when needed and will usually feel relieved to be free of the expectation to get better quickly. In working with families in this situation, it helps to emphasize their coping strengths, such as a good sense of humor or a history of working together to solve problems.

If the precipitating stressor mainly affects one family member (for example, job layoff or illness), the physician may discover that the depressed patient has great difficulty in asking for help from other family members. This person may always have been the stalwart, uncomplaining family member, the core of the family's strength in coping with the world. Asking for help may be impossible unless family roles are broadened and the family leadership becomes shared. A family with good flexibility may be able to adapt to the role changes by its own efforts or through primary care family counseling. However, if there is little adaptability, this change in family functioning may require family therapy. In that case, the primary care physician should identify the problem, set expectations for the need for change, and then seek consultation for the family with an experienced family therapist or a psychiatrist who understands family systems. In the meantime, the medical management of the patient's depression should continue if antidepressant medication has been started.

If the patient comes from a family with low levels of family cohesion (i.e., a disengaged family), the family physician is likely to be seeing the primary patient as an isolated individual with little visible support from other family members. A family interview—if it can be arranged —is of great importance here in order to inquire as to the family's awareness and feelings about their low level of cohesion. If they choose to continue in that pattern because of their greater comfort with a disengaged family style, the physician may have to accept interacting with the primary patient on an individual basis. Adaptation to the external stressor may then require support beyond the primary physician. Self-help groups, adult education, or church activities may provide adequate social support for the individual who is in a disengaged family. In these cases, the physician should not label the level of family cohesion as a problem unless it is identified as a problem by the patient or family.

If the family assessment reveals an enmeshed family, then the entire family unit or a particular enmeshed subsystem (such as mother–daughter) may have a flat affect and depressed appearance. Giving permission for other family members to express independent and perhaps different feelings about the situation may be helpful. It may be a family assumption that if one person in the family reacts to a stressor with depression, all family members must follow suit. Exploring the feelings and opinions of each family member will often be complicated by comments from the "family spokesperson." Permitting individuals to speak for themselves in the family sessions is a primary counseling strategy for this type of family. If the family strenuously resists the primary physician's attempts to allow for individual expression, the need for family therapy must be considered.

In many instances, the major stressor for the individual patient comes from chronic conflict within the family. A family interaction pattern may have become organized around one person as the identified patient in order to prevent meaningful discussion of family problems. A counseling plan in this situation would be to deemphasize the "sick" role for the identified patient and to identify clearly the source of discomfort within the family relationships. A common example is a mother who has been rearing children for the first 15 years of marriage and now seeks outside employment or educational opportunities. If the mother's depressed symptoms have been obvious for several months, it may take considerable effort on the part of the counselor to deemphasize her role as a patient and to focus on more generalized role changes within the family. The goal here is to keep her from a dead-end role that has progressed from child care provider to perpetual patient and has locked her husband into the equally uncomfortable role of perpetual caretaker. Exploring family members' dissatisfaction with these constricting roles can be an important step toward change. For a young family with a depressed spouse, the physician may be of great help by improving the family's adaptability through using internal and external resources. This may be as simple as suggesting competent babysitters, encouraging increased spouse discussions, encouraging some private time for a young couple to reestablish their own marital and sexual relationship, or helping the partners to define their autonomy apart from their own parents. This is an ideal setting for primary care family counseling to help young couples handle their present problems and to lessen the risk of future episodes of depression in one family member.

CONCLUSION

Generally, the family physician will be able to gauge the severity of depression-related family problems by limiting the attempts at primary care counseling to two or three family visits over 6 to 8 weeks. If no progress is noticed during this time, the best primary care intervention would be to seek more experienced help. During these initial attempts at primary care family counseling, the goals should be (1) to clarify individual boundaries in an enmeshed family; (2) to encourage patterns of mutual support in a disengaged family; (3) to mobilize outside supports for the patient and family; and (4) to change interaction patterns that perpetuate the depressed member's helpless role. Whether or not medication is used to control the uncomfortable symptoms of depression, primary care family counseling is useful to improve the patient's family and social context. The medical and family counseling strategies are neither mutually exclusive nor competitive. When used together wisely, they offer the epitome of biopsychosocial primary care.

APPENDIX: CASE EXAMPLES

The following examples are from Baird's practice.

DEPRESSION: CASE 1

DESCRIPTION

Mrs. W, a bright, usually energetic mother of four, presented to the office with a complaint of lethargy, poor appetite, and generally not feeling well for 2 to 3 months. She had seen other physicians recently for gastrointestinal (GI) distress and had negative X-rays of her stomach and colon, and normal blood tests. Yet she still had "no pep." Review of her medical history indicated that she had never before had a serious illness. Her only hospitalizations were for childbirth. Her children, aged 8 to 18, were all well, were not in trouble at school, had friends, and were socially active. Her husband was well, had no major illnesses, and was reported as helpful by Mrs. W. Neither she nor her husband drank much alcohol, and neither smoked. On physical examination, Mrs. W was of normal weight; vital signs and physical examination were entirely normal. She was intelligent, socially comfortable, and attractive. She and Baird discussed her findings at this and previous examinations. Mrs. W agreed that she *should* be well but did not *feel* well. Baird suggested that her diagnosis was depression but that he did not fully understand the context of her depression and what factors may have contributed to the depression. With further discussion, Baird found that there were no financial problems; the children did not seem to be in any unusual conflicts, nor were they discipline problems. Her husband seemed attentive and generally supportive. But she felt frustrated at the end of each day. She cared for everyone else all day long, but no one was saying "Thank you."

When she went shopping and was late returning home, no one would even start dinner. She had few activities outside her home and had no hobbies. When asked "Who takes care of you?," her response was "No one." Within 20 minutes both Mrs. W and Baird realized that she had not set her own needs as an important priority. She felt blue most days, but after she thought about things she felt angry—at herself and sometimes at other family members. She agreed to return in 2 weeks with her family and also agreed that she needed no medication. She felt much better after the interview and left with a faint smile.

As scheduled, Mrs. W arrived with her entire family. Discussion centered on how the members felt about (1) their self-described roles in the family, and (2) the mother's diagnosis of depression. The family mood was fairly bright. They poked fun at each other appropriately and did not outwardly resent coming to the office. They all agreed that they wanted the mother to get better. The youngest son felt somewhat responsible for the mother's illness, and this was discussed in a family setting. He was relieved to find that no one else agreed with him, and he immediately became more animated and cheerful. The family agreed that new rules of courtesy and respect for each other's needs were in order. It was apparent to them that it was especially important to respect the mother's needs that extended beyond her role as a mother. During the interview Mr. W was supportive and seemed flexible about changing some tasks and interaction patterns at home.

Over the next three months, Baird saw Mrs. W individually four times. Each time we concentrated upon her role in the family, her ability to see and change that role, and her feelings about her progress. She gradually improved, lost her bodily discomforts, and began smiling. Other family members had begun to help with family household chores, and none seemed upset about their new level of work activity. There were some initial complaints that the mother was not as "helpful as she had been." The teenagers did manage to collect their dirty clothes as requested; tables were set and cleared at mealtimes. The household ran fairly well even though the mother was occasionally absent, since she now had free time for other activities. Mr. and Mrs. W had a vacation alone for 3 days and returned with a renewed sense of joy in being a couple. In general, Mrs. W's depression and her family situation had improved after a total of five office visits that included one family interview. No medications were used. At this writing, Mrs. W no longer comes to the office except for routine gynecological exams and to accompany her children during their occasional acute illnesses.

COMMENTS ON CASE 1

This case was ideally suited for family-centered treatment without medication. The patient has been depression-free in the past, was well motivated, and had a generally supportive and well-functioning family. In DSM-III terms, her diagnosis was probably an adjustment disorder with depressed mood—or in more everyday family practice language, a mild depression of recent onset. The primary patient readily accepted responsibility for creating change and did not blame others for her problems. Although her "super mom" role had been developing for many years, the depressive symptoms were of relatively short duration. The family had not yet organized around these symptoms in an unyielding fashion. Not every patient who comes to the office with symptoms of depression has such a good prognosis; however, family physicians can be trained to recognize such persons, do an appropriate evaluation, engage the family in the treatment process, provide brief primary care counseling, and then withdraw in order to allow the family to resume its normal and hopefully improved functioning. In such cases, the treatment is brief, is cost-effective, avoids family scapegoats, and can often be done without medication. A missed diagnosis or inappropriate treatment could eventually result in more pronounced individual and family dysfunction.

DEPRESSION: CASE 2

DESCRIPTION

Mrs. J presented to the office with complaints of fatigue, listlessness, and despair. She no longer felt useful to her family. She and her husband had had marital therapy several years ago, and things had temporarily improved. Now she was feeling hopeless again. Mrs. J was 39 years old and had two girls and one boy, aged 15, 9, and 3, respectively. Her husband had a good job, and she had worked intermittently in the past, primarily to break the monotony. She grew up in another state with one older sister and one younger brother. Both of her parents were well, but had experienced many years of marital conflict. No one in her family had suffered any major psychiatric illnesses or chemical dependencies. Her mother was an adamant "teetotaler" and did not use alcohol.

Mrs. J stated that she was depressed and wanted help. She had been uncomfortable for 2 or 3 years and had been treated with several different antianxiety agents (benzodiazepines), which she was still taking as prescribed —three times a day. She denied alcohol use. Baird asked to see her together with her husband in the office. Her husband agreed to the joint interview when Baird called him, and he also volunteered that his wife had for several months been drinking large amounts of alcoholic beverages at home during the evenings.

When the couple and Baird met together, they reviewed the history of discomfort as described above. When the subject of medication and alcohol was broached, Mrs. J agreed that there was a problem. Mr. J had a very pessimistic outlook about chemical dependency, but both of them agreed that immediate formal chemical dependency treatment was appropriate before further treatment of the depression could be accomplished. Mrs. J entered a family-oriented treatment center within 2 weeks. Mr. J participated fully in the "family week"; he became more optimistic about chemical dependency and became aware that it was a family illness. Upon returning from the treatment center, Mrs. J was optimistic, sleeping better, and appreciative of the help that had been offered. She was no longer depressed and believed that the primary problem was chemical dependency. However, now she voiced concern for her husband's drinking behavior. She was involved in AA and understood that she was not responsible for his chemical or alcohol abuse, but felt that the issue should eventually be discussed.

Mr. J was involved in Al-Anon and was very comfortable there. He was happy that his spouse was much better, but now felt more uncomfortable about himself and became overly involved in his work role. After about 6 months, Mr. J attended a party and became quite drunk. This had happened several times in the past, but now the context of the event made it more noticeable: After all, his wife had just returned from "treatment." He was unable to work the next day due to the "flu," which was really just his hangover. Mr. and Mrs. J agreed to a follow-up family office visit. Mr. J agreed that he, too, was chemically dependent. He agreed to change from Al-Anon to AA meetings. The decision to seek formal chemical dependency inpatient treatment was delayed until his progress could be evaluated through outpatient chemical dependency counseling and group therapy. He immediately achieved sobriety and more slowly became aware of his extreme commitment to the work role. At this writing, group and couples therapy with a chemical dependency counselor and AA activities have been maintained. Neither Mr. or Mrs. J is on medication, and both have abstained from drinking since their individual confrontations. Mrs. J no longer feels listless, and Mr. J is much more comfortable. Both feel that they are "recovering" but that it will be a continual process. Neither sees a physician except for routine health maintenance. The children are functioning well in school and have been involved in the outpatient counseling program.

COMMENTS ON CASE 2

Mrs. J was the identified patient, but the family system was dysfunctional. The depression was real but secondary to a chemical dependency problem. The chemical dependency was treated first, and her depressive symptoms resolved. However, since her chemical dependency treatment involved her spouse, he eventually sought treatment for his chemical dependency problem as well. The family physician recognized the context of the depression in the index patient and sought appropriate help for this very complex and often rigid family problem. He did not advise simple discontinuance of medications or abstinence without formal chemical dependency treatment, because the family system had become organized around chemical and alcohol use. Swift and specific treatment was instituted as soon as the diagnosis of depression was accompanied by the diagnosis of chemical dependency. Treating the depression first on an individual basis would not have permitted appropriate attention to the dysfunctional family roles beyond the primary patient. Chemical dependency deserves the first priority, because the family-centered AA-based treatment approach has enough power to change rigid, long-standing family interaction patterns. The index patient presented for treatment first, but she was only the "tip of the iceberg." Appropriate intervention for her resulted in help for her spouse as well. At the time of her treatment, the primary physician had a strong feeling that her spouse also had problems with alcohol use, but he delayed his intervention until the family members gained some understanding of their involvement in the problem. It may have been overwhelming to approach both spouses' dependency problems at once; the resistance to this intervention may have been so great that nothing would have been accomplished. In this case, the symptoms of depression resolved relatively quick when the associated chemical dependency was treated. However, the total recovery process for the family system can be a slow struggle. Ongoing support was critically important. After the initial stages, the family physician remained involved but was not a central figure. Self-help groups, such as AA and Al-Anon, and formal chemical dependency counselors had the major role. The network of supportive systems aided the family physician and provided ongoing care.

DEPRESSION: CASE 3

DESCRIPTION

Mrs. D, a 64-year-old retired widow, presented to the office with complaints of dizziness, sleepless nights, poor appetite, weight loss, and fear of leaving her apartment. She reported no trouble getting to sleep, but did experience early morning awakening and a 10-pound weight loss over the past 6 months. She felt blue on some occasions, but was generally quite restless and fearful most of the day. Mrs. D related that she had been a teacher at a public grade school in a large urban school district for 15 years. She retired 2 years ago and soon thereafter was hospitalized for chest pain. At that time there was no confirmation of myocardial damage, and she had not had chest pain since that time. Because of her sudden illness, Mrs. D's sister invited her to stay in her local rural town for a few weeks of recovery. Mrs. D's sister was also single, now retired and very active socially with card clubs and senior citizen groups. After 1½ years Mrs. D moved to her own apartment near her sister. She was now feeling very afraid of leaving that apartment even to walk downtown or go to church; she had not done either activity for several months. Friends were becoming concerned and urged medical attention; thereupon Mrs. D presented to the office and saw her first physician.

The primary physician felt that she was agitated but primarily depressed, antidepressant medication was recommended, and a psychiatric consultation was urged. Mrs. D's sister strongly agreed with that idea, but Mrs. D was reluctant. She wanted some medication if it would help her to "relax," but refused antidepressant medications and consultation. The family physician reluctantly prescribed a low-dose antianxiety agent (a benzodiazepine) and followed the patient closely. After several months with no improvement, Mrs. D agreed under much pressure from her sister and friend to get psychiatric consultation. The consultant agreed with the diagnosis of agitated depression and recommended stopping the benzodiazepines and starting a tricyclic antidepressant. Mrs. D then returned to her primary physician, who changed her medications as directed. However, Mrs. D soon stopped her tricyclic antidepressant because she experienced an unpleasant dry mouth and drowsiness. Her physician again reluctantly stopped her new medication, returned to the previous benzodiazepine, and requested help from another family physician (Baird).

Mrs. D returned to the office with her sister as requested. Mrs. D was fidgeting, pacing the floor occasionally, and very unsure of her ability to improve. She was constantly apologizing for causing so much trouble. Her sister was confident, spoke freely, and often spoke for Mrs. D. The sister was frustrated over the lack of improvement Mrs. D had shown. She was becoming tired of doing everything for Mrs. D, from making meals to washing clothes to arranging for friends to visit.

During the first interview, Baird simply engaged both sisters in the treatment process and requested that the original consultant's recommendation of changing her medications be followed. Baird agreed to compromise and use a tricyclic antidepresant in combination with a low-dose benzodiazepine, a combination that he rarely uses. They agreed to that idea and to joint participation in the treatment process. Baird also requested help from the visiting clinical psychologist from the local mental health center, who could see them more frequently than he could. He cautioned that improvement would be largely due to their own efforts and only slightly due to the change in medication.

Initially, things went quite poorly. Mrs. D became more agitated, and her sister became more demanding and wanted something "done" about her. They finally agreed that everyone should "resign" from taking care of Mrs. D except for the mental health professionals. The sister was quite relieved. This worked well until one Sunday when Mrs. D became extremely agitated and expressed so much hopelessness that her friends practically carried her to the local emergency room. There she was treated with intravenous diazepam and was briefly admitted to the hospital by the emergency room physician. That crisis prompted a confrontation at which Baird requested that Mrs. D not be taken anywhere, including to the hospital, unless she specifically requested it.

Mrs. D continued to see the clinical psychologist, who prescribed increasingly independent tasks to be done as homework. Baird saw Mrs. D and Ms. X every 2 to 3 weeks to reinforce the concept that recovery was primarily Mrs. D's responsibility, not her sister's or the physician's. The goal was to increase the emotional boundaries between these two sisters. The clinical psychologist and Baird consulted with each other frequently, with Mrs. D's permission. The sister went on a long out-of-state trip, and Mrs. D rapidly improved. (Their boundaries were improved by physical separation.) She began to express anger at becoming so dependent upon her sister. Upon her return, the sister too began to express anger at Mrs. D's leaning on her so heavily. Together, Baird and the sisters explored the changes in Mrs. D's life: First, she had retired (a major life cycle event); then she had a sudden hospitalization (a major health event); and thereafter had moved from an urban to a rural location away from life long friends (a major social change). She had become quite helpless and dependent. The sister reported that she was "letting go" of Mrs. D and Mrs. D was now accepting the responsibility for her own recovery. After approximately 7 months of family-centered treatment, at first with visits every 2 weeks, then monthly, Mrs. D is feeling somewhat better. At this writing, she is driving her own car, visiting friends, and cautiously thinking of moving back to her urban environment. The sister has resumed her previously active and independent life style. The antidepressant was tapered off and discontinued about 10 months after the initial office visit, and has not been reinstituted during a 1-year follow-up. Both sisters receive routine health evaluations but do not consider themselves ill, nor are they under a specific care plan at this time.

COMMENTS ON CASE 3

Unlike the patient in Case 1, Mrs. D did not fit the criteria for a good prognosis. Unfortunately, that is not an unfamiliar situation for most family physicians. She had symptoms that qualified as a major depressive episode for over 1 year. She had suffered a series of major life stresses at the onset of her symptoms. Her family interaction pattern had become rigid and was organized around her symptoms. She and her sister had an enmeshed type of family cohesion. Her guarded prognosis warranted consultation and a therapeutic team approach.

The physician needed to take charge of the specific type and dose of medication being used. Since the consultant had an appropriate rationale for using an antidepressant medication, it was used cautiously but with full expectation of compliance. Flexibility as to the dose and changes needed because of side effects required decisions tailored to this individual patient.

However, the responsible physician accepted a leadership role and did not compromise reasonable therapeutic principles because of the patient's reluctance. The antianxiety medication proved unhelpful in the treatment of primary depression, although it did seem to relieve some of the short-term anxiety effects. A more sedating tricyclic antidepressant was selected, and in this case, a combination of the two drugs was tried. On occasion, stopping the antianxiety medication may alleviate some depressive symptoms, although it can be argued that a trial dose of benzodiazapine may uncover masked depression.

The *context* of this patient's depression was crucial. A psychiatric consultant may be too distant or too busy to appreciate the full reality of the patient's environment and the ecology of the symptoms. Perhaps a helpless role is accepted by the primary patient, but is someone else promoting and unknowingly perpetuating the role? It is not uncommon for family physicians to seek psychiatric consultation for depression, but they often want to implement the treatment plan themselves. In many areas of this country, the recommendations of a consultant would be to use a tricyclic antidepressant, a monoamine oxidase inhibitor, or, rarely, electroshock therapy. Then why are some patients returning to physicians' offices unimproved? Every family physician can list patients who never really seem to improve in spite of multiple, reasonable recommendations from consultants.

Perhaps physicians are asking the impossible from their consultants. It is the family physician's task to appreciate the context or ecology of the primary patient's illness in order to implement the appropriate treatment process fully. Medication and electroshock therapy may be effective for depressive disorders, but what can be done to alter the "ecological disorder" that may surround the depressed patient? Physicians are in the position to challenge family members and involve friends and community resources in an effort to promote healthy functioning. It is not enough that the primary patients are treated medically and no longer complaining (perhaps due to isolation), and thereby no longer upsetting friends and families. These persons may want to feel more complete, self-confident, and hopeful about the future. Family physicians based in primary patients' communities are in the best position to help this to occur. They can feel the texture of the patients' environment because they are living in the same community. They should fully utilize their advantage by considering the context of their patients' depression.

In this case, the primary physician was one member of a therapeutic team. It should be noted that the primary physician did not accept total responsibility for management of this problem. A consulting psychiatrist confirmed the diagnosis and the medical treatment plan. A clinical psychologist based in the local mental health center provided close therapeutic treatment and support. The emergency room physician responded to a crisis, even though the primary physician might have handled the situation differently. Finally, the primary patient and family were challenged to assume a major part of the responsibility and credit for recovery. The primary physician was not willing to reinforce the helpless role of the identified patient by accepting undue responsibility for the therapeutic outcome. Similarly, before prescribing the appropriate medication, the physician cautioned that improvement would only be partially due to the medication. Therefore, when the time came to taper off or stop the medication, the patient was confident of her ability to continue to function well. The psychological dependency upon the medication was thereby minimized.

15 TREATING ANXIETY IN A FAMILY CONTEXT

Anxiety is a feeling of apprehension, uncertainty, and fear. A normal reaction to certain physical and psychological stresses, anxiety has been called the "flight or fight" response to threatening stimuli. As all family physicians know, many physiological symptoms accompany anxiety. Increased adrenalin and sympathetic nervous discharge may result in hyperalertness, irritability, excitement, restlessness, and a fearful sensation. Accompanying physical symptoms may include dry mouth, flushing of the skin, dilated pupils, increased heart rate, increased respiratory rate, increased cardiac output, and systolic hypertension. Subjective complaints may include palpitations, shortness of breath and/or chest pain, inability to swallow comfortably, dizziness, and peripheral paresthesias. Similar sensations can be produced by injections of epinephrine, hyperthyroidism, extreme pain, and certain tumors that secrete catecholamine.

These multiple somatic complaints associated with anxiety make the initial assessment a complex task for a family physician. The diagnosis of anxiety may be accompanied by muscle contraction headaches, functional bowel syndrome, insomnia, globus hystericus, and others. The physician may easily be sidetracked into pursuing every biomedical symptom while ignoring the underlying anxiety state and its biopsychosocial context.

Formal diagnosis of an anxiety disorder can be guided by the criteria in DSM-III (American Psychiatric Association, 1980). DSM-III distinguishes between "phobic disorders" and "anxiety states" (or "anxiety neuroses"). Of the anxiety states, probably the most common one encountered in family practice is "generalized anxiety disorder." The other anxiety state disorders are "panic disorder," "obsessive–compulsive disorder," and "posttraumatic stress disorder." "Generalized anxiety disorder" is defined in DSM-III as generalized persistent anxiety of at least 1 month's duration without the specific symptoms (e.g., phobia) of the other anxiety conditions. In the majority of cases, the course of the illness is mild and the complications less severe than for depression and chemical dependency (Goodwin & Guze, 1979).

The DSM-III criteria for generalized anxiety disorder are as follows:

A. Generalized, persistent anxiety is manifested by symptoms from three of the following four categories:
   1. Motor tension: shakiness, jitteriness, jumpiness, trembling, tension, muscle aches, fatigability, inability to relax, eyelid twitch, furrowed brow, strained face, fidgeting, restlessness, easy startle.
   2. Automatic hyperactivity: sweating, heart pounding or racing, cold, clammy hands, dry mouth, dizziness, light-headedness, paresthesias (tingling in hands or feet), upset stomach, hot or cold spells, frequent urination, diarrhea, discomfort in the pit of the stomach, lump in the throat, flushing, pallor, high resting pulse and respiration rate.
   3. Apprehensive expectation: anxiety, worry, fear, rumination, and anticipation of misfortune to self and others.
   4. Vigilance and scanning: hyperattentiveness resulting in distractability, difficulty in concentrating, insomnia, feeling "on edge," irritability, impatience.
B. The anxious mood has been continuous for at least 1 month.
C. Not due to another mental disorder, such as a depressive disorder or schizophrenia.
D. At least 18 years of age.

"Panic disorder" may be diagnosed when the individual experiences at least three panic attacks during a 3-week period in situations not marked by great physical exertion or life-threatening events. "Panic attacks" are defined in DSM-III as discrete periods of apprehension or fear accompanied by at least four of the following symptoms: (1) dyspnea; (2) palpitations; (3) chest pain or discomfort; (4) choking or smothering sensations; (5) dizziness, vertigo, or unsteady feelings; (6) feelings of unreality; (7) paresthesias; (8) hot and cold flashes; (9) sweating; (10) faintness; (11) trembling or shaking; and (12) fear of dying, going crazy, or losing control. If panic attacks are associated with an underlying depression, the diagnosis of panic disorder is not made.

"Agoraphobia" is an anxiety disorder marked by fear and avoidance of being alone or in public places such as crowds, tunnels, bridges, and public transportation vehicles. The individual experiences increasing limitation of normal activities until the disorder dominates the individual's life. Agoraphobia is more common among women and is often—but not always—accompanied by panic attacks (American Psychiatric Association, 1980).

Finally, DSM-III distinguishes an adjustment disorder with anxious mood from a full-blown anxiety disorder. Adjustment–reaction anxiety is a maladaptive reaction (nervousness, worry, jitteriness) to an identifiable psychosocial stressor and presumably is self-limiting when the stressor ceases or the patient adjusts to a new situation. Thus it is important to distinguish generalized anxiety from anxiety connected with a central stressful event. In either case, the physician should evaluate the social context of the problem.

ASSESSMENT OF THE FAMILY CONTEXT OF ANXIETY

Since the feeling of anxiety is a common experience for many persons, the physician's first task is to discover why an individual presents to the office at a particular time with a specific complaint or a series of complaints. What are the multiple factors that have tipped the balance in favor of seeing a health care professional rather than consulting friends or the family's informal health care network? To discover what has triggered the patient into presenting to the office on that given day, the physician must view the patient in a systems context and explore dimensions beyond the physiological complaint that is usually given as an entry ticket into the health care system. The following discussion uses our four family assessment dimensions to explore the social context of anxiety problems.

STRESSORS

Because anxiety, like many other patient problems, has a multifactorial etiology, the family physician must approach the anxious patient with a plan that is more complex than diagnosing or excluding so-called "real organic disease." A good place to start is to assess the stressors that are affecting this individual in this family at this time. External stressors at times push everyone beyond the limits of coping. Job layoffs, occupational hazards (such as long hours or night shifts), accidental injuries, and financial crises may contribute to anxiety. Many external stressors are impossible to control but need to be understood in the context of this particular patient, family, and physician in order to understand the context of anxiety.

Sometimes chemical stressors significantly affect the severity of anxiety symptoms. For some persons, excessive caffeine ingestion in the form of coffee, tea, and chocolate or soft drinks may be of primary importance. Avoidance of these and other stimulant medications (such as No-Doz, cold medicines, and diet remedies) may be all that is necessary for the successful management of anxiety symptoms in some cases.

Fear of underlying serious illness should be addressed specifically as a possible internal stressor. A family history of specific illnesses such as heart disease and diabetes is an appropriate cause for concern for subsequent generations. In this case physicians can thoroughly assess the presenting complaint, offer a reasonably accurate prognosis, and suggest preventive measures for the concerned patient. In patients who repeatedly present with similar complaints that relate to familial disease, the physician would do well to ask for a family interview in order to understand the family's assumptions about their familial disease. Occasionally there may be a misunderstanding of normal physiology or a misinformed piece of folklore that has not been openly discussed with the physician. By addressing these issues directly but with compassion for the difficult task of changing long-held family myths, the physician can sometimes relieve the anxiety of the primary patient and the family. This is a good occasion for engaging the therapeutic triangle in order to improve physician effectiveness. By incorporating the family into the evaluation of anxiety, the physician may be able to address more directly the health-related assumptions that sometimes serve as avoidable sources of stress for the anxious patient. A family interview may also uncover the need for periodic medical rescreening for previously unnoticed illnesses that are part of the family's genetic heritage.

Family life cycle changes are a frequent source of anxiety for family members. By reviewing life cycle events such as a new marriage, birth of children, children leaving home, retirement, and role reversal with elderly parents, the physician and the primary patient may see anxiety symptoms as related to these life changes. If the anxiety symptoms seem to be related to life cycle changes, both the physician and the primary patient may wish to discuss adaptation to the new challenges facing the patient and family, instead of focusing primarily on the medical complaint. For example, a 35-year-old man may complain of palpitations while he is adjusting to an increasing professional workload, a second child, and the need to spend more time at home. For this patient, a thorough medical diagnostic evaluation is appropriate; however, a family interview will more clearly define the basic problem. Whether or not a serious cardiac problem is found, the family interview will help everyone understand the father's problem. His new health problem can be explained in terms of life cycle stress and/or in terms of any pathology that has been discovered.

FAMILY ADAPTABILITY

If the physician hopes to incorporate the family in the management of the presenting patient's anxiety, it is important to know whether the family is likely to cooperate with or to undermine the physician's attempts at treatment. By evaluating the family's history of adaptability, the physician may predict more accurately the family's response to the new challenge. A review of previously accomplished challenges along the life cycle is generally helpful. If this family has charted a successful course through earlier life challenges, it is more likely to be adaptable and has a better prognosis for cooperation with physician-requested changes. On the other hand, a poor record of coping with life cycle events such as marriage, early child rearing, or raising adolescents may indicate that the family will have difficulty cooperating with treatment because it lacks the internal resources to make important adjustments. As in the case of depression and chemical dependency, a long history of chronic anxiety is commonly associated with poor family adaptability. In this situation, the physician must be patient and set expectations appropriately. Change will be slow. An appropriate management strategy would involve community resources to help the family cope with the stress of a chronically anxious family member; a family therapist or family-oriented psychiatrist might become involved if the symptoms are severe. If the presenting patient has anxiety of recent onset and has a family with good adaptability, the family physician may start primary care counseling with a reasonable expectation of successful treatment of anxiety.

FAMILY COHESION

By understanding the presenting patient's social context in terms of family cohesion, the primary physician will sometimes discover the etiology of the anxiety and will usually make more accurate predictions about complications in treating the patient's anxiety. In an enmeshed family cohesion pattern, the physician is likely to get many phone calls from different persons complaining about anxiety symptoms, evaluation procedures, inconvenience associated with treatment plans, or all of these at once. It may become difficult to identify the most anxious patient in the family. In extreme cases of enmeshment, the primary care physician may wish to initiate immediate consultation or referral to a family therapist in order to help the family clarify interpersonal boundaries. At least, the physician should not be surprised at the intensity of other family members' reactions to the treatment of the presenting patient. During interviews with enmeshed families, it is particularly important for the physician to enforce self-responsibility and self-expression, rather than allowing one family member to speak for others. This alone may be helpful if the initial symptoms are not severely disturbing. If the appropriate treatment is reassurance that the identified symptoms are in fact physiologically normal, the physician may have to reassure all family members rather than just the presenting patient. One family session may prevent innumerable phone calls from other family members who cannot tolerate secondhand information. Progress should be observable after two or three family sessions. If not, the physician should consider consultation with a family therapist.

If the patient's family is difficult to contact and seems unconcerned about the presenting patient, the family might have a disengaged cohesion pattern. Like depression, anxiety may be a precursor of divorce and family breakup. A treatment plan that incorporates other family members may then take on the task of keeping the family intact (if the members want to stay together), as well as that of reducing the presenting patient's anxiety. This is a major therapeutic undertaking and may require referral to a family therapist. If the presenting patient decides that reduction of *individual* symptoms are his or her primary goal and that family cohesion is of secondary importance, then individual primary care counseling may be appropriate for the index patient without family participation. Just as for depression, one outcome of successful treatment may be divorce or separation. If the physician who undertakes such individually focused treatment in this context does not anticipate this outcome, he or she may repeatedly feel responsible for family disintegrations. This in turn may produce "professional casualties" and occupational dissatisfaction. Just as a surgeon must be aware of the probability and management of surgical complications, the family physician should be aware of complications of primary care counseling and should know how to predict and handle the aftermath of these complications.

INTERACTION PATTERNS

Are there recurring interaction patterns that relate directly to the patient's symptoms of anxiety? During the family interview, the family physician can observe and sometimes identify specific interaction patterns within the family that contribute to or maintain the patient's state of anxiety. If conflicts arise, are they resolved, or do they remain undiscussed only to resurface at unpredictable times? How do other people in the family react when the index patient complains of anxiety or related symptoms? Perhaps the pattern of interaction reinforces the index patient's complaint. For example, a 38-year-old mother of four may complain of anxiety and stomach cramps which improve when she rests in a quiet place. If family members respect her request for quiet solitude and if her symptoms then resolve relatively quickly, the anxiety symptoms may help stabilize the patient and family by permitting the busy mother/housewife a brief "time out" or temporary reprieve from young active children. In this context, the anxiety symptoms may not need specific treatment, and the family should be viewed as having found a way of coping with its situation. A better solution might be to have the mother state specifically her reasons for needing a brief rest rather than initiate the request with a physical complaint. In another example, a man presents with anxiety and dysphagia. A family interview shows that he has most of his swallowing difficulty the day following an argument in which he and his wife discuss his drinking. This cycle may repeat itself many times but might not be discovered without an interview with the spouse present. If recurring serious conflict or family violence seem to be associated with anxiety, the physician should review strenuously any alcohol or drug use associated with this conflict. The index patient may be the "symptom bearer" for the family suffering from chemical dependency.

THE ROLE OF ANTIANXIETY MEDICATIONS

Antianxiety medications, especially benzodiazepines, have proven useful in the short-term management of anxiety-related complaints (Rickels, 1977). It has been argued that short-term treatment with benzodiazepines is helpful in distinguishing between anxiety and depression, since if the patient does not improve, the physician should seriously consider treating depression as the underlying illness (Hollister, 1978). Do these medications actually decrease medical complaints related to anxiety? Johnson, Widmer, Cadoret, Troughton, and Wilson (1981) have found that the frequency of medical visits for anxiety-related somatic complaints actually increased with the use of antianxiety medications. However, if the patient's symptoms improve, the treatment recommended by the manufacturers is for a relatively short span of 2 to 4 weeks (*Physicians' Desk Reference*, 1981). If the symptoms are mild and of recent origin, and if the family system review suggests reasonable adaptability and cohesion together with no dysfunctional interaction patterns, the family physician can expect a good outcome, no matter what type of treatment is recommended. Therefore, are these medications really needed in these circumstances? If medication is used and the anxious patient improves with short-term treatment, under what circumstances should the medication be restarted (e.g., with recurrence of new or different symptoms, or only if symptoms are more severe)? If the symptoms soon recur, then perhaps the medical treatment was ineffective and therefore should not be instituted a second time. If symptoms are chronic and the physician is expecting long-term use of any treatment plan because of low adaptability or extreme enmeshment or disengagement in the family system, then consultation or referral may be in order. In those situations, medication would be only one part of the ongoing treatment plan.

A decision to continue antianxiety medications indefinitely suggests a long-term care problem that has serious implications for the patient and his or her family. If the consultant recommends continuing the medication, it is the family physician's task to consider the family context of that recommendation. A family physician is able to assemble the family, assess the impact of the medication upon the family, and determine more fully the personal and family impact of both the patient's symptoms and the proposed treatment plan. If the family system has become organized around the medication as much as around the anxiety symptoms, if patterns of interaction are rigid, and if other family members unconsciously contribute to the underlying symptoms and their problems, the physician must consider chemical dependency as a primary diagnosis. In spite of reassurances by experienced physicians (Abuzzahab, 1979; Hollister *et al.*, 1981), what starts out as anxiety can end up as chemical dependency with multiple negative impacts upon the family. If there is any doubt about the occurrence of this scenario, the physician should consult any local AA group or chemical dependency treatment center for confirmation of the existence of this problem (*FDA Drug Bulletin*, 1980). The use of these medications is extensive (Harsday & Karch, 1981). In 1978, there were 58 million prescriptions for diazapam and related compounds in the United States (*FDA Drug Bulletin*, 1980). Emergency room treatment for overdose often demonstrates alcohol ingestion and multiple drug use, including the use of benzodiazepines. These compounds may be pharmacologically safe to use in a laboratory or hospital and under close supervision, but some of the people for whom they are prescribed seem to be having trouble handling them.

Baird receives very few patient complaints about his rarely using benzodiazepines in an outpatient setting. If the reasons for nonuse are explained, and if the context of the symptoms is explored and is relatively well understood by the presenting patient and the family, very few patients or family members will request continuing medication. As family or other conflicts are resolved, or inevitable stressors such as death or chronic illness are accepted, the feeling of need for the antianxiety medication decreases or passes. The patient and family who have not received medication can learn coping mechanisms that will help them in the future, yet may not require ongoing physician involvement. The physician should contrast that outcome with the lesson learned with pharmacological intervention. The family has been taught that future life crises should be managed by physicians and their prescribed pills. This can diminish the family's sense of independence and self-esteem and can place the physician in an ordinately powerful position in the therapeutic triangle. *We propose that the overall impact of the long-term pharmacological management of anxiety is to undermine the family's adaptability and to promote an unrealistic physician role.* Ultimately, the physician grows weary, and the patient and family languish in incompetence.

TREATING ANXIETY IN A FAMILY CONTEXT

Family physicians can evaluate anxiety complaints in a family context and offer appropriate treatment which rarely requires the use of prescribed medications. Following is a list of suggestions for appropriate evaluation and management of anxiety.

1. *Do a thorough physical examination and plan for ongoing evaluation and reevaluation.* Subtle endocrine and other disorders may be unrecognizable at first but can be discovered if careful follow-up is included in the ongoing management of the patient and the family. Extensive use or abuse of caffeine or related stimulants should be reviewed thoroughly in the initial history and of course should be avoided by symptomatic patients.

2. *During the patient interview, assess the context of the symptoms with specific reference to internal and external stressors, family adaptability, family cohesion, and common family interaction patterns.* This will help you estimate the degree to which family members may contribute to anxiety symptoms and the extent to which they may successfully participate in the recovery process. How supportive is the patient's family or close friends? Is there at least one person with whom the patient can talk honestly and expect reasonably supportive listening?

3. *If symptoms are severe or persistent, assemble the family for further assessment and possibly for ongoing involvement in the treatment process.* Also use the family for monitoring treatment response.

4. *Assess the history of preexisting drug and alcohol use by the patient and family.* If chemical dependency exists in the primary patient or other family members, treat that first. We suggest from our clinical experience that anxiety complaints in young adults should make you particularly attuned to the possibility of chemical dependency. If these patients present with pain complaints as well as anxiety, the risk of chemical dependency is even higher (Ries, Bolkan, Katon, & Kleinman, 1981). Therefore, Baird rarely prescribes antianxiety medications for young people who complain of anxiety. A request for a specific antianxiety agent is an obvious clue to purposeful manipulation of the physician. However, the patient's convincing and subtle manipulations may be so well honed that almost any physician can be outwitted. A preferable response is to ask for a family interview to assess the primary patient's complaints further before you prescribe any antianxiety medications. If the patient has no family, then close friends or other available supportive persons can be included. If no "family" can be found, then the diagnosis may be social isolation, not anxiety. This is definitely not treatable with medication. Through this process of assembling the family, chemical and alcohol use can be more accurately assessed.

5. *Look strenuously for underlying depression in the index patient with anxiety.* Underlying depression is sometimes unmasked by initial treatment with benzodiazepines, in which case the patient's symptoms may get worse rather than better. Whether the benzodiazepines precipitate depression or merely uncover it is debatable (*Patient Care*, 1981).

6. *If marital, sexual, or child behavior problems or other specific issues are present, treat them systematically as part of the ongoing management of anxiety, through primary care family counseling.* The patient's anxiety may relent when these family problems are resolved. It is particularly important

to relieve the anxious person of the "helpless patient" role in the family if meaningful family problem solving is to be undertaken.

7. *Sometimes it is the primary patient's task to accept relatively unacceptable circumstances such as death, divorce, chronic illness, or other significant emotional losses.* These tasks do not require medication but do require the physician's or therapist's time and understanding. Reviewing these challenges with the entire family is the most appropriate way in which to help the family system to stabilize around a new reality and the patient to recover emotional equilibrium.

8. *Whether or not pharmacological treatment is recommended, non-pharmacological treatment should be included in the treatment of anxiety.* This includes instituting a regular and sensible exercise program, instructing the patient to avoid caffeine and other stimulants, and explaining uncomfortable physiological symptoms such as hyperventilation and globus hystericus. Sometimes understanding the physiology of these symptoms in lay terms is more helpful to the patient and family than are continued, repeated evaluations. If insomnia is a presenting complaint, instituting bedtime rituals such as gradual relaxation, warm milk, or reading can be helpful. An explanation that "sleeping" medications are of little help after several weeks is sometimes comforting to the patient who is ambivalent about using medication. For all of these self-help treatments, the responsibility should be on the anxious patient for his or her own progress, with the family and the physician playing supportive roles. You can work against overprotective family responses by helping all family members identify their own individual needs and wants at this time in the family's life.

9. *If antianxiety agents are used, the benzodiazepines are probably the safest, pharmacologically.* However, they must be used in the context of the family and the surrounding ecology of the patient, and only for a brief time.

10. *Chronic anxiety or anxiety in the context of a dysfunctional family will probably require a team approach.* A family therapist or family-oriented psychiatrist working together with the family physician may constitute the ideal treatment team.

CONCLUSION

Because anxiety so frequently manifests itself in physical symptoms, most anxious patients present to their family physician with concerns about their bodies. The psychosocial context of these complaints often holds the key to accurate diagnosis and meaningful treatment. Since anxiety disorders are not ordinarily severe or highly disruptive of the patient's life style, primary care management is frequently the optimal treatment response. In this chapter, we argue for assessing the family context of anxiety and for enlisting the family in therapeutic plan. When long-term management of anxiety is required, primary care family counseling offers the physician an alternative to the extended use of antianxiety medications, which might undermine individual and family functioning.

APPENDIX: CASE EXAMPLES

These case examples are from Baird's practice.

ANXIETY: CASE 1

DESCRIPTION

Mrs. C was a 74-year-old widow who had severe coronary artery disease. She had had two previous myocardial infarctions and was now readmitted to the hospital with chest pain. She had chronic premature ventricular contractions and angina pectoris, plus congestive heart failure and diabetes. She had been evaluated for coronary artery bypass surgery previously, but was not accepted because of poor ventricular function and a massively dilated heart. She took multiple medications for controlling ventricular arrhythmias, for control of congestive heart failure, for reduction of her anxiety and insomnia, and for treatment of constant esophageal reflux and aerophagia.

She lived in constant fear of the next heart attack, slept very poorly, was constantly belching, and generally felt miserable. Her nearby family, which included three daughters and one son, was at wits' end. Almost weekly they would be called by their mother while she was experiencing chest pain and anticipating another infarction. This was typically accompanied by a feeling of impending doom. The family member would rush her to the physician, who would try to decide if the patient should be admitted to the hospital for the umpteenth time to rule out another myocardial infarction. This uncomfortable scenario had been building in tempo for about 2 years.

With this admission to the hospital, there was no evidence of myocardial damage. The family was asked to come to the hospital for a "family conference." All of Mrs. C's children and their spouses arrived on time and were eager to participate. Baird and the family reviewed the history of this very uncomfortable situation. How did everyone feel? "Exhausted," "Wrung out," and "Fearful of each day" were their responses. Mrs. C felt the same. She could no longer talk much with friends, play the piano, or enjoy family visits, which were usually centered around the cardiac crisis. What was the worst that could happen? Mrs. C's response was that she would rather die of a myocardial infarction than continually be taken to the brink and then come back. There were many tears. With a little help, the entire family expressed their mixed feelings about their plight. All loved Mrs. C very much, but all were exhausted and felt that their lives had become unpleasant and unfairly burdened. They agreed with Mrs. C that death was preferable and probably less cruel than what had been happening. This was the first time that they had all sat down and discussed their situation, and they considered it a good beginning. Mrs. C remained in the hospital for several more days while she started a walking and exercise program. Her goal was to be able to play her beloved piano, even briefly. When she had chest pains, she sat down and rested and took nitroglycerine as advised. She rested when fatigued, and adjusted her walking accordingly. Her antianxiety medications and sleeping pills were tapered off. Her belching nearly ceased. She and her physician had 10- to 15-minute talks each day during hospital rounds, at which time they discussed her progress and the reality of death. Eventually she accepted the fact that she was going to die someday from heart disease, but she was determined to enjoy each day until then. She began to sleep better and generally seemed to be happy for the first time in years. She was discharged in good condition on far fewer medications than before admission.

During the next several months, all of Mrs. C's antianxiety and sleeping medications were discontinued. She continued to have angina pectoris with exercise, but the pains were relieved by nitroglycerin. Her family visits became more cheerful and were not precipitated by anginal attacks. Over the next 1½ years Mrs. C suffered two more myocardial infarctions. She was admitted to the hospital only those two times. This was a dramatic decrease in hospital admissions from the previous 2 years. In fact, she only called for help when the pain was very severe and did not resolve after nitroglycerin and rest. She was able to play the piano, although only for brief periods. At Mrs. C's last admission to the hospital she was smiling upon arrival—"Here we go again," she said cheerfully. She died about 48 hours later from irreversible complications on her fifth myocardial infarction. Her family and her physician were proud of her courageous approach to an unrelenting disease and mourned her death appropriately.

COMMENTS ON CASE 1

Mrs. C's anxiety was reality-based. She had severe coronary artery disease that would eventually be fatal. She and her family were living in constant fear of not responding quickly enough to save her life. The major intervention was to see her anxiety in that context. Once she and her family accepted the inevitable reality of her death (and in some sense everyone's death), they could go on with the business of living each day. She no longer needed antianxiety medications; she could resume a meaningful relationship with her family; and eventually she died with great dignity. Her family was released from the responsibility of saving her from an inevitable fate. They felt pride, relief, and normal grief at her death. The family system was adapting well before her death and has continued to do so at this writing, with no increase in routine or other medical visits.

ANXIETY: CASE 2

DESCRIPTION

Mrs. R presented to the office with a complaint of constant "jitters." She was always tense and had been seeing physicians frequently for the past 8½ months for various complaints. Her particular complaint now was that when she and her husband went out to eat—their primary form of entertainment— the food stuck in her dry mouth and she could not eat. After several months of this without any relief, she came in for help. She had already been treated with several kinds of antianxiety medications, but none seemed to help. She had trouble falling asleep, but also awakened early and could not return to sleep. She seemed to become very upset when writing out checks and now could not sign her name without becoming light-headed and short of breath. A brief family history was taken. Mr. and Mrs. R had two children who lived far away. Mr. R had had a laryngectomy about 1 year ago and had had to speak with a voice resonator since then. Every 3 months he returned to a large referral center for a laryngoscopy and a bronscopy to make sure that there was no recurrence of this disease. Previously he was a heavy smoker, but he had quit smoking at the time of his initial surgery.

How had things changed since his diagnosis and surgery? Mr. R used to talk forcefully and often. He had always managed the family finances and business details. He had continued his outside relationships and friendships, but his communication was now difficult, even though he had become a skilled resonance speaker. He had always been the more confident partner, with Mrs. R being more anxious and retiring. Whenever Mr. R tried to teach his wife about the family financial matters, Mrs. R became very uncomfortable and left the room. Baird asked Mrs. R to return to the office in one week with her husband.

In the first conjoint interview, Mr. R spoke quite well with his external resonator and seemed confident. Mrs. R was literally trembling. Together, Baird and the Rs reviewed his medical problems. He had been told that recurrence of his tumor was quite possible, but each examination so far had been negative for recurrent disease. Each return was quite dramatic: Mr. R would have a partial anesthesia and bronscopy while Mrs. R waited alone in a large waiting room. At the end of each procedure, the endoscopist would sit with Mrs. R and explain the results. For several nights before the last two visits, Mrs. R was unable to go to sleep.

They had not discussed what Mrs. R would do if her husband died from this disease, and they both felt nervous about his long-term future. After some discussion, Mrs. R agreed to stop the current antianxiety medications by tapering them off over several weeks. Baird's diagnosis was depression and nonacceptance of a difficult situation. She accepted a trial of a tricyclic antidepressant to be taken at bedtime. Baird and the Rs agreed to have conjoint office visits every two weeks, at which time they would review progress and plan new strategy.

Through the next several visits, Mr. R began to express his frustrations about his disease, the operation, and his future. He needed help from Mrs. R but had never dared to ask for it for fear of overburdening his wife. Now he began to rely on his wife more for support. At first Mrs. R could still not write checks or eat in restaurants, but this pattern changed slowly. Initially she had the dry mouth caused by the medication, which seemed to aggravate her eating problems. She accepted these side effects when they were explained to her carefully. The return visits to the endoscopist proved less threatening after Mrs. R found a good friend to accompany her on these visits. After about 2 weeks her sleeping pattern had improved. Slowly she began to write checks and was actually able to sign them. Finally their weekly trips to restaurants resumed a cheerful tone, and eating was no problem. After 4 months Mrs. and Mr. R. were back to enjoying themselves and their friends. After 6 months she requested that her medication be tapered off. This was accomplished slowly but with no difficulty over a 5-week period.

During the next year Mrs. R rarely saw a physician. Then she returned to the office feeling upset and anxious again. Her teenaged nephew had originally asked to spend several days with Mr. and Mrs. R, but he had now been there for 1 month and showed no signs of leaving. After we discussed the situation, Mrs. R decided that she was actually quite angry but had never expressed that feeling to her nephew. She readily decided to return home and ask the overstayed visitor to leave so that she could resume her normal life style. She did just that. Since that time she has been feeling quite well, eating and sleeping normally, and staying away from the office except for periodic checkups. Mr. R's periodic evaluations have shown no recurrent tumor over the past 3½ years.

COMMENTS ON CASE 2

Mrs. R was anxious and depressed. Her fears of losing her husband and being alone were normal, but she had become disabled by them. Over the years she and her husband had formed rigid roles, with her husband as the confident and strong one and she as the more dependent and helpless one. They were able to become more adaptable in sharing both strength and dependency. They could then face a difficult reality and accept it. When the antianxiety medications did not improve her symptoms, they were slowly stopped. Then masked depression was diagnosed and treated with tricyclic antidepressants. Although the initial antianxiety agent was prescribed by a different physician, Baird, too, might have tried that at first; this person was literally trembling. However, these medications were easily tapered off and changed, since they had not noticeably helped the patient. The context of her symptoms was explored with her spouse and understood by the family and her physician. Then appropriate changes in the interaction pattern of the family were initiated and supported during relatively brief office visits of 20 to 30 minutes each. A more supportive environment was created for the agonizing wait for the declaration of tumor versus no tumor at Mr. R's periodic examinations. Finally, Mrs. R became more assertive of and responsive to her own needs. The result of this individual and family system was improved short-term functioning and better long-term adaptability.

Anxiety: Case 3

DESCRIPTION

Mrs. H presented with vague complaints of chest pain that started about 3 weeks before her coming to the office. She was 44 years old; she had four children aged 14 to 23, with one son and one daughter currently in high school. She was married to an attentive, physically healthy husband and had many outside activities that she enjoyed. None of her family members were ill, and she considered herself in relatively good health until the symptoms began. She stated that none of her pains had been terribly severe, but she was quite worried about their origin. Her father had died at age 62 from heart disease, and no older siblings had any cardiac disease as yet. Further review of systems was negative. It was noted that she did not smoke and was physically active. About 1 month ago, she had decided to return to work at an office where she had worked before she was married. She said that she was feeling anxious about that and wondered if it had anything to do with her current symptoms.

Mrs. H's physical exam was entirely normal. A chest X-ray, resting electrocardiogram, complete blood count, and urinalysis were normal. No other laboratory tests were ordered. When the results of these tests were explained to Mrs. H, she accepted this limited data as sufficiently reassuring. Together Mrs. H and her physician agreed on a treatment plan that included (1) regular exercise—a dance exercise class and periodic walks; (2) expression of her feelings to her husband; (3) avoidance of caffeine and related stimulants; and (4) return to the office for an exercise electrocardiogram or other tests if her symptoms continued. She left the office reassured, smiling, and eager to discuss her evaluation and treatment plan with her husband. No further office visit was scheduled, and the physician did not call or ask for a conjoint visit with the patient's husband. Mrs. H returned to work and followed the treatment plan conscientiously. She called about 2 months after the initial evaluation to report freedom from any symptoms and gratitude for the interaction with her physician. Her insurance company wrote a letter to complain about the charges made for the extended office visit, but no complaint was registered about the laboratory fees. A brief letter of rebuttal laid that matter to rest and resulted in a full payment. At this writing Mrs. H has been working for 2 years. Her only physician visits have been for routine gynecological exams, at which time her progress has been reported as good.

COMMENTS ON CASE 3

Mrs. H was an excellent candidate for brief office counseling. She had good individual resources and readily believed that roles and relationship issues were important factors that contributed to her physiologic symptoms. Her complaint was evaluated in a family systems context but did not require intervention with anyone beyond the primary patient. She had anxiety symptoms of recent origin and had previously been in good health. Her family system seemed supportive when it was assessed through her individual interview. Follow-up assessment plans were available, but were not needed. No medications were used to relieve her symptoms, and she improved very rapidly. Her life style has been changed moderately to enable her to tolerate future stresses without professional intervention.

16 IMPLEMENTING A FAMILY-SYSTEMS-ORIENTED MEDICAL PRACTICE

The proof of the primary care family model we have proposed in this book lies in its practical application to the physician's office and hospital practice. Many young physicians begin their practice with high ideals of personalized, humanistic care, only to find themselves burdened with too many patients, concerned about lagging behind their partners financially because of too many undercompensated counseling sessions, and overwhelmed at times by trying to handle difficult psychosocial problems without adequate consultation and support. In this chapter we discuss what family physicians need to do to survive—and even to enjoy—a family-centered medical practice. The chapter ends with an extended case example of the development of Baird's own practice in rural Minnesota.

ESTABLISHING A FAMILY-ORIENTED SERVICE NETWORK

The typical medical system is not set up in a fashion conducive to working with families. It is important that the physician interested in doing primary care family work take a systematic approach to establishing a supportive network that promotes and makes possible a medical practice with a family emphasis. Prior to leaving a training center, it is extremely helpful to develop a close relationship with an experienced family therapist or other similar person experienced in family systems thinking. This should be a close enough relationship to allow consultations and case review by telephone once the family physician is out in practice. If a physician is already in practice, learning about family systems, and trying to implement a family-centered practice, he or she should try to locate a supportive, experienced family-systems-oriented practitioner. Without this close initial support, it will be extremely difficult to change a local medical system enough to allow family-oriented delivery of care.

If the physician is practicing in a group, enough trust must be developed with other physicians in that group and local community to allow the delivery of health care in a slightly different manner than may be the usual custom. This is best done slowly by establishing a trusting relationship with other physicians and health care professionals. Low-key case discussion and hallway consultations are helpful ways to build this trust. Family-systems-oriented physicians can lend curbstone consultations about their particular area of interest, just as they might receive such consultations from a partner about an orthopedic problem. Each physician has strengths and weaknesses; a family-systems-oriented physician who is willing to learn from colleagues in some areas may be able to provide help to these colleagues in the family area. In a solo practice, the family physician will have more control over the office environment, but may have to establish working relationships with other physicians through continuing education meetings, hospital conferences, and other informal settings. However this is accomplished, the physician doing family counseling will definitely need the support of the surrounding community, especially of other physicians.

Office personnel may initially be quite confused by a physician's request to see the entire family. Everyone from the receptionist to the insurance clerk to the physician's primary nurse should understand the need to see more than one person during some office visits. Their initial confusion or lack of support can be alleviated if the physician will take the time to explain a family systems approach to the delivery of primary care. This can be done in brief meetings or informal ways, but it is essential in order to establish a systems-oriented practice. The primary nurse will be the crucial, supportive link. This person can be included in case reviews of families being seen, or can be included in family interview sessions. The front office personnel and receptionist need to be warned ahead of time that four, five, or ten family members may arrive for an office visit, so that there is no look of surprise and dismay among the staff when the family arrives *en masse*.

The hospital setting will be equally unsupportive unless the family physician is willing to present this new approach to the delivery of health care in a nonthreatening and educational manner. Very little support is forthcoming from angry demands for cooperation from hospital personnel as the physician stalks down the hallways. The concept of seeing whole families at times of illness and crisis will seem reasonable to most health care professionals, but the approach must be explained and its rationale defended in order for them to give full support. A hospital-based inservice program on the primary care of families through primary care counseling will usually be well received. It would be especially helpful to invite everyone from maintenance personnel to dietary staff and nurses to such a conference. The broader the understanding, the greater the support that is likely to be developed. Furthermore, such a broad-based educational effort would emphasize the systems approach to the delivery of health care in a consistent manner. A hospital system is as important to the delivery of family-centered care as are the physician and the individual family system. A second helpful step is to ask any nurse who is primarily involved with a hospitalized patient to attend family meetings. This person can be debriefed after the family meeting and in that way can be incorporated into the supportive network.

Support within a *community* can be developed by initiating contact with anyone who sees a family in a professional manner. Mental health professionals of almost any kind, local police officers, county attorneys, county sheriffs, court services officers, and school officials are usually pleasantly surprised to have a physician-initiated meeting to discuss their common goals of helping families and the ways in which they can work together in a more efficient manner. Community self-help groups will be key links in a supportive family systems network, especially Al-Anon, Alateen, battered women's groups, weight loss groups, and exercise groups. Any physician showing interest in these types of organizations will be much appreciated by the community and by the organizations. Close links with these self-help organizations are important, especially for treating problems that are primarily behavioral in nature and require life style changes. Unless these resource groups are contacted and supported, the primary physician may not be able to use them with full confidence and full cooperation. Any effort spent in this direction will yield multiple benefits to an office-based practice by making the community aspect of therapy more secure and efficient. The level of community involvement can be expanded beyond the local community to state and national political activities that promote legislation favoring family survival. This activity may be beyond the scope of most family physicians, but may have profound effects on lawmakers and other government officials when they consider legislation with major impact upon families.

Perhaps the most useful support for the physician would come from a close association with a trained family therapist who could be incorporated into an office practice. This is still a rare occurrence, but it may be the ideal way to coordinate the delivery of comprehensive care to families. In that setting, the family physician could observe families and make preliminary assessments. Therapeutic contracts could be established as a normal part of office practice. The family physician could assemble families for further assessment and primary care counseling with families or individuals. If needed, the in-house family therapist could be utilized for formal family therapy or consultations on the preceding steps. Although this arrangement would provide a most supportive environment for the delivery of primary care to families, well-trained family therapists are not always available.

Finally, it would also be extremely useful for family physicians interested in delivering primary care family counseling to gather at formal and informal educational sessions to build their own network of support.

PRACTICAL ISSUES IN THE
PRIMARY CARE OF FAMILIES

The classic medical environment is established with the expectation of seeing the single patient for a brief period of time in a small office room. Considerations of seating capacity in the waiting room and in a consultation room are critical to allow the physician to interview a whole family. Obviously families cannot be interviewed while they are standing in a 4 foot $\times$ 8 foot room or when they are distracted by office noises. Occasionally examination rooms can be changed to allow adequate seating by simply removing an examination table. A physician's willingness to sacrifice an examination room for holding family interviews is a good practical test of his or her commitment to the primary care of families. Without adequate seating it is simply impossible to see families, and the discussion of family-centered care becomes moot.

In primary care, there is great pressure for physicians to gauge their professional competence by the number of individual patients seen daily. Generally the physician's income is somewhat proportional to the number of patients seen; stature among other physicians, in turn, may be gauged by income. While not ignoring this harsh reality, we believe that physicians can see families in a busy office practice and not be penalized either financially or in the smooth running of an office practice. Even a major emphasis on the primary care of families would result in perhaps one or two family interviews or spouse dyad interviews daily, requiring 15 to 30 minutes (or occasionally 45 minutes) each. A physician who charges appropriately for this professional time spent with the patient and family will not suffer financially. However, it may be necessary for the physician to see families primarily when he or she is not responsible for all of the emergencies in a given practice in a day. Families may also have to understand that there will be occasional interruptions, but these interruptions can be limited if planned family interviews are scheduled for the least busy time of day.

Insurance companies will often cover medically associated charges for anxiety and depression, but may be reluctant to cover any diagnosis that begins with the word "family," such as "family discord," "family disruption," "family violence," or "family stress." Therefore, when the physician or insurance specialist in a clinic is filling out claim forms, it may be useful to consider an accurate diagnosis that translates to computer terms. Most companies will cover for professional time spent with patients if the diagnosis is a routine one such as anxiety or depression, and if the plan of action and the expected length of therapy can be reasonably estimated. Most charges for family therapy from nonphysician therapists are not covered; however, for physicians delivering primary care family counseling, time spent with patients may often be reimbursed through standard insurance mechanisms. We hope that this inequity toward nonphysician therapists will be corrected in the future.

As all physicians know, technical procedures are much better rewarded in financial terms than are verbal forms of intervention and therapy. However, physicians delivering primary care counseling services to families need not suffer economic penalties if they discipline their time spent with families and if they do not underestimate the value of primary care counseling by undercharging for this service. For some reason, it seems easy for most physicians to charge for office chest X-rays, electrocardiograms, and lab tests with no apologies, while it is difficult to charge appropriately for 30 minutes spent with a family or individual patient. Any physician who has set up a supportive network and who is delivering primary care to families with a family systems orientation will begin to see outcomes that demonstrate the value of this approach in human terms. Therefore, it is important not to undermine the entire process by undervaluing the service in economic terms and thereby eventually precluding its continued use.

Since it will not be common for physicians to set aside a whole hour for family counseling, and since most such counseling will be short-term, the financial impact upon patients and families should not be excessive. After initial assessment and setting up a therapeutic contract or other steps along the continuum of primary care counseling, the follow-up visits are apt to be brief, often 15 to 30 minutes. Since family physicians will rarely be seeing people and families weekly and over long periods of time such as a family therapist might do, the total cost of primary care counseling would be lower than would seem apparent from considering only the per-minute physician fee. Brief follow-up interviews and counseling sessions can be incorporated easily into a normal fee structure and will be competitive with other mental health services. In a hospital setting, there will usually be little difficulty in convincing insurance companies or families that time spent in consultation is worthwhile and cost effective.

PROTECTING THE PHYSICIAN WHO DELIVERS
PRIMARY CARE COUNSELING

A cardinal rule for primary care counseling is that it should not injure the physician/counselor. If the physician develops skill in delivering primary care counseling to a practice population, it is highly probable that he or she will develop a reputation for unusual effectiveness in the delivery of health care. This may lead to an overloaded schedule and unrealistic work load. What can be done to protect this physician?

First, a systems perspective in the delivery of health care demands that the physician resign from the all-knowing, always-caring, and always-available role as a family physician. These attributes may be admired by television audiences, but are detrimental to the physician's well-being and family survival. Second, the physician must demonstrate by example the importance of a family perspective. There is a hollow ring to a physician's request for an individual patient to incorporate the family into the treatment plan if the physician cannot rely on family resources for handling the complex issues generated by a busy career. The physician is very much part of the physician–patient–family triangle. If the physician is dysfunctional, obviously the triangular relationship loses its strength and vitality. Therefore, the emotional and family health of the physician is of utmost importance. This is not to say that family physicians delivering this type of care will be immune from family conflicts or unheavals. However, the physician must respect the time and energy that will be needed to maintain adequate family cohesion and adaptability. Third, if the physician's personal life patterns become dysfunctional, there must be a supportive environment from which help can be gained. Extended family, friends, professional associates, and trusted but more distant consultants can be organized in a fashion that is supportive and therapeutic if needed.

CONCLUSION

The major purpose of this book is to help physicians deliver care in a family context and through a systems orientation. Throughout this discussion, we emphasize that there must be limits to a physician's involvement and risk taking. A network approach will allow the physician to set limits on individual involvement and risk taking by transferring part of the care of the family to other individuals and organizations. A full understanding of a systems perspective suggests that it is not the physician's role to be solely responsible for patient and family outcomes. The large social context of patient care—beginning with the therapeutic triangle—suggests that many factors beyond the physician are important in determining outcome. This allows the physician to become only partially involved when personal energy levels or outside pressures circumscribe full involvement. Community resources are often more important and more effective in helping families than are the physician's own efforts in the office; in these cases, the physician's crucial task is to help patients get access to these resources. When viewed as part of a network of helping resources, the physician's role becomes less burdensome, more effective, and immeasurably more enjoyable.

APPENDIX: FAMILY-ORIENTED MEDICAL PRACTICE—
BAIRD DESCRIBES HIS OWN EXPERIENCE

My personal experience in implementing a family-systems-based medical practice in a small community demonstrates the multiple impacts of this type of health care delivery system on the community, on the health care system— and on the physician. It could not work without broad-based support that takes time to develop.

My story probably begins with the period before I entered medical school. I grew up in a small town in which the medical model was the classic small-town general practitioner (who, by the way, is still delivering very personalized, excellent health care in that community). I left my home town of Dodge Center, Minnesota, to enter Macalester College in St. Paul with an overriding interest in participating in intercollegiate football on a team that was of modest enough caliber to allow me to play. About midway through my sophomore year I began to understand that there must be priorities beyond football. I seemed to be functioning as an informal counselor in the dorm. I thought that pursuing a medical–counseling career would be interesting. When I discussed this with the chaplain he offered me encouragement, but cautioned me about the impracticality of a physician's spending meaningful conversation time with patients. This seemed to be a rare event in his opinion and probably not feasible. As I finished college, I became heavily involved in the environmental movement and was an eager participant in organizing activities for the first Earth Day in 1970. I entered graduate school and pursued a Master's of Science in environmental health, which was completed in 1971. Part way through that experience, I discovered that I would rather be in medicine and entered medical school in the fall of 1971.

In the second year of medical school, I met a rare professor, John Verby, who seemed to be interested in the family aspects of medicine (and, in fact, wondered if I was spending enough time with my own spouse). He was and is a director of the Rural Physician Association Program of the University of Minnesota. He invited me to participate in the next year's rural program; I considered this an unlikely prospect because my wife was from an urban area and, I felt, would not enjoy rural life. Much to my surprise, she thought it would be a wonderful opportunity to experience a year in rural Minnesota. So we accepted that 1-year educational experience in the small town of Wabasha, Minnesota. During my year in an apprenticeship-type learning environment in a small clinic, it became apparent to me that the diagnoses discussed in medical school often related only indirectly to the patient's discomforts. It seemed that people were unhappy or dissatisfied more with relationships than with physical ailments. During that year, we were introduced to the concepts of psychological medicine and family systems thinking through a team of consultants that included Elof (Gus)

Nelson, STD, Donald Cassata, PhD, and John Verby, MD. I then returned to the University of Minnesota for the fourth year of medical school and entered a family practice residency at the University of Minnesota with an interest in continuing the family therapy training.

During the family practice residency I spent most of my available free time seeking supervision in interviewing families and couples with the staff at Bethesda Hospital in St. Paul and through the University of Minnesota family practice teaching staff. I was allowed the flexibility of reducing my time in several surgical rotations to spend those days in the graduate school classes on various topics in psychiatry, psychology, and human sexuality. Most of my training in family therapy was accomplished in one-to-one supervision and videotaping of interviews with couples and families. As I expressed interest in pursuing family-centered practice in a small town, I was advised by at least one consultant that this would be impossible because of the complex nature of the task and my proximity to the patients in a small town. I still consider that advice pertinent but feel that it is overly pessimistic. Long before leaving the residency, I was convinced that delivering family-centered care was possible and enjoyable. As a medical student, I had decided to return to Wabasha as a place to practice and during the residency had recruited three young physicians who were already in practice by the time I returned there in 1978.

I was surprised to find upon entering practice that the medical system was not set up in a fashion that permitted seeing families or even couples. My first experience in seeing families was in a hospital setting, usually for interventions and problems of chemical dependency in which the dependent person was the hospitalized patient. When I called a family meeting, I had to explain to the nurses what I was doing and why I was seeing more than one person. (Initially, interviews were held in the nurses' lounge.) After this initial confusion, I began to invite nurses into the interview sessions, a practice that ultimately generated a more supportive atmosphere. After the family interviews, I would debrief with the nurses and we would share our reactions. Just as I had done during my initial and ongoing training in family systems thinking, the nurses became introspective and began to bring up issues about their own families, which I tried to discuss in a supportive way. We found family interviewing space that did not conflict with nurses' activities, and their support gradually increased. An in-service session, offered to all nurses as well as any other members of the hospital staff, on the topic of family involvement in management and treatment of alcoholism generated increased respect and support for the family systems approach.

In the office, my initial contact with the primary nurse resulted in cautious tolerance for seeing families for 30 to 45 minutes during my early weeks in practice. Initially this was not a hindrance to patient flow, because as a new physician I was not overwhelmingly busy for the first several months. After interviewing the families alone, I would review the case materials with the nurse and we would discuss general topics. Just like the hospital staff members, the clinic staff members became interested in their own family issues, and we discussed these concerns in a supportive manner. Sometimes this caused increased stress on the staff, but mostly it has seemed to be a healthy process.

My medical partners were initially very cautious about what seemed a rather unusual approach to many different kinds of medical problems for which I would see couples and families. They were trustful of me because of my previous long-term contact with the clinic, but they were experienced enough to view my approach with appropriate skepticism. I am quite sure that a person entering an entirely new environment with no prior relationship with the medical delivery personnel would need to take a cautious and patient approach in order not to change the delivery system too quickly. In most places, the delivery system in place is functioning in a manner that does provide some satisfaction to both the deliverers of health care and the patient population. A new method of delivery must be demonstrated to be at least as effective as the old method before enthusiasm can be expected or would be appropriate.

After about 8 months of generally cool reception for the family systems approach, I was becoming somewhat discouraged. The nurses and physicians closest to me were generally supportive, but there was no real evidence of any patients' or families' changing to a noticeable degree during those early months. At about that point, I went to a conference at the University of Minnesota at which Carl Whitaker presented his unique style of family therapy. Although I would not attempt to emulate Whitaker's style precisely, I did leave the conference with a new confidence in the validity of the family systems approach. I was also cautioned by Whitaker to relax and enjoy my style of practice in order to allow greater effectiveness and a greater likelihood that I would continue to function with a systems perspective. Whether it was coincidence or whether Whitaker's influence was therapeutic, positive results seemed to become more apparent to me. Families began to return from family-centered chemical dependency treatment with an enthusiasm for sobriety and an improved family functioning that had not been seen in the community previously. Other psychosocial issues, such as depression and anxiety, that had been chronic problems for patients and physicians seemed to improve; my own confidence, as well as that of my partners, began to grow. Soon I was asked questions about problem patients by my partners in a supportive tone and in a context in which I was a consultant. As my first year in practice passed, I began to feel confident that a family systems approach was feasible and rewarding.

With help from several people in the community, I was able to arrange meetings with county sheriffs, social service workers, local police officers, and anyone else who saw families at times of stress or trouble. Relatively few had ever met other than at times of a specific family's crisis, and they seemed interested that a physician would lend support to such a meeting. This generated more support and closer worker relationships with many community professionals whom I would need in order to offer community-based support to families. The result was a more cohesive community network that offered support both to families and to me in sharing the work load and responsibility for difficult cases.

As I entered the second year in practice, it became apparent that there were impacts on the health delivery system in general and specifically on the health care personnel. The number of referrals to our in-house clinical psychologist, who was trained primarily to treat individuals, decreased. My medical colleagues had gained such enthusiasm for a family-centered approach that individual consultations with patients were no longer requested. We decided to discontinue the services of our clinical psychologist.

The other physicians in the group were now becoming more interested in a family-centered approach to medical care. Informal and formal discussion about our own families became more frequent. Occasionally this resulted in clarifying major life decisions. Outside therapeutic resources were utilized in some cases. I think all of us have changed and benefited from these interactions.

My work load and earned income are now similar to those of many family physicians. I am accustomed, like the other family physicians in our group, to seeing 20 to 30 patients on most days. On call days I may see as many as 35 to 40 patients, but that is unusual. I see couples for 15 to 45 minutes once or twice daily, and I encounter problems related to chemical dependency every day. My average contact with persons who are chemically dependent or with family members of dependent persons is still occurring at a rate of about 7 to 8% of office visits. Some days, as many as 6 out of 30 patient contacts are of that nature. I see whole families once a week or less, usually for about 45 minutes.

I have found in my relatively brief experience of practicing medicine that I make my worst mistakes not only by coming to late diagnoses for unusual diseases (the nemesis of primary care), but more commonly by not maintaining a healthy patient–family–physician therapeutic triangle. I find that if I do not communicate clearly and often with family members with significant psychosocial problems and with serious straightforward medical problems, it is possible for me as a physician to become the "villain" in a family system. Continued contact with family members prevents that problem but does not happen without some effort on my part.

I am currently afforded excellent support from my partners, who periodically confront me when I need it and occasionally "throw me out of the office" when I seem overcommitted to my work role. The local community respects my personal free time reasonably well and offers excellent support for my efforts to intervene in multiple problems that families face. My main support is my wife and family; our time together is precious to me. We continue to struggle with work and community commitments that compete for our "family time." Although that conflict is unending, we are optimistic and happy with our present course. The preface to this volume outlines my contact with Bill Doherty, who has afforded me increasing support during the past 2 years. I continue to get support from my friends at the University of Minnesota and now from contacts on a national level at professional meetings.

As my experience has demonstrated, it is possible to deliver primary care to families with the use of a family systems model. This approach has ramifications within the medical delivery system and the persons and families that make up that system. These consequences should not be underestimated as family physicians attempt to apply this model in other communties. I believe that a healthy medical delivery system based on the family model will demonstrate increased effectiveness over the years and will continue to develop its own supportive network in family medicine and beyond.

REFERENCES

Abuzzahab, F. Twenty-five years of psychopharmacology. *Minnesota Medicine*, 1979, *62*, 8.

Albert, J. J., Kosa, J., & Haggerty, R. J. A month of illness and health care among low-income families. *Health Reports*, 82, *8*, 705–713.

American Psychiatric Association. *Diagnostic and statistical manual of mental disorders* (3rd ed.). Washington, D.C.: Author, 1980.

Balint, M. *The doctor, his patient, and the illness* (2nd ed.). New York: Pitman, 1964.

Barnard, C. P. *Families, alcoholism, and therapy.* Springfield, Ill.: Charles C Thomas, 1981.

Bauman, M. H., & Grace, N. T. Family process and family practice. *Journal of Family Practice*, 1977, *4*, 1135–1137.

Becker, M. H., Drachman, R. H., & Kirscht, J. P. Motivations as predictors of health behavior. *Health Services Reports*, 1972, *87*, 852–861.

Becker, M. H., & Maiman, L. Sociobehavioral determinants of compliance with health and medical care recommendations. *Medical Care*, 1975, *13*, 10–24.

Bielski, R. J., & Friedel, R. O. Prediction of tricyclic antidepressant response. *Archives of General Psychiatry*, 1976, *33*, 1479–1489.

Bloom, B. L., Asher, S. J., & White, S. W. Marital disruption as a stressor: A review and analysis. *Psychological Bulletin*, 1978, *85*, 867–894.

Bodin, A. M. The interactional view: Family therapy approaches of the Mental Research Institute. In A. S. Gurman & D. P. Kniskern (Eds.), *Handbook of family therapy.* New York: Brunner/Mazel, 1981.

Bothwell, S., & Weissman, M. Social impairments four years after an acute depressive episode. *American Journal of Orthopsychiatry*, 1977, *47*, 231–237.

Bowen, M. *Family therapy in clinical practice.* New York: Jason Aronson, 1978.

Boyd, J. H., & Weissman, M. M. Epidemiology of affective disorders. *Archives of General Psychiatry*, 1981, *38*, 1039–1046.

Briggs, T., Malerich, J., Hafner, J., Magee, T., & Michaelson, J. *Detection of the alcoholic patient in the acute care setting.* Foundation for Health Care Evaluation, Minneapolis, Minn., 1980.

Bronfenbrenner, U. *The ecology of human development.* Cambridge, Mass.: Harvard University Press, 1979.

Brown, G. W., & Harris, T. *Social origins of depression.* New York: Free Press, 1978.

285

Brownell, K. D., Heckerman, C. L., Westlake, R. J., Hayes, S. C., & Monti, P. M. The effect of couples training and partner cooperativeness in the behavioral treatment of obesity. *Behaviour Research and Therapy*, 1978, *16*, 323–333.

Bruhn, J. G. Effects of chronic illness on the family. *Journal of Family Practice*, 1977, *4*, 1057–1060.

Cadoret, R. J., Widmer, R. B., & Troughton, E. P. Somatic complaints: Harbinger of depression in primary care. *Journal of Affective Disorders*, 1980, *2*, 61–70.

Caldwell, R., Cobb, S., Dowling, M. D., & Jongh, D. The dropout problem in antihypertensive therapy. *Journal of Chronic Diseases*, 1970, *22*, 579–592.

Caplan, R. D., von Harrison, R., Wellons, R. V., & French, J. R. P. *Social support and patient adherence: Experimental and survey findings* (final report to the National Heart, Lung, and Blood Institute, Grant H1 18418-03). Ann Arbor, Mich.: Institute for Social Research, 1979.

Carter, E. A., & McGoldrick, M. The family life cycle and family therapy: An overview. In E. A. Carter & M. McGoldrick (Eds.), *The family life cycle: A framework for family therapy*. New York: Gardner Press, 1980.

Cassata, D. M., & Kirkman-Liff, B. Mental health activities of family physicians. *Journal of Family Practice*, 1981, *12*, 683–692.

Charney, E., Bynum, R., Eldridge, D., MacWhinney, J. B., McNabb, N., Scheiner, D., Sumpter, E., & Iker, H. How well do patients take oral penicillin? A collaborative study in private practice. *Pediatrics*, 1967, *34*, 188–195.

Clark, W. B., & Midonik, L. *Alcoholic use and alcohol problems among United States adults: Results of the 1979 national survey*. Report prepared for the National Institute on Alcohol Abuse and Alcoholism (Contract No. ADM 281-79-0022), 1980.

Clarke-Stewart, K. A. Popular primers for parents. *American Psychologist*, 1978, *33*, 359–369.

Council on Mental Health. Medical school education on abuse of alcohol and other psychoactive drugs. *Journal of the American Medical Association*, 1972, *219*, 1746–1749.

Criteria Committee, National Council on Alcoholism. Criteria for the diagnosis of alcoholism. *Annals of Internal Medicine*, 1972, *77*, 249–258.

Cromwell, R. E., Olson, D. H., & Fournier, D. G. Diagnosis and evaluation in marital and family counseling. In D. H. Olson (Ed.), *Treating relationships*. Lake Mills, Iowa: Graphic, 1976.

Dingle, J. H., Badger, G., & Jordon, W. S., Jr. *Illness in the home*. Cleveland: Case Western Reserve University Press, 1964.

Doherty, W. J. Cognitive processes in intimate conflict: I. Extending attribution theory. *American Journal of Family Therapy*, 1981, *9*, 1–13. (a)

Doherty, W. J. Cognitive processes in intimate conflict: II. Efficacy and learned helplessness. *American Journal of Family Therapy*, 1981, *9*, 35–44. (b)

Doherty, W. J. Involving the reluctant father in family therapy. In A. S. Gurman (Ed.), *Questions and answers in the practice of family therapy*. New York: Brunner/Mazel, 1981. (c)

Doherty, W. J., & Ryder, R. G. Parent effectiveness training (P.E.T.): Criticisms and caveats. *Journal of Marital and Family Therapy*, 1980, *6*, 409–419.

Doherty, W. J., Schrott, H., Metcalf, L., & Vailas, L. *Spouse support and spouse health beliefs in patient adherence*. Paper presented at the Society of Teachers of Family Medicine meeting, Chicago, May 1982.

Doherty, W. J., & Walker, B. Marriage Encounter casualties: A preliminary investigation. *American Journal of Family Therapy*, 1982, *10*, 15–25.

Donovan, J. E., & Jessor, R. *Problem drinking among adolescents: A social-psychological study of a national sample*. Report prepared for National Institute on Alcohol Abuse and Alcoholism (Contract No. ADM 281-75-0028), 1976.

Earp, J. A., & Ory, M. G. The effects of social support and health professional visits on patient adherence to hypertension regimens. *Preventive Medicine*, 1979, *8*, 155.

Eckardt, M. J., Harford, T. C., Kaelber, C. T., Parker, E. S., Rosenthal, L. S., Ryback, P. S., Salmoiraghi, G. C., Vanderveen, E., & Warren, K. R. Health hazards associated with alcohol consumption. *Journal of the American Medical Association*, 1981, *246*, 648–666.

Engel, G. L. The need for a new medical model: A challenge for biomedicine. *Science*, 1977, *196*, 129–136.

Ewing, J. Some recent attempts to institute controlled drinking patterns in patients resistant to Alcoholics Anonymous. *Annals of the New York Academy of Science*, 1974, *233*, 147–154.

FDA Drug Bulletin. Prescribing of minor tranquilizers. *FDA Drug Bulletin*, 1980, *10*, 2–3.

France, R. D., Weddington, W. W., & Houpt, J. L. Referral of patients from primary care physicians to a community mental health center. *Journal of Nervous and Mental Diseases*, 1978, *166*, 594–598.

Friedman, A. Interaction of drug therapy with marital therapy in depressed patients. *Archives of General Psychiatry*, 1975, *32*, 619–637.

Geyman, J. P. The family as the object of care in family practice. *Journal of Family Practice*, 1977, *5*, 571–577.

Glick, P. C. Updating the life cycle of the family. *Journal of Marriage and the Family*, 1977, *39*, 5–13.

Glick, P. C. *The future of the American family* (Current Population Reports, Special Studies Series P-23, No. 78). Washington, D.C.: U.S. Government Printing Office, 1979.

Goodwin, D. W. *Is alcoholism hereditary?* New York: Oxford University Press, 1976.

Goodwin, D. W., & Guze, S. B. *Psychiatric diagnosis* (2nd ed.). New York: Oxford University Press, 1979.

Grolnick, L. Evaluation and treatment effect disturbances within a familly context. In A. S. Gurman (Ed.), *Questions and answers in the practice of family therapy*. New York: Brunner/Mazel, 1981.

Gunby, P. Air controller strike spotlights job stress. *Journal of the American Medical Association*, 1981, *246*, 1632–1633.

Gurman, A. S., & Kniskern, D. P. Research on marital and family therapy: Progress, perspective, and prospect. In S. L. Garfield & A. E. Bergin (Eds.), *Handbook of psychotherapy and behavior change: An empirical analysis* (2nd ed.). New York: Wiley, 1978.

Gurman, A. S., & Kniskern, D. P. (Eds.). *Handbook of family therapy*. New York: Brunner/Mazel, 1981.

Haley, J. *Problem-solving therapy*. San Francisco: Jossey-Bass, 1976.

Haley, J. *Leaving home*. New York: McGraw-Hill, 1980.

Harsday, J., & Karch, F. Benzodiazepine prescribing in a family medicine center. *Journal of the American Medical Association*, 1981, *246*, 1321–1325.

Haynes, R. B. Strategies to improve compliance with referrals, appointments, and prescribed medical regimens. In R. B. Haynes, D. W. Taylor, & D. L. Sackett (Eds.), *Compliance in health care*. Baltimore: Johns Hopkins University Press, 1979.

Haynes, R. B., Taylor, D. W., & Sackett, D. L. (Eds.). *Compliance in health care*. Baltimore: Johns Hopkins University Press, 1979.

Heinzelmann, F., & Bagley, R. W. Response to physical activity programs and their effects on health behavior. *Public Health Reports*, 1970, *85*, 905–911.

Hollister, L. E. *Clinical pharmacology of psychotherapeutic drugs*. New York: Churchill-Livingstone, 1978.

Hollister, L. E., Conley, F. K., Britt, R. H., & Shuen, L. Long-term use of diazepam. *Journal of the American Medical Association*, 1981, *246*, 1568–1570.

Hubbell, J. Danger! Prescription drug abuse. *Reader's Digest*, April 1980, pp. 100–104.

Ireton, H. R., & Cassata, D. M. Psychological systems review. *Journal of Family Practice*, 1976, *3*, 70–74.

Jackson, J., & Bressler, R. Prescribing tricyclic antidepressants. *Drug Therapy*, December 1981, pp. 87–96.

Jacobson, N. S., & Margolin, G. *Marital therapy.* New York: Brunner/Mazel, 1979.

Johnson, R. Widmer, R., Cadoret, R., Troughton, E., & Wilson, J. *Use of minor tranquilizers in a primary care practice.* Unpublished manuscript. The University of Iowa, 1981.

Journal of the American Medical Association, Editorial. Susceptibility to dependence on alcohol. *Journal of the American Medical Association,* 1975, *233,* 124–127.

Kaplan, H. S. *The new sex therapy.* New York: Brunner/Mazel, 1974.

Kaplan, H. S. *The illustrated manual of sex therapy.* New York: Quadrangle, 1978.

Kasl, S. V., & Cobb, S. Health behavior, illness behavior, and sick role behavior. *Archives of Environmental Health,* 1966, *12,* 246–266.

Katon, W., Williamson, P., & Ries, R. A prospective study of 60 consecutive psychiatric consultations in a family medicine clinic. *Journal of Family Practice,* 1981, *13,* 47–55.

Kaufman, E., & Kaufmann, P. N. (Eds.). *Family therapy of drug and alcohol abuse.* New York: Gardner Press, 1979.

Klemme, H. Alcoholism: "Not me" reassurances may bring trouble. *Minneapolis Star,* September 12, 1977.

Korsch, B. M., & Negrette, V. F. Doctor–patient communication. *Scientific American,* 1972, *227,* 66–74.

Kovacs, M., Rush, A. J., Beck, A. T., & Hollon, S. D. Depressed outpatients treated with cognitive therapy or pharmacotherapy. *Archives of General Psychiatry,* 1981, *38,* 33–39.

Lester, M. E., & Doherty, W. J. Couples' long-term evaluations of their Marriage Encounter experience. *Journal of Marital and Family Therapy,* 1983, *9.*

Levine, D. M., Green, L. W., Deeds, S. G., Chualow, J., Russell, R. P., & Finlay, J. Health education for hypertensive patients. *Journal of the American Medical Association,* 1979, *241,* 1700–1703.

Levy, R. L. The role of social support in patient compliance: A selective review. In *Patient compliance to prescribed antihypertensive medication regimens* (Department of Health, Education and Welfare, Public Health Service, NIH Publication No. 81-2102). Washington, D.C.: U.S. Government Printing Office, 1980.

Litman, T. J. The family as a basic unit in health and medical care: A social–behavioral overview. *Social Science and Medicine,* 1974, 495–519.

Lloyd, C. Life events and depressive disorder reviewed: II. Events as precipitating factors. *Archives of General Psychiatry,* 1980, *37,* 541–548.

Macklin, E. D. Review of research on nonmarital cohabitation in the United States. In B. I. Murstein (Ed.), *Exploring intimate life styles.* New York: Springer, 1978.

Masters, W. H., & Johnson, V. E. *Human sexual inadequacy.* Boston: Little, Brown, 1970.

McCubbin, H. I., Joy, C. B., Cauble, A. E., Comeau, J. K., Patterson, J. M., & Needle, R. H. Family stress and coping: A decade review. *Journal of Marriage and the Family,* 1980, *42,* 855–871.

McKenney, J. M., Slining, J. M., Henderson, H. R., Devins, D., & Barr, M. The effect of clinical pharmacy services on patients with essential hypertension. *Circulation,* 1973, *48,* 1104–1111.

Medalie, J. H., & Goldbourt, U. Angina pectoris among 10,000 men: II. Psychosocial and other risk factors as evidenced in a multivariate analysis of a five-year incidence study. *American Journal of Medicine,* 1976, *60,* 910–921.

Medalie, J. H., Kitson, G. C., & Zyzanski, S. J. A family epidemiological model: A practice and research concept for family medicine. *Journal of Family Practice,* 1981, *12,* 79–87.

Medalie, J. H., Snyder, M., Groen, J. J., Neufeld, H. N., Goldbourt, U., & Riss, E. Angina pectoris among 10,000 men: Five-year incidence and univariate analysis. *American Journal of Medicine,* 1973, *55,* 583–594.

Meyer, R. J., & Haggerty, R. J. Streptococcal infections in families: Factors altering individual susceptibility. *Pediatrics,* 1962, *29,* 539–549.

Minuchin, S. *Families and family therapy.* Cambridge, Mass.: Harvard University Press, 1974.

Minuchin, S., & Fishman, H. C. *Family therapy techniques.* Cambridge, Mass.: Harvard University Press, 1981.

Minuchin, S., Rosman, B. L., & Baker, L. *Psychosomatic families: Anorexia nervosa in context.* Cambridge, Mass.: Harvard University Press, 1978.

Morris, J. B., & Beck, A. T. The efficacy of antidepressant drugs: A review of research (1958 to 1972). *Archives of General Psychiatry,* 1974, *30,* 667–674.

Murphy, G. E., Woodruff, R. A., Jr., Herjanic, J., & Super, G. Variability of the clinical course of primary affective disorder. *Archives of General Psychiatry,* 1974, *30,* 757–761.

National Center for Health Statistics. *Hospital discharge survey.* Washington, D.C.: U.S. Government Printing Office, 1975.

Olson, D. H. Marital and family therapy: Integrative review and critique. *Journal of Marriage and the Family,* 1970, *32,* 501–538.

Olson, D. H., Sprenkle, D. H., & Russell, C. Circumplex model of marital and family systems: I. Cohesion and adaptability dimensions, family types, and clinical applications. *Family Process,* 1979, *18,* 3–28.

Osterweis, M., Bush, P. J., & Zuckerman, A. F. Family context as a predictor of individual medicine use. *Social Science and Medicine,* 1979, *13A,* 287–291.

Patient Care. When stress tips the balance: Anxiety versus depression. *Patient Care,* 1981, *15,* 149–171.

Pattison, E. M., Headley, E. B., Gleser, G. C., & Gohschalk, L. A. Abstinence and normal drinking: An assessment of changes in drinking patterns in alcoholics after treatment. *Quarterly Journal of Studies on Alcohol,* 1968, *29,* 610–633.

Pattison, E. M., & Anderson, R. C. Family health care. *Public Health Review,* 1978, *7,* 83–134.

Pearce, J. W., LeBow, M. D., & Orchard, J. Role of spouse involvement in the behavioral treatment of overweight women. *Journal of Consulting and Clinical Psychology,* 1981, *49,* 236–244.

Pevanik, J. S., Jasinski, D. R., & Haretzin, C. A. Abrupt withdrawal from therapeutically administered diazepam. *Archives of General Psychiatry,* 1978, *25,* 995–998.

Physicians' desk reference (35th ed.). Oradell, N.J.: Litton Industries, 1981.

Rakel, R. E. *Principles of family medicine.* Philadelphia: W. B. Saunders, 1977.

Ransom, D.C., & Massad, R. J. Family structure and function. In R. E. Rakel & H. F. Conn (Eds.), *Family practice* (2nd ed.). Philadelphia: W. B. Saunders, 1978.

Rickels, K. Drugs in the symptomatic treatment of neurotic anxiety. *Clinical Therapeutics,* 1977, *1,* 106–117.

Ries, R., Bolkan, J., Katon, W., & Kleinman, A. The medical care abuser: Differential diagnosis and management. *Journal of Family Practice,* 1981, *13,* 257–265.

Rollins, B. C., & Cannon, K. L. Marital satisfaction over the family life cycle: A reevaluation. *Journal of Marriage and the Family,* 1974, *36,* 271–282.

Rounsaville, B. J., Klerman, J. D., & Weissman, M. M. Do psychotherapy and pharmacotherapy for depression conflict? Empirical evidence from a clinical trial. *Archives of General Psychiatry,* 1981, *38,* 24–29.

Rounsaville, B. J., Weissman, M. M., Prusoff, B. A., & Herceg-Baron, R. L. Marital disputes and treatment outcome in depressed women. *Comprehensive Psychiatry,* 1979, *20,* 483–490.

Russell, C. S. Transition to parenthood: Problems and gratifications. *Journal of Marriage and the Family,* 1974, *36,* 294–302.

Ryder, R. G., Kafka, J. S., & Olson, D. H. Separating and joining influences in courtship and early marriage. *American Journal of Orthopsychiatry,* 1971, *41,* 450–464.

Saalwaechter, J. J., & Heinrichs, R. Family interviews: Shortcut or drawback? *Patient Care,* September 15, 1976, pp. 95–103.

Saccone, A. J., & Israel, A. C. Effects of experimenter versus significant other-controlled reinforcement and choice of target behavior on weight loss. *Behavior Therapy,* 1978, *9,* 271–278.

Sackett, D. L., Haynes, R. B., Gibson, E. S., Hackett, B. C., Taylor, D. W., Roberts, R. S., & Johnson, A. L. Randomized clinical trial of strategies for improving medication compliance in primary hypertension. *Lancet*, 1975, *1*, 1205-1207.

Sackett, D. L., Haynes, R. B., Gibson, E. S., & Johnson, A. The problem of compliance with antihypertensive therapy. *Practice Cardiology*, 1976, *2*, 35-39.

Seixas, F. A. Definition of alcoholism. *Annals of Internal Medicine*, 1976, *85*, 764.

Selvini-Palazzoli, M., Boscolo, L., Cecchin, G., & Prata, G. The problem of the referring person. *Journal of Marital and Family Therapy*, 1980, *6*, 3-9.

Smilkstein, G. The family APGAR: A proposal for a family function test and its use by physicians. *Journal of Family Practice*, 1978, *6*, 1231-1239.

Smilkstein, G. Assessment of family function. In G. M. Rosen, J. P. Geymen, & R. H. Layton (Eds.), *Behavioral science in family practice*. New York: Appleton-Century-Crofts, 1980.

Steidl, J. H., Finkelstein, F. O., Wexler, J. P., Feigenbaum, H., Kitsen, J., Kliger, A. S., & Quinlan, D. M. Medical regimens and family functioning. *Archives of General Psychiatry*, 1980, *37*, 1025-1027.

Steinberg, H., Torem, M., & Saravay, S. M. An analysis of physician resistance to psychiatric consultations. *Archives of General Psychiatry*, 1980, *37*, 1007-1012.

Steinglass, P. Experimenting with family treatment approaches to alcoholism, 1950-1975: A review. *Family Process*, 1976, *15*, 97-123.

Steinglass, P. Family therapy in alcoholism. In B. Kissin & H. Begleiter (Eds.), *The biology of alcoholism* (Vol. 5), *Treatment and rehabilitation of the chronic alcoholic*). New York: Plenum, 1977.

Steinglass, P. A life history model of the alcoholic family. *Family Process*, 1980, *19*, 211-226.

Steinglass, P., Davis, D. I., & Berenson, D. Observations of conjointly hospitalized "alcoholic couples" during sobriety and intoxication: Implications for theory and therapy. *Family Process*, 1977, *16*, 1-16.

Stuart, R. B. *Helping couples change: A social learning approach to marital therapy*. New York: Guilford Press, 1980.

Stuart, R. B., & Davis, B. *Slim chance in a fat world: Behavioral control of obesity*. Champaign, Ill.: Research Press, 1972.

Stunkard, A. J., & Penick, S. B. Behavior modification in the treatment of obesity: The problem of maintaining weight loss. *Archives of General Psychiatry*, 1979, *36*, 801-806.

Taylor, R. Categories of care in family medicine. *Family Medicine*, 1981, *13*, 7-9.

U.S. Bureau of the Census. *Characteristics of children and youth* (Current Population Reports, Special Studies Series P-23, No. 66). Washington, D.C.: U.S. Government Printing Office, 1978.

U.S. Bureau of the Census. *Divorce, child custody, and child support* (Current Population Reports, Special Studies Series P-23, No. 84). Washington, D.C.: U.S. Government Printing Office, 1979.

U.S. Bureau of the Census. *Marital status and living arrangements: March 1978* (Current Population Reports, Series P-20, No. 388). Washington, D.C.: U.S. Government Printing Office, 1979.

U.S. Bureau of the Census. *Population characteristics* (Current Population Reports, Series P-20, No. 341). Washington, D.C.: U.S. Government Printing Office, 1979.

U.S. Bureau of the Census. *Population characteristics* (Current Population Reports, Series P-20, No. 349). Washington, D.C.: U.S. Government Printing Office, 1980.

Usdin, G. Introduction. In G. Usdin (Ed.), *Depression: Clinical, biological, and psychological perspectives*. New York: Brunner/Mazel, 1977.

Watzlawick, P. Introduction. In P. Watzlawick & J. H. Weakland (Eds.), *The interactional view*. New York: Norton, 1977.

Watzlawick, P., Beavin, J. H., & Jackson, D. D. *Pragmatics of human communication*. New York: Norton, 1967.

Watzlawick, P., & Weakland, J. H. (Eds.). *The interactional view*. New York: Norton, 1977.

Watzlawick, P., Weakland, J., & Fisch, R. *Change: Principles of problem formation and problem resolution*. New York: Norton, 1974.

Weakland, J. H., Fisch, R., Watzlawick, P., & Bodin, A. M. Brief therapy: Focused problem resolution. *Family Process*, 1974, *13*, 141–168.

Wegescheider, S. *Another chance: Hope and help for the alcoholic family*. Palo Alto, Calif.: Science & Behavior Books, 1981.

Weinberg, J. R. Interview technique for diagnosing alcoholism. *American Family Physician*, 1974, *9*, 107–115.

Weinberg, J. R. Assessing drinking problems by history. *Postgraduate Medicine*, 1976, *59*, 87–90.

Weissman, M. M. The psychological treatment of depression: Evidence for the efficacy of psychotherapy alone, in comparison with, and in combination with pharmacotherapy. *Archives of General Psychiatry*, 1979, *36*, 1261–1269.

Weissman, M. M., Kasl, S. V., & Klerman, G. L. Follow-up of depressed women after maintenance treatment. *American Journal of Psychiatry*, 1976, *133*, 757–760.

Weissman, M. M., Klerman, G. L., Prusoff, B. A., Sholomskas, M. A., & Padian, N. Depressed outpatients: Results one year after treatment with drug and/or interpersonal psychotherapy. *Archives of General Psychiatry*, 1981, *38*, 51–55.

Weissman, M. M., & Paykel, E. S. *The depressed woman: A study of social relationships*. Chicago: University of Chicago Press, 1974.

Whitaker, C. A., & Keith, D. V. Symbolic-experiential family therapy. In A. S. Gurman & D. P. Kniskern (Eds.), *Handbook of family therapy*. New York: Brunner/Mazel, 1981.

Widmer, R. B., & Cadoret, R. J. Depression in primary care: Changes in pattern of patient visits and complaints during a developing depression. *Journal of Family Practice*, 1978, *7*, 293–302.

Widmer, R. B., Cadoret, R. J., & North, C. S. Depression in family practice: Some effects on spouses and children. *Journal of Family Practice*, 1980, *10*, 45–51.

Wilber, J. A., & Barrows, J. S. Reducing elevated blood pressure: Experience found in a community. *Minnesota Medicine*, 1969, *52*, 1303–1305.

Wilber, J. A., & Barrows, J. S. Hypertension—a community problem. *American Journal of Medicine*, 1972, *52*, 653–663.

Wiseman, J. P. The "home treatment": The first steps in trying to cope with an alcoholic husband. *Family Relations*, 1980, *29*, 541–549.

Worby, C., & Gerard, R. Family dynamics. In R. E. Rakel & H. F. Conn (Eds.), *Family practice* (2nd ed.). Philadelphia: W. B. Saunders, 1978.

Zarafonetis, C. Drug abuse. In C. Zarafonetis (Ed.), *Proceedings of the International Conference on Drug Abuse*. Philadelphia: Lea & Febiger, 1972.

AUTHOR INDEX

SUBJECT INDEX